Glaucoma - Recent Advances and New Perspectives

Edited by Pinakin Gunvant Davey

Published in London, United Kingdom

Glaucoma - Recent Advances and New Perspectives
http://dx.doi.org/10.5772/intechopen.98102
Edited by Pinakin Gunvant Davey

Contributors
Xiaolong Shi, Li Tang, Chao Tang, Ying Wang, Hilda Petrs-Silva, Mariana Santana Dias, Victor Guedes de Araujo, Rafael Lani-Louzada, Vinicius Toledo Ribas, Rafael Linden, Julie Pegu, Suneeta Dubey, Prerna Garg, Shanu Mittal, Tripti Johri, Surbhi Arora, Sean J. McCafferty, Khin P. Kilgore, Jason M. Levine, Govindasamy Kumaramanickavel, Siddhita Amit Jadhav, Sugirdhana Parthiban Ramsait, Pinakin Gunvant Davey, Najam A. A. Sharif, Pinakin Gunvant Gunvant Davey, Jason D. Duncan

First published in London, United Kingdom, 2023 by IntechOpen
IntechOpen is the global imprint of INTECHOPEN LIMITED, registered in England and Wales, registration number: 11086078, 5 Princes Gate Court, London, SW7 2QJ, United Kingdom

British Library Cataloguing-in-Publication Data
A catalogue record for this book is available from the British Library

Additional hard and PDF copies can be obtained from orders@intechopen.com

Glaucoma - Recent Advances and New Perspectives
Edited by Pinakin Gunvant Davey
p. cm.
Print ISBN 978-1-80355-534-8
Online ISBN 978-1-80355-535-5
eBook (PDF) ISBN 978-1-80355-536-2

For EU product safety concerns:
IN TECH d.o.o., Prolaz Marije Krucifikse Kozulić 3, 51000 Rijeka, Croatia,
info@intechopen.com or visit our website at intechopen.com.

Meet the editor

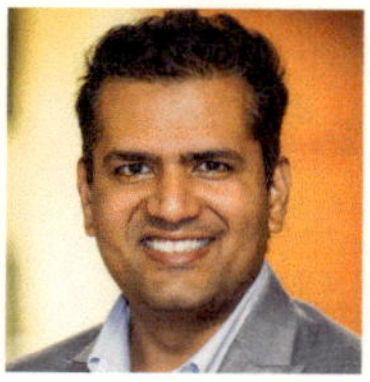

Dr. Pinakin Gunvant Davey is a tenured full professor and the director of clinical research at Western University of Health Sciences, California, USA. He earned his OD from Southern College of Optometry, Tennessee, USA, and a Ph.D. from Anglia Ruskin University, Cambridge, England. His three-year post-doctoral research fellowship at the University of Louisville, Kentucky, USA was focused on improving imaging techniques in glaucoma. His current research is focused on retinal physiology and glaucoma, particularly improving visual function in disease states. He has authored more than 75 international publications and has given more than 500 conference and invited presentations both nationally and internationally. He is a fellow of the Association for Research in Vision and Ophthalmology (ARVO) and the American Academy of Optometry (AAO) and a member of the Optometric Glaucoma Society.

Contents

Preface

Glaucoma, the leading cause of irreversible blindness, has long challenged eyecare providers and posed a substantial socioeconomic burden. Although glaucoma does not directly lead to increased mortality, it does cause blindness, which many consider a fate worse than death. This was apparent in a National Institutes of Health survey in which terminally ill cancer patients said it was not dying but losing sight that they feared the most. With that in mind, physicians should focus their efforts on preserving patients' sight.

This book looks at various aspects of cutting-edge research and hypotheses in glaucoma. Given that diagnostic delays and dilemmas are significant problems, state-of-the-art devices are needed to identify patients promptly. Efforts must be made to develop new technologies and strategies to aid and accelerate the diagnostic process. Tonometry to measure intraocular pressure, a continuous variable with ultra-short-term and long-term variations, is pivotal to the management of glaucoma. Although there are expensive devices that may provide a much more accurate intraocular pressure estimate than that provided by the Goldmann applanation tonometer, the simplicity, and genius of the CATS tonometer to modify the Goldmann applanation tonometer cannot be underestimated, as discussed in this book.

To do the same thing repeatedly and expect better outcomes is the definition of insanity. We are stuck in that rut, and the advances in glaucoma testing, particularly genetic testing, are a welcome addition. However, it is fair to say that the eyecare field is far from ready to make serious decisions based on genetic testing in glaucoma. As such, this book also addresses potential biomarkers in primary open-angle glaucoma.

New medications and surgical techniques can ensure that eyecare providers help glaucoma patients maintain quality of life and valuable functional vision. With the growing population and increased life expectancy, it is assumed that the incidence and prevalence of glaucoma will increase. Thus, we must continue looking for alternative treatment methods and ways to control this "deadly" disease. We have a long way to go in personalized and preventative medicine for glaucoma. In animal and epidemiological studies, there is evidence that nutritional elements and status may be associated with decreased glaucoma progression. It is sometimes as simple as increased use of carotenoids or water-soluble vitamins that have shown benefits. What is needed is more clinical trials and testing. In the meantime, we are likely to see a growth in adjunctive therapies that, along with intraocular pressure-lowering medications and surgical techniques, will enhance the survivability of retinal ganglion cells. Indeed, the final frontier will be the regeneration of the retinal ganglion cells, which has eluded us for the last few decades; however, there is "hope," and philosophically speaking, hope makes the world go round.

I want to thank all the authors and the staff at IntechOpen for continuing the grand effort to "democratize science" and making knowledge and information readily available and freely accessible to anyone who wishes to obtain it.

No great work is ever completed without a great support network; I am the luckiest to have that. I want to thank Publishing and Processing Manager Karla Skuliber for her assistance in completing this project. To Payal, my dear wife, thank you for putting up with my insane work schedule. To Ved and Jash, my dear children, you are my energy source. To my parents, Gunvant Davey and Minaben Davey, I am what I am because of your efforts, and thank you for all you continue to do for us. To my brother Karthikai Davey and my sister Darshna Vyas, you have always been there for me, day or night, and I am grateful to have you in my life.

I want to dedicate this book to my professor and mentor, Daniel O'Leary. Professor O'Leary has dedicated his life to the growth of science and the progress of the careers of his students. I am blessed and honored to have him in my life and eternally grateful for his guidance and teaching.

Pinakin Gunvant Davey
College of Optometry,
Western University of Health Sciences,
Pomona, USA

Section 1

Introduction

Chapter 1

Introductory Chapter: Glaucoma Beyond 2020

Pinakin Gunvant Davey and Jason D. Duncan

1. Introduction

Glaucoma is an optic neuropathy and possibly the most common optic neuropathy seen in the clinical care of general eye care physicians [1, 2]. Glaucomatous optic neuropathy has distinct structural changes visible on the optic nerve head. Thus, it has become a hallmark of the disease, making the optic nerve head a biomarker for evaluation. Although the optic nerve head and retinal nerve fiber changes are visible through dilated fundus evaluation, the objectivity, repeatability, and micron-level resolution provided by imaging technology have been extremely welcome in the last few decades. Imaging devices have become pivotal to glaucoma evaluation and follow-up care. The natural course of history has led to multimodal devices becoming a standard that can serve multiple functions in the clinical care of various anterior-segment and posterior-segment diseases, including glaucoma.

2. Diagnostic advances in glaucoma

The cause of open-angle glaucoma still eludes us; however, we know numerous risk factors are related to glaucoma, like age, race, intraocular pressure, and perfusion pressure, to name a few [1, 2]. Of all the risk factors associated with glaucoma, intraocular pressure is the modifiable risk factor that all treatment and management modalities focus on; intraocular pressure is the most critical risk factor [3–5]. Tonometry is used routinely in all eye examinations, and various forms exist, with the Goldmann applanation tonometer being the "gold standard" in clinical practice. Various ocular, systemic, patient, and examiner-related issues influence the outcome of intraocular pressure measurements [3, 4, 6]. The Goldmann applanation tonometer is far free of errors, yet it remains the "gold standard" because it is the most commonly used device in the clinics [3]. The main inaccuracies in the Goldmann applanation tonometer measurements are due to the variations in biomechanical properties of the cornea, particularly the central corneal thickness, which varies significantly in humans [3–6]. Numerous attempts have been made to create correction equations that adjust the Goldmann applanation tonometer measured IOP measurements to account for the corneal biomechanics [6]. These correction factors or equations lead to further errors and are unsuitable for individual patient care. At best, using multiparameter equations, we can get the IOP adjusted in a population and obtain IOP values that will decrease the effect of corneal biomechanics in clinical studies [6].

The world glaucoma consensus series in 2007 declared that the Ocular Response Analyzer and the Dynamic Contour Tonometer are better at measuring intraocular pressure when compared to the intraocular pressure measured using the Goldmann applanation tonometer [7]. These devices are less influenced due to corneal parameters. Yet these devices are not standard of care in clinical practice. There is a real need for home tonometry and to democratize intraocular pressure measurements [8]. Accurate intraocular pressure measurements are highly dependent on the eye care providers' equipment and skill. There is a need for IOP to be measured by nurses and nurse practitioners, and primary care physicians. It will be ideal if technician-independent automated devices capable of measuring IOP are housed in supermarkets, pharmacies, or other community locations. Having tonometers available to the public could provide access to IOP measurements away from eye care providers' offices, and aid the issue of underdiagnosis of the disease. Access to these automated testing options can and also potentially offer between-office visits IOP measurements for patients already on treatment for the disease. In the same spirit of obtaining multiple measurements of IOP, there is a need for at-home IOP monitoring. The iCare home tonometer is FDA-cleared for measurements of IOP at home, and has been shown to have clinical utility, however, is still an expensive device and not always affordable [9]. Contact lens devices like the Triggerfish have shown some clinical utility and gained some traction. But the accuracy in identifying nocturnal acrophase is less than ideal and probably identifiable in 60–65% of the patients. Although the benefits of home tonometry are intuitive, the exact socioeconomic benefits of these remain to be ascertained [10].

Imaging devices have become a mainstay in any clinic, and optical coherence tomography (OCT) has revolutionized eye care. These devices have undergone a lot of transition since their introduction in early 1990s. Today multimodal devices that image and measure anterior- and posterior-segment of the eye and perform ophthalmic photography are commonplace [11]. More recently, due to high scan capture rate (70–120 K scans per second), these devices have been able to provide superficial and deep vasculature measurements. These are clinically valuable measures, and their use as a diagnostic or prognostic indicator is increasing [12, 13]. At-home testing using OCT is a close reality in the retina space, and once the model is successful, its glaucoma implementation is a possible logical extension [14]. We will need to see if the at-home monitoring of glaucoma using OCT enhances detection of progression of glaucoma.

Similarly, the visual field devices have seen some software upgrades with more tests concentrating on the macular region in addition to the damage seen in the peripheral fields [15, 16]. Devices like Octopus Perimeter have had G-protocol in glaucoma for a while and provide clinically meaningful information that could enhance our understanding of structure and function correlation [17]. Visual fields have seen some fundamental transformations in recent years. From large devices that perform one function, the virtual reality perimeters provide the comfort of patients performing tests independently in a waiting room [18–20]. Additionally, the device allows coupling with a few entrance tests like pupillary testing, visual acuity testing, color vision, and multi-modality testing helps in having greater functionality. These tests have been compared to the Humphrey Visual Field Analyzer [18–20]. Early results indicate that these can have an excellent correlation to Humphrey Visual Fields, but as expected, their agreement is less than ideal [18–20]. We are only experiencing the tip of the iceberg when evaluating the potential of virtual reality testing technology. A lot more innovation is yet to come; perhaps at-home monitoring of visual function in glaucoma would be the next phase in developing this technology.

3. Advances in medical management

In the last few years, we have seen a flurry of updates in the medical management of glaucoma, with new medications like latanoprostene bunod and rhokinase inhibitors getting approved [21]. These new drugs based on new mechanisms of action or working on multiple modes of action like uveoscleral pathway, trabecular meshwork, or lowering episcleral venous pressure and lowering intraocular pressure have provided physicians with a greater armamentarium in managing glaucoma. Further, the last decade also saw the approval of the first prostaglandin fixed-combination agent in USA [21]. The approval of fixed-combination agents with the prostaglandin group of drugs was long overdue as various fixed-combination agents are available in other countries and have been used successfully. More recently, it is particularly exciting to see the approval of EP2 receptor agents, specifically prostaglandin agents, in USA [22]. Omidenepag isopropyl 0.002% was approved in Japan in 2018 [23]. Given that Omidenepag isopropyl is an EP2 receptor prodrug instead of the FP receptor prostaglandin, one could expect that specific side effects affecting FP receptor class agents may be less in this new EP-receptor drug [24]. Early indicators show that the new EP2 receptor prodrug will likely not have or show decreased changes to iris pigmentation and prostaglandin-related periorbitopathy [24].

The issues of patient adherence and compliance to the medications and instructions of physicians hinder the use of medications for any chronic disease. The management of glaucoma is no exception to this. Glaucoma medications usually come in multi-dose units and require preservatives to prevent contamination and the growth of microorganisms. When used chronically, these preserved medications can lead to an iatrogenic dry eye syndrome [25]. To alleviate this problem, preservative-free options are available. To further improve comfort for the patient, implantable devices that can dissolve over time and provide continuous medication to the eye are available. A bimatoprost intracameral implant was recently approved [26]. It was realized that multiple injections could lead to decreased endothelial cell count and corneal decompensation [26]. Thus, it was approved for only one-time application and provided reasonable control in IOP for 15 weeks [26].

Similarly, the Travoprost Implantable devices are under investigation. The iDose Travoprost implant is titanium travoprost-eluting intracameral delivery system [27]. Its phase 2 studies have shown 8.0–8.5 mmHg (32–33%) reduction in IOP depending on whether a fast or slow system was used. The phase 3 results are not yet published but are expected this year [27]. The intracameral implants and delivery systems will likely immediately decrease the patient-related compliance and persistence issues in glaucoma but, in the long-term will help improve the dry eye and anterior-segment issues that affect patients on topical medications. A final but perhaps most important benefit will improve the quality of life in patients with glaucoma.

4. New frontiers in glaucoma

Neuroprotection has been a holy grail that still eludes us [28]. One of the most extensive clinical trials in ophthalmology was the Memantine Eye Study which explored the efficacy of oral memantine as a neuroprotective agent in open-angle glaucoma at risk for progression. The study failed to meet its endpoint, and daily treatment with memantine over 48 months did not prevent glaucomatous progression [29]. Some drugs and agents have the potential as neuroprotective agents. For example, brimonidine has shown early indications as neuroprotective agent but has not advanced to clinical trials or successful outcomes [28]. There is indeed a need for treatments that could be used as a standalone or adjunctive therapy to IOP-lowering modalities, given that patients progress despite successful IOP lowering. To this accord, nutritional supplements potentially have a role to play as an adjunctive therapy [30]. The nutritional agents that are explored are antioxidants or agents that could increase blood flow to the optic nerve that could be beneficial as an IOP-independent mechanism/technique to aid the survival of retinal ganglion cells. Recent evidence substantiates that sustained oxidative stress and compromised antioxidant defenses are critical drivers in the onset of glaucomatous neurodegeneration. Overwhelming oxidative injury is likely attributed to compounding mitochondrial dysfunction that worsens with age-related processes, causing the aberrant formation of free radical species. Thus, a compromised systemic antioxidant capacity exacerbates further oxidative insult in glaucoma, leading to apoptosis, neuroinflammation, and subsequent tissue injury. These mechanisms have been tested in laboratory and small-scale studies but need further evaluation with large-scale randomized controlled clinical trials [30].

Selective laser trabeculoplasty has enjoyed second-line therapy status for a while and was occasionally used as a first-line agent. More recently, the LIGHT trials propelled it as a solid first-line option and have shown that it can provide good IOP lowering in a substantial group of participants [31]. Over 50% of the participants obtained and maintained their requisite IOP levels with one 360-degree treatment, and around 74% maintained target IOP levels with two treatments [31]. It would not be surprising if the results of this study were to be a paradigm shift in managing patients with glaucoma. Given the excellent success rate of the Selective Laser Trabeculoplasty, it is very appropriate that the Transscleral Selective Laser Trabeculoplasty that does not need gonioscopy will be highly welcome and should aid in lowering variability between physicians and reduce complications post-SLT [32].

It will be ideal if all glaucoma management is achievable by IOP-lowering agents or laser procedures, however, given the complexity and heterogeneity of the disease it is unlikely to be true even with the best of the medications and technology. Surgical interventions remain a mainstay when robust IOP lowering is desired. Trabeculectomy is necessary for patients for whom very low IOPs are desired, there are substantial post-operative risks. Further, the success of trabeculectomy depends on the skill of the operating surgeon and requires advanced sub-specialty training in ophthalmology. The Minimally Invasive Glaucoma Surgery (MIGS) fulfills the role of surgical intervention that may be coupled with or without cataract extraction and does not cause a substantial increase in risk greater than that of the cataract extraction itself [33–35]. With these tenets, numerous MIGS devices that target various routes of outflow have been introduced. These have seen tremendous success in decreasing the IOP successfully and reducing the dependence on IOP-lowering medications post-surgery. In the field of MIGS we indeed expect a lot of advances.

Glaucoma is known for a long time, and it is fair to take stock of the current situation and ask "Where are we now"? One way is to compare glaucoma with other known chronic diseases. One of the chronic diseases that glaucoma often gets compared to is diabetes. The comparison is fair as both diseases require regular monitoring and continuous treatment, no cure is known for the diseases, but they both can be kept under control with appropriate monitoring and medications. To this accord, diabetes management has always been a little ahead of glaucoma management. Patients with diabetes have had options of at-home monitoring, continuous glucose monitoring, insulin pumps available long before such options were available for glaucoma. With the numerous changes that we are seeing in both the diagnostic and treatment, glaucoma management beyond the year 2020 is looking particularly attractive. With the new treatment options for medications and surgical modalities being launched regularly, we are perhaps entering a Golden age of glaucoma. We should not celebrate or rejoice prematurely. A lot will be needed before these new modalities become a standard of care. But perhaps paraphrasing the words of Winston Churchill best expresses the current sentiment, "this is not the beginning, this is not the end, but it is perhaps the end of the beginning".

Author details

Pinakin Gunvant Davey[1*] and Jason D. Duncan[2]

1 College of Optometry, Western University of Health Sciences, Pomona, California, USA

2 Southern College of Optometry, Memphis, Tennessee, USA

*Address all correspondence to: contact@pinakin-davey.com

References

[1] Kang JM, Tanna AP. Glaucoma. The Medical Clinics of North America. 2021;**105**(3):493-510. DOI: 10.1016/j.mcna.2021.01.004. Epub 2021 Apr 2

[2] Weinreb RN, Aung T, Medeiros FA. The pathophysiology and treatment of glaucoma: A review. Journal of the American Medical Association. 2014;**311**(18):1901-1911. DOI: 10.1001/jama.2014.3192

[3] Gunvant P, O'Leary DJ, Baskaran M, Broadway DC, Watkins RJ, Vijaya L. Evaluation of tonometric correction factors. Journal of Glaucoma. 2005;**14**(5):337-343. DOI: 10.1097/01.ijg.0000176940.81799.33

[4] Elsheikh A, Gunvant P, Jones SW, Pye D, Garway-Heath D. Correction factors for Goldmann tonometry. Journal of Glaucoma. 2013;**22**(2):156-163. DOI: 10.1097/IJG.0b013e3182312010

[5] Gunvant P, Baskaran M, Vijaya L, Joseph IS, Watkins RJ, Nallapothula M, et al. Effect of corneal parameters on measurements using the pulsatile ocular blood flow tonograph and Goldmann applanation tonometer. The British Journal of Ophthalmology. 2004;**88**(4):518-522. DOI: 10.1136/bjo.2003.019331

[6] Davey PG, Elsheikh A, Garway-Heath DF. Clinical evaluation of multiparameter correction equations for Goldmann applanation tonometry. Eye (London, England). 2013;**27**(5):621-629. DOI: 10.1038/eye.2013.23. Epub 2013 Mar 15

[7] Weinreb RN, Brandt JD, Garway-Heath D, Medeiros F. Intraocular Pressure Volume 4 of Consensus Series, World Glaucoma Association. Amsterdam, The Netherlands: Kugler Publications; 2007. ISSN 2590-1915. ISBN 9062992137

[8] Davey P, Nouri K, Zaczyk S. Assessing the need and benefits of home tonometers in the management of patients with glaucoma. Clinical Optometry (Auckl). 2013;**5**:19-27. DOI: 10.2147/OPTO.S31705

[9] Scott AT, Kanaster K, Kaizer AM, Young CC, Pantcheva MB, Ertel MK, et al. The utility of iCare HOME tonometry for detection of therapy-related intraocular pressure changes in glaucoma and ocular hypertension. Ophthalmology Glaucoma. 2022;**5**(1):85-93. DOI: 10.1016/j.ogla.2021.05.007. Epub 2021 May 31

[10] Mansouri K, Medeiros FA, Tafreshi A, Weinreb RN. Continuous 24-hour monitoring of intraocular pressure patterns with a contact lens sensor: Safety, tolerability, and reproducibility in patients with glaucoma. Archives of Ophthalmology. 2012;**130**(12):1534-1539. DOI: 10.1001/archophthalmol.2012.2280

[11] Chaglasian M, Fingeret M, Davey PG, Huang WC, Leung D, Ng E, et al. The development of a reference database with the Topcon 3D OCT-1 maestro. Clinical Ophthalmology. 2018;**12**:849-857. DOI: 10.2147/OPTH.S155229

[12] Kashani AH, Chen CL, Gahm JK, Zheng F, Richter GM, Rosenfeld PJ, et al. Optical coherence tomography angiography: A comprehensive review of current methods and clinical applications. Progress in Retinal and Eye Research. 2017;**60**:66-100. DOI: 10.1016/j.preteyeres.2017.07.002. Epub 2017 Jul 29

[13] Rao HL, Pradhan ZS, Suh MH, Moghimi S, Mansouri K, Weinreb RN. Opticalcoherencetomographyangiography in glaucoma. Journal of Glaucoma. 2020;**29**(4):312-321. DOI: 10.1097/IJG.0000000000001463

[14] Liu Y, Holekamp NM, Heier JS. Prospective, longitudinal study: Daily self-imaging with home OCT for Neovascular age-related macular degeneration. Ophthalmology Retina. 2022;**6**(7):575-585. DOI: 10.1016/j.oret.2022.02.011. Epub 2022 Feb 28

[15] Le CT, Fiksel J, Ramulu P, Yohannan J. Differences in visual field loss pattern when transitioning from SITA standard to SITA faster. Scientific Reports. 2022;**12**(1):7001. DOI: 10.1038/s41598-022-11044-8

[16] Lavanya R, Riyazuddin M, Dasari S, Puttaiah NK, Venugopal JP, Pradhan ZS, et al. A comparison of the visual field parameters of SITA faster and SITA standard strategies in glaucoma. Journal of Glaucoma. 2020;**29**(9):783-788. DOI: 10.1097/IJG.0000000000001551

[17] Cui QN, Gogt P, Lam JM, Siraj S, Hark LA, Myers JS, et al. Validation and reproducibility of the Heidelberg edge perimeter in the detection of glaucomatous visual field defects. International Journal of Ophthalmology. 2019;**12**(4):577-581. DOI: 10.18240/ijo.2019.04.08

[18] Greenfield JA, Deiner M, Nguyen A, Wollstein G, Damato B, Backus BT, et al. Virtual reality Oculokinetic Perimetry test reproducibility and relationship to conventional Perimetry and OCT. Ophthalmology Science. 2021;**2**(1):100105. DOI: 10.1016/j.xops.2021.100105

[19] Groth SL, Linton EF, Brown EN, Makadia F, Donahue SP. Evaluation of virtual reality Perimetry and standard automated Perimetry in Normal children. Translational Vision Science & Technology. 2023;**12**(1):6. DOI: 10.1167/tvst.12.1.6

[20] Razeghinejad R, Gonzalez-Garcia A, Myers JS, Katz LJ. Preliminary report on a novel virtual reality perimeter compared with standard automated Perimetry. Journal of Glaucoma. 2021;**30**(1):17-23. DOI: 10.1097/IJG.0000000000001670

[21] Mehran NA, Sinha S, Razeghinejad R. New glaucoma medications: Latanoprostene bunod, netarsudil, and fixed combination netarsudil-latanoprost. Eye (London, England). 2020;**34**(1):72-88. DOI: 10.1038/s41433-019-0671-0. Epub 2019 Nov 6

[22] Aihara M, Lu F, Kawata H, Iwata A, Odani-Kawabata N, Shams NK. Omidenepag isopropyl versus Latanoprost in primary open-angle glaucoma and ocular hypertension: The phase 3 AYAME study. American Journal of Ophthalmology. 2020;**220**:53-63. DOI: 10.1016/j.ajo.2020.06.003. Epub 2020 Jun 10. Erratum in: Am J Ophthalmol. 2021 Nov;231:211

[23] Duggan S. Omidenepag isopropyl ophthalmic solution 0.002%: First global approval. Drugs. 2018;**78**(18):1925-1929. DOI: 10.1007/s40265-018-1016-1

[24] Inoue K, Shiokawa M, Katakura S, Tsuruoka M, Kunimatsu-Sanuki S, Shimizu K, et al. Periocular adverse reactions to Omidenepag isopropyl. American Journal of Ophthalmology. 2022;**237**:114-121. DOI: 10.1016/j.ajo.2021.12.011. Epub 2021 Dec 20

[25] Konstas AG, Labbé A, Katsanos A, Meier-Gibbons F, Irkec M, Boboridis KG, et al. The treatment of glaucoma using topical preservative-free agents: An evaluation of safety

and tolerability. Expert Opinion on Drug Safety. 2021;**20**(4):453-466. DOI: 10.1080/14740338.2021.1873947. Epub 2021 Jan 21

[26] Sirinek PE, Lin MM. Intracameral sustained release bimatoprost implants (Durysta). Seminars in Ophthalmology. 2022;**37**(3):385-390. DOI: 10.1080/08820538.2021.1985145. Epub 2021 Sep 29

[27] Kesav NP, Young CEC, Ertel MK, Seibold LK, Kahook MY. Sustained-release drug delivery systems for the treatment of glaucoma. International Journal of Ophthalmology. 2021;**14**(1):148-159. DOI: 10.18240/ijo.2021.01.21

[28] Doozandeh A, Yazdani S. Neuroprotection in glaucoma. J. Ophthalmic Vis. Res. 2016;**11**(2):209-220. DOI: 10.4103/2008-322X.183923

[29] Weinreb RN, Liebmann JM, Cioffi GA, Goldberg I, Brandt JD, Johnson CA, et al. Oral Memantine for the treatment of glaucoma: Design and results of 2 randomized, placebo-controlled, phase 3 studies. Ophthalmology. 2018;**125**(12):1874-1885. DOI: 10.1016/j.ophtha.2018.06.017. Epub 2018 Aug 3

[30] Lem DW, Gierhart DL, Davey PG. Carotenoids in the Management of Glaucoma: A systematic review of the evidence. Nutrients. 2021;**13**(6):1949. DOI: 10.3390/nu13061949

[31] Gazzard G, Konstantakopoulou E, Garway-Heath D, Garg A, Vickerstaff V, Hunter R, et al. Selective laser trabeculoplasty versus eye drops for first-line treatment of ocular hypertension and glaucoma (LiGHT): A multicentre randomised controlled trial. Lancet. 2019;**393**(10180):1505-1516. DOI: 10.1016/S0140-6736(18)32213-X. Epub 2019 Mar 9. Erratum in: Lancet. 2019 Jul 6;394(10192):e1

[32] Geffen N, Ofir S, Belkin A, Segev F, Barkana Y, Kaplan Messas A, et al. Transscleral selective laser Trabeculoplasty without a Gonioscopy lens. Journal of Glaucoma. 2017;**26**(3):201-207. DOI: 10.1097/IJG.0000000000000464

[33] Mai DD, Ingram Z, Oberfeld B, Solá-Del VD. Combined microinvasive glaucoma surgery - a review of the literature and future directions. Seminars in Ophthalmology. 2023:1-8. DOI: 10.1080/08820538.2023.2181665 [Epub ahead of print]

[34] Aref AA, Parker PR, Chen MY. Microinvasive glaucoma surgeries: Critical summary of clinical trial data with and without phacoemulsification. Current Opinion in Ophthalmology. 2023;**34**(2):146-151. DOI: 10.1097/ICU.0000000000000923. Epub 2022 Nov 7

[35] Cantor L, Lindfield D, Ghinelli F, Świder AW, Torelli F, Steeds C, et al. Systematic literature review of clinical, economic, and humanistic outcomes following minimally invasive glaucoma surgery or selective laser Trabeculoplasty for the treatment of open-angle glaucoma with or without cataract extraction. Clinical Ophthalmology. 2023;**17**:85-101. DOI: 10.2147/OPTH.S389406. Epub 2021 May 31

Section 2

The Basics of Glaucoma

Chapter 2

The Molecular Mechanisms of Trabecular Meshwork Damage in POAG and Treatment Advances

Li Tang, Chao Tang, Ying Wang and Xiaolong Shi

Abstract

Primary open-angle glaucoma (POAG) is the leading cause of irreversible blindness affecting over 60 million people worldwide. Elevated intraocular pressure (IOP) due to dysfunction of trabecular meshwork (TM) is the most significant and the only known modifiable risk factor for POAG. Although, glaucomatous TM damage is known to be mainly responsible for IOP elevation, none of the current treatments target TM pathology. This is partly due to an incomplete understanding of the pathophysiological mechanisms of TM damage. In this review, we summarized pathological changes of TM damage in POAG and our current knowledge of the mechanisms of glaucomatous TM damage, particularly focusing on linking the genetic factors of POAG (e.g., mutations and variants in POAG risk genes, risk loci, dysregulation of gene expression) to molecular pathways of pathogenesis in TM. In terms of treatment, reduction of IOP is the mainstream strategy that can be achieved by medical, laser or surgical treatment. IOP lowering drugs, laser or surgery can lower IOP, but do not reverse or restore the oxidative stress or other TM damage in POAG. Additionally, antioxidants, *ginkgo biloba* extract and nutrients could be a promising treatment for POAG.

Keywords: primary open-angle glaucoma (POAG), trabecular meshwork (TM), intraocular pressure (IOP), pathophysiological mechanisms, oxidative stress, autophagy

1. Introduction

Glaucoma is a complex progressive neurodegenerative eye disease characterized by progressive loss of retinal ganglion cells (RGCs) axons [1]. It is the leading cause of irreversible blindness worldwide. Primary open-angle glaucoma (POAG) is the most prevalent form of glaucoma and is responsible for ~90% of all cases. POAG is a multi-tissue disease that targets, in ascending order, the TM, the optic nerve head, the lateral geniculate nuclei and the visual cortex [1]. As is known to us, TM dysfunction induces impaired aqueous humor (AH) drainage, elevated IOP and alterations of the optic nerve head and the visual field defects in POAG [2–5].

As the drainage of the AH outflow pathway, TM cells (TMCs) are constantly exposed to different types of stress such as mechanical, oxidative, and phagocytic stress during their lifetime. TMCs have cellular defense mechanisms including the antioxidant system, proteolytic system, and regulation of stress-responsive genes that allow them to cope with daily challenges. Since TMCs are known to be highly differentiated cells characterized by a low renewal rate, injured cells are not readily replaced and damage is not diluted through cell division, leading to the progressive acceleration of TM damage resulting in glaucoma [6, 7].

Although, significant advances in ophthalmologic knowledge and practice have been made, the mechanisms responsible for TM damage are not yet completely understood. Current treatment for POAG revolves around controlling IOP by drug, laser or surgical treatment, rather than preventing, reducing or repairing TM damage. Therefore, up to now, there is no effective treatment able to ensure healing. In this review, we summarize our current knowledge of the pathological mechanisms of glaucomatous TM damage, particularly focusing on linking the genetic factors of POAG (e.g., mutations and variants in POAG risk genes, risk loci, dysregulation of gene expression) to molecular pathways of pathogenesis in TM.

2. Anatomical structure and biomarkers of TM and AH outflow pathway

The TM is a highly specialized tissue with a small size (100–150 μg, containing approximately 200,000–300,000 cells) located at the angle formed by the cornea and the iris in anterior chamber (AC) [8]. The TM consists of three regions: the uveal meshwork (UM) which is adjacent to the anterior chamber, corneoscleral meshwork (CM) which is located at the middle layer, and juxtacanalicular tissue (JCT) which is made up of TM cells embedded in the extracellular matrix. The JCT is adjacent to the inner wall of Schlemm's canal (SC) and is considered to offer the major resistance to the AH outflow (**Figure 1**). The AH is generated in the ciliary processes from arterial blood. Then AH reaches the anterior chamber from the posterior chamber by passing the pupil and flows out through the TM. After crossing the TM, AH reaches Schlemm's canal, which drains directly to the aqueous veins. The TM is the main pathway (called the conventional pathway) for modulating AH outflow resistance. Approximately 10% of the remaining AH leaves the anterior chamber through the uveoscleral pathway (unconventional pathway).

Previously, AQP1, MGP, CHI3L1, TIMP3 and MYOC were used as typical TM markers. However, their application is hindered due to their limited specificity for distinguishing diverse cell types in a tissue. Larger-scale single-cell sequencing combining the *in situ* immunohistochemistry is a powerful strategy for revealing substantial cell markers for distinguishing different cell types in tissues. Recently, Patel et al. [9] and Zyl et al. [10] used single-cell RNA sequencing (scRNAseq) to identify the cell types in the human trabecular meshwork and the surrounding tissues, providing new insights into the cell types that comprise these pathways. Zyl et al. identified 19 cell types in these tissues with distinct molecular markers to define them using scRNAseq. The results of some key genes were validated in tissue by in situ hybridization or immunostaining. Among 19 cell types, 8 cell types (Clusters 3, 5, 8, 16, 15, 9,7, and 18) belong the conventional outflow pathway. Of them, cell types of Clusters 3, 5, and 8 are within the filtering TM region, with high expression levels of MYOC, MGP, PDPN, and RARRES1. Clusters 3 and 5 are distinguished by preferential expression of FABP4 and TMEFF2, respectively, each of which marked a subset of beam cells, Beam A and Beam B. Other clusters, such as Cluster 16, 15, 9, 7, and 18 correspond to cells adjacent to the filtering TM region with several new markers [10].

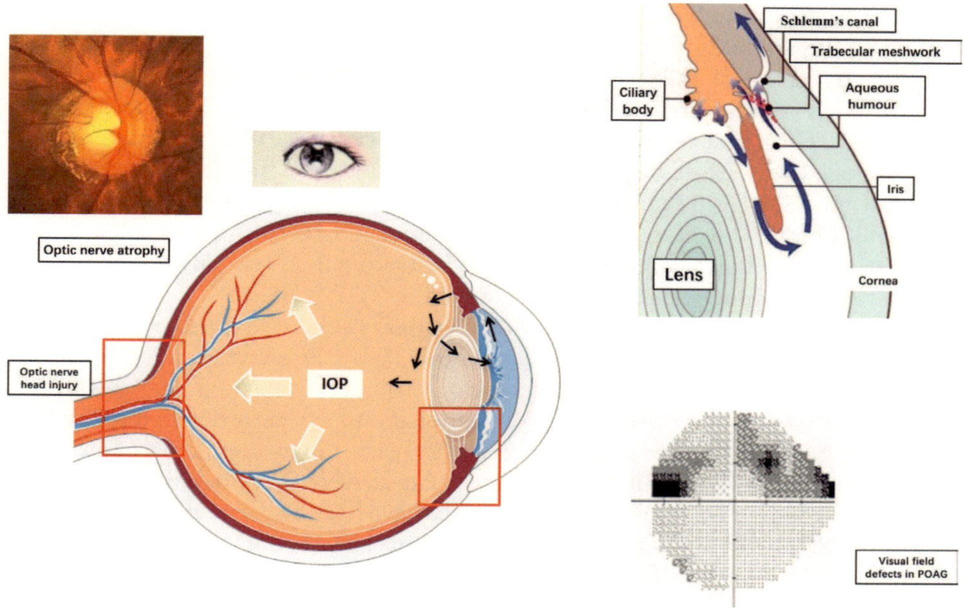

Figure 1.
The whole eye and the TM tissue were shown in both two-dimensionally and three-dimensionally to explain the AH outflow pathway. Normal IOP is required to maintain the proper physiological function and the structure of the globe of the eye. The IOP state critically depends on the balance between the inflow and outflow of AH. Malfunction of TM induces elevated IOP and alterations of the optic nerve head and the visual field defects. The TM consists of endothelial cells immersed in their fundamental substance. AH flows through the TM in both the intercellular route and the transcellular route.

3. Pathological changes of TM damage in POAG

3.1 Abnormal accumulation of extracellular matrix (ECM) components in glaucomatous TM

In POAG, TMCs undergo a series of molecular and morphological alterations which lead to a gradual decrease in their cell number and IOP elevation. The increase of IOP, in turn, results in other pathological alterations that further impair cell homeostasis, leading to a vicious circle [11].

TM fibrosis is a key pathological characteristic of POAG [12, 13]. Fibrosis results in increased ECM deposits both in the TM and in the lamina cribrosa (LC). Both aberrant stiffness of TMCs and abnormal accumulation of ECM components contribute to TM fibrosis, leading to AH outflow resistance and elevated IOP [13]. During the process of POAG, the TM displays several alterations on morphologies and functions, including cell loss, increased heterogeneity of TM cellularity, increased accumulation of ECM, reduced adhesion of TMCs to ECM, formation of cross-linked actin networks, endothelial dysregulation, changes in the cytoskeleton, altered motility, reduced adhesion of TMCs to ECM, subclinical inflammation, progressive senescence and outflow impairment [11–15]. TM damage might trigger cross-linked proteins formation within aging tissues with malfunctioning proteolytic and ECM remodeling, as well as apoptosis and cell loss [13]. The AH proteome profile also undergoes dramatic changes, reflecting cellular and molecular damage to the TM [14, 16].

Transforming growth factor-β (TGF-β) signaling is widely recognized as a core pathway of fibrosis. TGF-β2 expression is increased in the AH and TM of POAG eyes [12]. Activation of TGF-β2 signaling causes a significant increase in oxidative stress in TMCs [17]. Several studies have demonstrated that TGF-β is involved in TM damage: (1) TGF-β induces mitochondrial ROS generation, (2) ROS are required for TGF-β induced gene expression downstream of Smad3 phosphorylation and nuclear translocation, (3) TGF-β induced transcription of nicotinamide adenine dinucleotide phosphate (NADPH) oxidase 4 requires mitochondrial ROS forming a feedback loop leading to increased intracellular ROS, and (4) blocking ROS generation markedly reduces TM profibrotic gene expression induced by TGF-β [18, 19].

Clinical evidence also suggests that POAG patients exhibit features of impaired NO signaling. NO is produced in vascular endothelia by the enzyme endothelial NO synthase (eNOS). The previous studies have confirmed that eNOS is an important protein in IOP regulation through the conventional outflow pathway. In the TMCs, NO has a critical role on the relaxation of TM [20]. The down-regulation of eNOS activity and reduced availability of NO is associated with POAG. In animal model studies, increased eNOS levels in the mouse TM have been associated with a reduction of IOP [21]. Stamer et al. [21] reported that mice overexpressing NOS3 had lower IOP and increased outflow facility than wild type in mice. Conversely, increased IOP and reduced outflow facility were observed in the NOS3 KO mice [22]. Furthermore, exogenous NO donor compounds can reduce IOP and increase outflow facility in several animal models [23]. Recently, Patel et al. [23] show that fluid flow-induced shear stress activates TRPV4TM channels and induces eNOS-mediated NO production. The activity of TRPV4TM channels is impaired in glaucoma that render TM cells are insensitive to fluid flow-induced shear stress. TRPV4 channel activator can lowers IOP and improve outflow facility by increasing eNOS activity and production of NO in TM cells. This indicates an important role for TRPV4-eNOS signaling in IOP regulation. In addition, studies have also demonstrated the association of polymorphisms in the NOS3 gene, which encodes eNOS, with the development of glaucoma [24].

4. Pathophysiological mechanisms of TM damage: implications for POAG pathogenesis

It is well known that several factors, including aging, genetic factors, environmental factors, and metabolites, involved in the onset and development of TM damage in POAG. Moreover, several mechanisms are triggered, leading to TM damage.

4.1 Oxidative stress

Oxidative stress is the exact and the most concerned mechanism leading to DNA, mitochondrial, and ECM damage in the TM and contributing to POAG pathogenesis [25, 26]. Several studies have demonstrated that TMCs are the most sensitive cell types to oxidant damage [25, 26]. The ability of TMCs to fight oxidative damage is critical to their survival and functions. Under normal circumstances, TM is exposed to a constant low level of oxidative stress and the expression of antioxidant enzymes makes TMC relatively resistant to oxidative damage. Excessive accumulation of reactive oxygen species (ROS) or an imbalance between oxidants and antioxidants may lead to oxidative stress in TMCs [27, 28]. The progress of POAG may be accompanied by a decrease in the antioxidant capacity of TMCs. Also, free radicals cause a gradual increase in oxidative damage, cytoskeletal changes and ECM accumulation in TMCs [29]. Oxidative damage to ECM adhesion results in damage to TM integrity, TM cell adhesion, and finally leads to cell loss [30]. As well, oxidative stress could damage the TMCs proliferation and migration function [17].

4.2 Inflammation

Inflammation is known to be increased in POAG patients [18, 19, 31]. The study revealed that cellular infiltration of immunocompetent cells (CD3+ and CD45+ cells) exists around the collector channels of the TM pathway in POAG [31]. Increased levels of inflammatory mediators, such as TGF-β1, TNF-α, and interleukins (e.g., IL-1α, IL-1β, IL-6, IL-8, IL-10, IL-20 family) were found in the TMCs and the AH of POAG patients and animal models [31–33]. These inflammatory mediators can induce changes in the ECM and the TMCs cytoskeleton, and have been shown to be associated with the pathogenesis of POAG [33]. Some factors, such as IL-1α, which is highly expressed in TMCs, can up-regulate the expression of other inflammatory mediators [31–33]. The up-regulation of inflammatory mediators, e.g., IL-1α, and IL-1β, induced by oxidative stress in TMCs were reported [34]. In addition, both NF-κB and arachidonic acid are inflammatory components that are known to be activated in the TMCs to protect against oxidative stress in POAG eyes [35, 36]. Along with the continued activation of inflammatory responses, TM exhibits decreased cellularity and irreversible damage. Prostaglandin analogues converted from arachidonic acid are currently used for the treatment of POAG. These prostaglandin analogues reduce IOP by increasing the outflow of AH [37, 38]. These results reinforce the association between inflammation and POAG pathogenesis.

4.3 Vascular dysregulation and hypoxia

Primary vascular dysregulation (PVD) is another potential mechanism of POAG pathogenesis. Most POAG patients have signs of decreased ocular blood flow and ocular ischemia in the eye, indicating that hemodynamic factors are also involved in the POAG process [39–41]. In POAG eyes, oxygen tension in the tissue often falls temporarily and very mildly. This fall occurs repeatedly over years and leads to a preconditional adaptation, making the TMCs more resistant to coming oxygen fall. When the oxygen fall exceeds a certain critical value, reperfusion damage occurs. If the oxygen drop lasts longer or greater, it can cause tissue infarction. In POAG, reperfusion damage is very mild but recurrent as well [41]. Recurrently mild reperfusion induces chronic oxidative stress and inflammation, which harms a diversity of molecules and reduces cellular survival. IOP fluctuation is more damaging than a stably increased IOP [42]. All POAG patients with elevated IOP or normal IOP suffer from autoregulation disorders [43], for which the main cause is PVD contributing via ischemia, hypoxia and oxidative stress to TM damage. Meanwhile, systemic oxidative stress is also associated with decreased ocular blood flow [44]. In addition, nitric oxide (NO) is an endothelium-derived relaxing factor, which improves ocular blood flow [20]. In patients with glaucoma, decreased NO production has been found in AH of POAG patients compared with controls [45].

4.4 Endoplasmic reticulum (ER) stress

Recent studies have revealed the role of chronic ER dysfunction of TM in the POAG process [46]. The ER is a vast membranous network and interacts with the ribosome, Golgi bodies, proteasomes and mitochondria. ER is a central organelle for of synthesis, modification, folding and maturation of proteins. Accumulation of unfolded and misfolded proteins in the ER would trigger activation of the unfolded protein response (UPR) pathways [2, 47]. UPR could be activated by increased protein synthesis, inhibition of protein glycosylation, the presence of mutant or misfolded proteins, imbalance of ER calcium levels, energy deprivation, hypoxia, pathogens or pathogen and toxins. PERK, a type I ER transmembrane kinase, is activated by ER stress. The activation of PERK leads to phosphorylation of the eukaryotic translation initiation factor (eIF2α), resulting in translational repression. On the other hand, under ER stress condition, transcription factor 4 (ATF4) is upregulated that leading to the increase of C/EBP homologous protein (CHOP) [47]. The activation of PERK-ATF4-CHOP persists during chronic ER stress and triggers cell death [2, 47, 48]. Expression of either ATF4 or CHOP promotes aberrant TMCs protein synthesis and ER client protein load, leading to ECM accumulation and TM dysfunction. The damaged ER activates inflammation via NF-κB, mitochondrial damages, and enhanced TM cell apoptosis, which leads to elevated IOP [48].

4.5 Proteolytic system malfunction and compromised autophagy

The normal function of the proteolytic system in TM plays a role in preventing POAG. Misfolded and mutated newly synthesized proteins are rapidly degraded to prevent the toxicity caused by protein accumulation [49]. The major proteolytic system includes the ubiquitin-proteasome system (UPS) and autophagy. PERK, IRE1α and ATF6α that are the three ER stress sensors that can regulate UPS and autophagy during the ER stress [50]. The protein degradation process regulated by UPR has great significance for the maintenance of normal function of TM. In most cases, the degradation of excessive proteins protects TMCs with stress survival from apoptosis [51, 52].

Autophagy is a fundamental process for the degradation or recycling of intracellular components, which promotes cell survival or promotes cell death in an environment-dependent manner [49]. On one hand, basal autophagy under physiological conditions is a cellular self-protection mechanism, protecting cell survival in the absence of energy or nutrients and responding to cytotoxic insults, which is critical to maintain cell homeostasis in synthesis, degradation and recycling of cell compounds [49, 50]. On the other hand, excessive stress-induced autophagy may cause cellular stress in turn and promote apoptosis or autophagic cell death [50–53]. Autophagy selectively eliminates unwanted, potentially harmful cytosolic material, such as damaged mitochondria or protein aggregates. It is apparent that autophagy is impaired in TM pathologies [50].

Acute stress can initiate autophagosome formations and autophagic degradation [54]. However, the TM pathological processes of POAG are long-term chronic procedures instead of acute changes. When TM cells are chronically exposed to oxidative or other stress, significant functional damage to their lysosome system has been observed. The accumulation of nondegradable ECM resulting from impaired autophagy accelerates cell senescence [55]. These harmful processes contribute to TM structural and functional alterations. Porter et al. [54] revealed the activation of autophagy responding to chronic oxidative stress in TMCs is mTOR-dependent.

4.6 Aging

Oxidant stress, inflammation, ischemia, hypoxia ER stress, protein aggregation, metabolic block and other stress events as well as impaired cellular repairability, have been found to be involved in the induction of senescence of TM [56]. Senescent TM tissue presents an alternated morphological and molecular phenotype, including TM becomes more pigmented, the scleral spur becomes more evident, the trabeculae become flatter and gradually merges into each other, and the occurrence of the denudation of trabecular areas [57]. The increase in thickness of the sheaths of the elastic-like fibers is also observed in the cribriform layer of TM during the aging. The molecular alterations in TM during the aging include increased anti-apoptotic gene expression, chronic activation of the DNA-damage response (DDR), increased activity of the β-galactosidase associated with senescence (SA-β-Gal), lipofuscin accumulations in lysosomes, lysosomes accumulations, increased number of defective mitochondria and the activation of unfolded protein response (UPR) in the endoplasmic reticulum (ER). Moreover, a reduced ATP release in response to mechanical stress and a severe dysregulation of calcium homeostasis which can contribute to TM age-related damage were observed in TM senescent cells [58]. Decreased cellularity is another character in aging TM tissue. An approximately 60% of reduction is observed in TM cellularity associated with aging from 0 to 80 years, indicating there are fewer TM cells in aged glaucomatous human eyes compared to young, healthy human tissue [58].

5. Abnormal intercellular communication

Extracellular vesicles (EVs) allow the exchange of nucleotides, proteins and lipids between cells and mediate intracellular communication, which may play a key role in TM function and the POAG pathogenesis [59]. EVs are important constituents of the AH, which participates in the communication between the non-pigmented ciliary epithelium (NPCE) and the TM [60]. AH carrying EVs is produced by the NPCE and flows into the posterior chamber, which then moves into the anterior chamber and is finally drained through the TM and into the venous system [61]. Intercellular communication can be achieved by EVs membrane proteins that interact with the TMCs through endocytosis, phagocytosis or act as ligands for cell surface receptors on TMCs [62–64]. Interestingly, when TM is exposed to EVs, its ability to resist oxidative stress is enhanced [65]. EVs-mediated cell-to-cell communications between NPCE and TMCs are involved in the IOP regulation. When TMCs receive the wrong signal carried by EV from NPCE, TMCs will not be able to respond sensitively to maintain IOP homeostasis. Recurrent incorrect response patterns may lead to TM dysfunction and morphologic alterations. The canonical Wnt signaling may involved in the regulation of IOP and in the effects of NPCE-derived EVs on TMCs [65].

6. Pathogenic genes associated with trabecular meshwork damage in POAG

A substantial fraction of glaucoma cases is influenced by genetic factors. About 5–10% of POAG is currently attributed to single-gene (e.g., MYOC, CYP1B1, GLIS3, LOXL1, LTBP2, PITX2, EFEMP1 and OPTN) or Mendelian forms of glaucoma [66–69]. Many of the remaining cases of POAG may due to the combined effects of multiple genes and the interactions of gene-environment. Genome-wide association studies (GWAS) have demonstrated many genomic loci are associated with POAG risk, including CDKN2B-AS1, TMCO1, CAV1, CAV2, SIX1, SIX6, AFAP1, ABCA1,

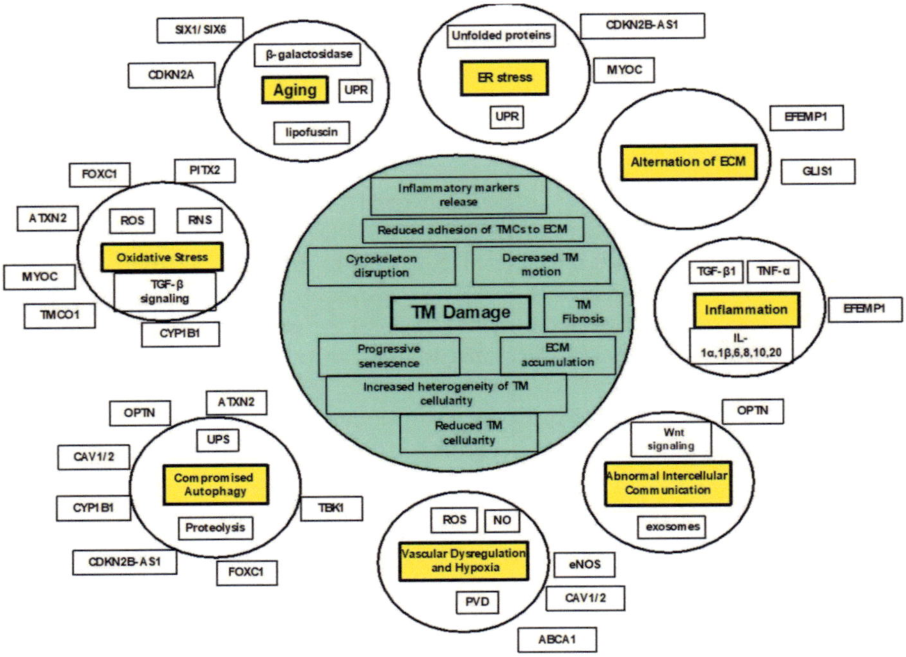

Figure 2.
Histopathological characters of trabecular meshwork (TM) damage in POAG. Implications for POAG pathogenesis: pathophysiological mechanisms of TM damage driven by oxidative stress and mitochondrial dysfunction, inflammation, vascular dysregulation and hypoxia, compromised autophagy, endoplasmic reticulum (ER) stress, abnormal intercellular communication and aging.

TXNRD2, FOXC1/GMDS, ATXN2, FNDC3B, ABO, PMM2, ATOH7, TMCO1, and GAS7 [69]. Recently, a large multi-ethnic meta-analysis of genome-wide association studies identified 127 POAG risk loci, and of which 44 loci were previously unreported [70]. These genetic risk factors affect the development of POAG through a variety of pathological processes (**Figure 2**). Here we focus on several genes involved in the maintenance of TM functions and pathological processes of POAG.

6.1 MYOC

MYOC is the first gene identified to be involved in POAG. MYOC encodes the secreted protein myocilin, which is highly expressed in the TM cells. Mutations in MYOC were found with a high prevalence rate in patients with POAG of various populations. However, studies demonstrate that overexpression or knockout of Myoc in mice does not cause glaucoma, hinting a gain-of-function mechanism may be involved [71, 72]. Accumulating evidences indicate that mutant Myoc is misfolded and accumulates within TM cells, which promote ER stress [73, 74]. The ER stress activates the UPR signal, which protects the TM cells, corrects misfolding, prevents translation of misfolded proteins, prevents translation of misfolded proteins and degrades misfolded proteins. However, excessive and sustained ER stress can trigger apoptosis in the TMCs, which then leads to an increase in resistance to AH outflow and elevated IOP, and, ultimately, glaucoma.

6.2 GLIS1 and GLIS3

GLI-similar 1-3 (GLIS1-3) constitute a subfamily of Krüppel-like zinc finger proteins that are involved in multiple biological processes by acting either as activators or repressors of gene transcription [75]. GLIS2 plays a critical role in the kidney and GLIS2 dysfunction leads to nephronophthisis, an end-stage, cystic renal disease [75]. GLIS3 plays a critical role in the regulation of multiple biological processes and is a key regulator of pancreatic β cell generation and maturation, insulin gene expression, thyroid hormone biosynthesis, spermatogenesis, and the maintenance of normal kidney functions [75]. GLIS3 genes have been associated with the increased risk of several diseases including glaucoma [75, 76]. GWAS studies have identified several SNP located in GLIS3, e.g., rs2224492 [76], rs736893 [77] and rs6476827 [78], associated with increased risk of POAG or raised IOP.

A previous study showed that GLIS1 significantly promotes the reprogramming of somatic cells into induced pluripotent stem cells (iPSCs) [75]. Recently, Gharahkhani et al. [70] conducted a large multi-ethnic meta-analysis of genome-wide association studies and identified more novel loci for POAG risk, including GLIS1 locus (rs941125). The study by Nair et al. [79] demonstrates that the mice lacking GLIS1 developed enlarged eyes and a long-lasting increase in IOP. The study revealed that low levels of GLIS1 induce the degeneration of the TM, leading to inefficient drainage of the AH in mice. In addition, they showed that GLIS1 regulates the expression of several glaucoma-associated genes, e.g., MYOC, LTBP2, LOXL1, TGFBR3, ADAMTS10, CYP1B1, EFEMP1, MMP2, and several ECM-related genes including collagen I, IV, ADAMTS10, FBN2, LOXL1–4, and VI families, LTBP2, a regulator of TGFβ signaling and ECM deposition. In addition, the researchers also identified rs941125 at GLIS1 gene in humans are linked to risk of POAG. All these results indicate that GLIS1 is a key regulator in TMCs and a risk gene of glaucoma.

6.3 FOXC1

FOXC1 belongs to the Forkhead box (FOX) family of transcription factors and it is expressed in the adult eye including the TM. FOXC1 has been identified as a susceptibility locus for POAG and elevated IOP in several GWAS studies [76, 78, 80]. Mutations in the FOXC1 gene can cause Axenfeld-Rieger syndrome (ARS), a developmental disorder affecting structures in the anterior segment of the eye with an increase in IOP [80]. More than half of ARS patients with FOXC1 mutations will develop earlier-onset glaucoma. FOXC1 is expressed in ocular tissues including TM. Several genes that have TM relevant functions including miR-204, OLFM3, CXCL6, MEIS2, LDLRAD2, CLOCK and ITGb1 expressions was affected by FOXC1 in TM cells [81]. FOXC1 has been demonstrated to be a critical regulator for stress response [82]. The TM is the most sensitive tissue of the anterior segment of the eye to oxidative stress. Studies demonstrate that reduced FOXC1 expression increases cell death in cultured TM cells in response to oxidative stress, suggesting FOXC1 have a role in preventing cell death under both normal and oxidative stress conditions [82, 83]. HSPA6, a member of the heat-shock 70 family of proteins, has been identified as a target gene of FOXC1 [83]. HSPA6 protein is induced under severe oxidative stress conditions, has a protective function in TM cells. A decrease in FOXC1 results in the repression of several anti-apoptotic genes, including FOXO1A [82]. FOXO1A is a key protein in cellular stress response and apoptotic pathways, its expression is directly regulated by FOXC1 in TM cells [82]. Studies have shown that the FOXC1 gene also was involved in the regulation of prostaglandin receptor genes [84]. Doucette et al. [84] confirmed that FOXC1 binds to enhancer element of EP3 gene prostaglandin receptor (PTGER3) and activates PTGER3 expression. Other prostaglandin receptor genes EP1 (PTGER1), EP2 (PTGER2), EP4 (PTGER4), and FP (PTGFR) were altered when FOXC1 was knocked down in culture TM cells. This study provides a clue to explain why some glaucomatous patients do not respond to treatment of Prostaglandin analogs. Prostaglandin analogs (e.g., latanoprost, bimatoprost, travoprost, and tafluprost) are the frontline medications used to lower IOP in glaucomatous patients. However, about 30% of patients do not respond to these medications. Furthermore, 50–60% of patients with secondary glaucoma caused by FOXC1-mediated ARS did not respond to these medications. FOXC1 mutation or reduction of expression leads to the dysregulation of the prostaglandin signaling pathway, which probably account for the lacking of response to prostaglandin-based medications [84].

6.4 ATXN2

ATXN2 is a ubiquitous RNA-binding protein with a polyglutamine (polyQ) CAG repeat in its coding region. ATXN2 has roles in regulating many cellular processes, including stress granule formation, starvation and stress response, translation, RNA processing, metabolism, mitochondrial function, and calcium signaling [85, 86]. Expansions of polyglutamine repeat of ATXN2 have been implicated in spinocerebellar ataxia 2 (SCA2) and amyotrophic lateral sclerosis (ALS) [83]. In addition to causing SCA2 and increasing the risk of developing ALS, mutations in ATXN2 may play a role in a handful of other diseases, including Parkinson's disease (PD), spinocerebellar ataxia type I (SCA1), Machado-Joseph Disease (SCA3), tauopathies, POAG, obesity and type I diabetes [85, 86].

In eukaryotic cells, various cellular stresses (e.g., starvation, heat shock, ER stress, oxidative stress) elicit the formation of cytoplasmic stress granules (SGs) as a part of the homeostatic response [87]. SGs contain non-translating mRNAs, translation initiation factors, and RBPs, which protect cells from damaging signals and suppress general translation. SG formation is beneficial for cell survival by preventing the accumulation of misfolded proteins and mutant proteins. Furthermore, upon the environmental stresses, SGs sequester several apoptosis regulatory factors into granules and thereby inhibit stress-induced cell death signaling. Since TM cells are exposed to various stresses simultaneously during their lifetime, the formation of SGs under multiple stress conditions is important for the function maintenance of TM cells.

Mutations of ATXN2 have been linked to impaired formation of stress granule in normotensive glaucoma, primary open-angle glaucoma, SCA2, and ALS [85]. ATXN2, ATXN2L, and their associating proteins have been identified as key components of mammalian SGs. Depletion of ATXN2 suppresses the SGs formation. ATXN2 repeat expansions impair the assembly of stress granule, leading to stress-granule-induced cytotoxicity and neurodegeneration. Studies show that inhibition of SGs assembly could promote apoptosis of cells [88]. Clearing of SGs involves in the autophagy pathway. Polyglutamine expansions in ATXN2 have been associated with autophagic and mitochondrial dysfunction in several neurodegenerative diseases. The study finds that the SCA2 cells expressing expanded ataxin-2 are particularly susceptible to autophagic inhibition when cells were treated with autophagy inhibitor chloroquine [89]. This treatment led to more apoptosis in SCA2 cells compare to controls, hinting that the SCA2 cells are more susceptible for autophagic inhibition [89]. This could be explained that ATXN2 is an inhibitor of mTOR signaling [90]. MTOR has been characterized as a negative regulator of autophagy [91]. This suggests that mutation of ATXN2 may lead to compromised autophagy by reducing inhibition of mTOR signaling.

Besides, GWAS study have identified ATXN2 were associated with risk for POAG [78, 79]. Expression analysis reveals that ATXN2 is expressed in the cornea, trabecular meshwork, ciliary body, retina and optic nerve [92]. It has the strongest expression in RGCs [92] and this result is confirmed by the expression profile from scRNAseq [10]. The expression of ATXN2 in key POAG-relevant ocular tissues supports its potential role in autophagy and stress granule formation in response to ocular hypertension.

6.5 EFEMP1

EFEMP1 encodes fibulin-3, an extracellular matrix protein that serves to modulate cellular behavior and functions by connecting and integrating multiple partner molecules in the extracellular compartment. It is expressed in the retina and RPE, involved in age-related macular degeneration (AMD) [93, 94]. A GWAS identified copy number variation (CNV) at NPHP1 and EFEMP1 as potential candidates for the association of inherited retinal degenerative diseases [95]. The EFEMP1 gene was located within the GLC1H locus on chromosome 2p (2p15-p16). A report located a genetic locus (GLC1H) for adult-onset POAG maps to the 2p15-p16 region with linkage analysis in an Afro-Caribbean (Jamaican) population [96]. In another study, a region on chr2 (chr2: 46.4 M–65.6 M) was located that contributed to POAG with family-linkage analysis studies in Chinese [97, 98], which is overlapped with the 2p15-p16 region. A study identified a novel missense variant (p.Arg140Trp) in exon 5 of the gene coding for EFEMP1 that cosegregated with POAG in an African-American family [99]. Recently several GWAS studies have demonstrated that EFEMP1 is associated with increased risk for increased IOP for POAG [66, 78, 100]. In addition, mutations in EFEMP1 also were identified in sporadic POAG patients [68]. EFEMP1 is regulated by GLIS1 in TM cells [79]. Altered cell-ECM interaction or abnormal ECM organization was observed in Glis1-KO mice [79]. Furthermore, analysis of single-cell sequencing revealed that EFEMP1 is high expressed in Fibroblast, JCT and BeamB in TM region [10], indicating EFEMP1 plays a critical regulatory role in maintaining the structural integrity and functionality of the TM. As described in the previous section, TGF-β2 is significantly increased in the AH of patients with POAG. Expression analysis showed that EFEMP1 can be downregulated by TGF-β2 in cultured HTM cells [101], indicating the function of EFEMP1 may be impaired in TM in some POAG patients.

6.6 LOXL1

LOXL1 is a member of the lysyl oxidase family involving in extracellular matrix formation. This enzyme is required for linking collagen and elastin in connective tissues and catalyzing the polymerization of tropoelastin to form the mature elastin polymer. Previously, it was thought that the LOXL1 gene was associated only with XFG [102]. The allele T for the intronic SNP (rs2165241), and the allele G for both coding SNPs (rs1048661 and rs3825942) are associated with a higher risk of XFS and XFG in the studied population [102]. It seems that low levels of LOXL1 expression could predispose to XFS. No association was seen with POAG in that study. However, several recent GWAS studies in different ethnic populations have demonstrated that LOXL1 was associated with risk for POAG [70, 103–105].

LOXL1 expression is detected in ocular tissues such as lamina cribrosa, lens epithelium, cornea, ciliary muscle, and trabecular meshwork, all of which are mainly involved in the formation of the extracellular matrix. Profile of expression from scRNAseq revealed LOXL1 is predominantly expressed in TM (BeamB, JCT, and BeamA) [10]. In TM cells, LOXL1 is regulated by GLIS1. When GLIS1 was knocked down by shRNA lentivirus in HTM cells, the expression of LOXL1 was reduced [102]. ChIP-Seq analyses revealed that LOXL1 is directly regulated by GLIS1 protein binding to its promoter [79].

Glaucoma is age-related disease in human. Recent research suggests that epigenetics, especially DNA methylation, plays a critical role in aging. One proposed cause of aging is the disruption of epigenetic-sensitive molecular networks, which lead to decreased tissue function. Several evidences of LOXL1 epigenetic silencing by promoter methylation were reported in cancer and Cutis Laxa, a disorder of connective tissue [106–108]. Ye et al. reported that the promoter region of the LOXL1 gene was hypermethylated in patients with Pseudoexfoliation Glaucoma (PXFG) compared with controls, leading to a reduced expression of its protein product and downstream impaired elastic fiber homeostasis [107]. Similarly, Greene et al. [109] also discovered that the LOXL1 promoter methylation was increased in patients with PXFG compared to Control. These results indicated that hypermethylation of CpG islands in the LOXL1 gene may function as an essential mechanism in the pathogenesis of PXFG Glaucoma. In addition, the rare variant that probably impacts the function of LOXL1 protein was discovered in sporadic cases of POAG [68]. In our recent report, we found a rare variant (p.Cys448Phe) occurred in the LOXL1 protein lysyl oxidase domain [68]. This site is a conserved residue since the 443–456 sites are highly conserved in this domain, and several copper ion binding sites (His449, His451, and H453) are located in this region. It is worth noting that Cys448 and Cys497 will form a disulfide bond and the alternation of amino acid (from Cys to Phe) may lead to breakage of the S–S bond. These multiple lines of evidence indicate that the loss or decrease of LOXL1 function is related to Glaucoma, and it may also be an important risk factor for POAG.

7. Treatment

Different worldwide treatment recommendations and guidelines exist for the management of POAG [110–113]. IOP is the main modifiable risk factor proven to alter the disease course in these guidelines. IOP lowering can be achieved by medication, laser or surgery (either alone or in combination). Moreover, nutrients in the foods that we consume every day can alter gene expression in cells, thereby exerting a beneficial or harmful physiological effect. Lifestyle, exercise, and nutrients therefore play a key role in eye health and could be used as an adjuvant in POAG therapy [114, 115].

Re-cellularization of the trabecular meshwork (TM) using stem cells is a potential novel treatment for POAG. Recent experimental studies demonstrated the potential effectiveness of regenerative therapies using iPSCs or TM progenitor cells in restoring TM tissue and reducing IOP. however, the potential plasticity and the lack of definitive cell markers for TM cells compound the biological challenge. Morphological and differential gene expression of TM cells located within different regions made it difficult to regenerate [116]. Here, we will not describe the detail of these novel therapies.

7.1 IOP-lowering drugs

Topical IOP-lowering medications have long been the POAG treatment and are widely used. The prostaglandin analogues reduce IOP by increasing the outflow of AH, primarily through the uveoscleral pathway [37]. They have also been shown to remodel ECM within the TM and reduce outflow resistance [38]. Prostaglandins became the first-line medication for POAG because of their IOP-lowering efficacy, once daily application and minimal systemic side-effects. Long-term use of PGA has been reported to decrease the central corneal thickness due to activation of corneal stromal matrix metalloproteinases (MMPs) [117–120]. The other ophthalmic medication classes used in clinical practice include the beta-adrenergic blocking agents, the alpha-2 adrenergic agonists, and the carbonic anhydrase inhibitors [118, 119]. They can cause multiple ocular and systemic side-effects with poor compliance, which limits their clinical use.

Newer medical treatments are in development, including trabodenoson (a highly selective adenosine-1 receptor agonist), netarsudil (a Rho-kinase inhibitor and norepinephrine transporter inhibitor), latanoprostene bunod (a modified prostaglandin analogue), ONO-9054 (a novel non-selective prostanoid receptor agonist, dual EP3 and FP agonist) and others. Theoretically, most of these medicines are IOP-lowering treatments with new mechanisms of action, better efficacy, tolerability and convenience. The results of clinical trials including phase 3 trials were concluded successively [120–130].

As novel candidates for POAG, the ATP channel openers have been reported to protect the retinal ganglion cells during ischemic stress and glutamate-induced toxicity suggesting a neuroprotective property for this drug class [131].

7.2 Lasers

Selective laser trabeculoplasty (SLT) is a viable alternative ophthalmic treatment when patients experience ocular or systemic side effects due to medication. SLT is relatively safe and well-tolerated with low complication rates [132]. Recently, the laser in glaucoma and ocular hypertension (LiGHT) study [133] has evaluated treatment-naive patients with POAG or ocular hypertension randomly allocated to receive either initial primary SLT or initial topical medication. The LiGHT study demonstrates that there is no difference in health-related quality of life (HRQL) between primary SLT and initial topical medication at 36 months. It provides good IOP control, at a lower cost and allowed almost 74% of patients to be successfully controlled without drops for at least 3 years after starting treatment. The study demonstrates that SLT is safe and effective as a first-line treatment for POAG and should be offered as an alternative to IOP-lowering topical medication. Other laser trabeculoplasty procedures include Micropulse Diode Laser Trabeculoplasty (MDMT), Titanium Sapphire Laser Trabeculoplasty (TLT) and Pattern Scanning Laser Trabeculoplasty (PSLT) [132, 133]. Some small studies have compared their efficacy against SLT and found their potential advantages. However, larger studies are required to support whether any of them provide extra advantages over existing SLT.

7.3 Surgery

Several different glaucoma IOP-lowering surgeries exist, including penetrating (trabeculectomy, tube surgery, etc.), and non-penetrating surgery (deep sclerectomy, visco-canalostomy, and canaloplasty, etc.). Their use in clinical practice should consider not only the evidence of lowering intraocular pressure and the safety of each operation, but also the individual patient's status. The decreases of IOP often were observed after cataract surgery [134, 135]. Cataract surgery has been described as the single best glaucoma surgery due to its IOP-lowering effect. Thus, clinicians may serve phacoemulsification as a valid treatment option for newly diagnosed POAG. The incisional operation generally achieves greater IOP lowering compared to medication and is usually performed if IOP lowering is insufficient by medication or laser [135]. But it may be a viable first option in those newly diagnosed POAG patients with a poor compliance or intolerant to medication. The Treatment of Advanced Glaucoma Study (TAGS) is currently investigating whether the surgical intervention could be the first treatment option in newly diagnosed advanced POAG [136].

7.4 *Ginkgo biloba* extract

G. biloba has been used as traditional herbal medicine for hundreds of years in China [137]. *G. biloba* extract (GBE) contains two groups of active substances: flavonoid glycosides including quercetin, rutin, and terpene lactones including ginkgolides A, B, C, and bilobalide [137, 138]. All these substances are now widely used as dietary supplements for decades in the world [137]. It has been used as a brain tonic to enhance memory, to decrease mental fatigue, and to improve concentration. Additionally, it is used to treat vertigo, tinnitus and vitiligo, to improve visual and auditory acuity, and in various neurological and psychological disorders such as dementia, cognitive decline and functional disability [137]. GBE has also beneficial effects on the cardiovascular system and has been claimed to prevent atherosclerosis [139]. Currently, its application in glaucoma is garnering much attention [140]. Flavonoids that are often found in *G. biloba* could increase ocular blood flow and potentially delay the progression of vision loss [141]. Several properties of GBE can be useful in the treatment of POAG by protecting TM and other non-IOP risk factors. GBE has been shown to act as an antioxidant and free radical scavenger, a membrane stabilizer, an inhibitor of the platelet-activating factor, a vasodilator, and a regulator of metabolism [142]. Several experimental studies have demonstrated the efficacy of GBE in reducing free-radical damage and lipid peroxidation and protecting the vascular endothelium [143, 144]. GBE may increase microvascular blood flow of various tissues including the eyes, brain and others, perhaps by reducing the viscosity of the blood. GBE has been found to increase perfusion in skin and nail bed capillaries without changing laboratory coagulation parameters [38]. Indeed, a study showed that GBE could improve ocular blood flow, without affecting blood pressure, heart rate or IOP [145]. Another study demonstrated that GBE significantly suppressed steroid-induced IOP elevation and prevent TMCs from damage in animal model [146]. GBE was also proved to protect the retina and macule from degeneration as well [147]. We speculate that there might be some synergy effects between GBE and drugs or other support substances. It seems that GBE increases their concentration in ocular through increasing ocular blood flow, that seems to be a "targeted drug delivery".

7.5 Nutrition with antioxidative properties

Antioxidants can be grouped into two categories: enzymatic and nonenzymatic [148–150]. The enzymatic antioxidants, including superoxide dismutase, catalase, glutathione reductase, glutathione peroxidase and glutathione-S-transferase to scavenge the ROS in the body.

7.5.1 The enzymatic antioxidants

Disorders of glutathione peroxidase (Gpx) and nitric oxide synthase (NOS) are associated with glaucoma. Gpx can regulate ROS, while the NOS can produce nitrogen species (RNS). Lower plasma levels of both glutathione and glutathione peroxidase were found in POAG patients compared to controls [151]. In contrast, a significant increase in glutathione peroxidase activity in the AH and plasma of POAG patients have been reported by others [148, 149]. This divergence might be caused by the fact that antioxidant defense is decreased in patients with glaucoma, which results in an increase in the activity of antioxidant enzymes in an attempt to counteract the damage caused by ROS.

Ingested nitrate is turned into the vasodilator NO which improves ocular blood flow [148–150]. NO is also produced by the endothelium of the TM. The abnormal function of TMCs is associated with reduced NO bioavailability. The TM experiences physiological shear stress which triggers NO production. These cells may get lost as glaucoma progresses.

7.5.2 The nonenzymatic antioxidants

Non-enzymatic antioxidants including vitamins, carotenoids, polyphenols and flavonoids were intensively studied in POAG pathology [148]. Intake of vitamin A, C, E, B3 (nicotinamide), showed a beneficial association with glaucoma, improve inner retinal function [152–154]. Low vitamin D has been identified by some studies as an independent risk factor for glaucoma [155]. Vitamin D probably serves as an anti-inflammatory agent in the oxidative stress-driven pathogenesis of POAG. Coenzyme Q acts as another antioxidant similar to vitamins and was suggested to have the neuroprotective efficacy in glaucoma models [156]. In clinical studies, increased levels of carotenoids in macular pigment can help improve visual performance in glaucoma patients [157]. Astaxanthin features some important biologic properties, mostly represented by the strong antioxidant, anti-inflammatory and antiapoptotic activities. Both astaxanthin and saffron might be efficacious in the prevention and treatment of glaucoma [158, 159].

Polyphenols are plant-derived organic substances. Polyphenols can be divided into different subclasses, according to the number of phenolic rings present in their structure [160]. They comprise 4 families: simple phenolic acids, stilbenes (e.g., resveratrol), coumarins and flavonoids. Flavonoids include anthoxanthins, flavanones, flavanonols, flavans and anthocyanins. Flavonoids are widespread in nature, being found in a vast range of plants, including citrus fruits, grapes, tomatoes, berries and green tea; more than 5000 compounds that exert beneficial effects on health are known. These substances can protect cells or mitochondria from oxidative stress through different mechanisms and could offer therapeutic benefits to POAG patients [160].

Quercetin is a natural flavanol antioxidant and it has been reported to have notable curative effects on the treatment of glaucoma [161]. Baicalein has antioxidant and anti-inflammatory properties and can improve the treatment of glaucoma [162]. Curcumin reduces the inflammatory response by inhibiting the release of TNF-α and C-reactive protein and induces the expression of antioxidant enzymes or cytoprotective proteins [163, 164]. Resveratrol has been shown to increase the survival of retinal ganglion cells following ischemia-reperfusion injury for glaucoma in a study [165]. Meanwhile, resveratrol protects optic nerve head astrocytes from oxidative stress-Induced cell death through inhibiting the activation of caspase-3 activation, the dephosphorylation Ser 422 of Tau and the formation of misfolded protein aggregates [166]. Hesperidin, betalain and trehalose exert protective effects against glaucoma [167–169]. Polyphenols reduce inflammation through several mechanisms, such as reducing the expression of cytokines like IL-2, IL-6 and TNF-alpha [160]. Salidroside could inhibit TGF-β2-induced ECM expression in TMCs, and lower IOP which was elevated by TGF-β2 overexpression in mouse model [170]. Myricetin, is present in apples, oranges, berries, and vegetables. As a flavonoid, it can reduce oxidative stress and improve ocular blood flow in POAG. In POAG TMC, myricetin can substantially down-regulate the expression of TGFβ1/β2 [171, 172]. Myricetin effectively prevented IOP elevation and decreased IL-1α, IL-1β, IL-6, Il-8 and TNF-α) in the AH and TMCs in glaucoma rat model [172]. The results of these suggest that the intake of antioxidants in the diet could reduce the risk of glaucoma. The evidence is not conclusive; thus, more researches and long-term observations are required to evaluate the role of nutritional supplementation in glaucoma. The systemic status of these antioxidants in the tear, aqueous and vitreous fluid, as well as plasma, is a prospective gap in research.

7.5.3 Omega 3 fatty acids

Omega-3 (ω-3) fatty acids belong to the long-chain polyunsaturated fatty acid (PUFA) family. They have several properties that make them a potential adjuvant therapeutic agent in POAG. The first is that derivatives of ω-3 are the eicosanoids. These include the prostaglandin analogues, which are known for their IOP-lowering effect [38, 173]. Meanwhile, ω-3 exerts a highly protective effect on endothelial cells [174]. Omega-3 PUFA could reduce blood viscosity, probably because they improve the deformability of the red blood cells [175]. The anti-inflammatory properties of Omega-3 have also been demonstrated, which may have therapeutic potential for chronic inflammatory diseases such as glaucoma [176]. A high omega-3:6 ratio is recommended. Wang et al. [177] found that increasing the daily dietary intake of PUFA, including ω-3 fatty acids, was associated with a significant decrease in the probability of POAG. Finally, oral omega-3 supplementation for 3 months has been seen to significantly reduce IOP in normotensive adults [178] and in pseudoexfoliative glaucoma [179].

8. Conclusion

More and more evidences show that the onset of glaucoma is a result of the interaction of age, external environmental factors and genetic factors. The external environmental factors gradually impair the function of some key genes in the TM cell through a variety of ways, including decreased gene expression by cytokines, or epigenetic modification, which gradually change the phenotype of cells. Similarly, genetic factors (e.g., mutations of gene or polymorphism of POAG-associated genes) also lead to the gradual function impair in TM cells by influencing key regulatory pathways. There are some common signal pathways affected by genetic factors and environmental factors. Thus, the detailed characterization of the molecular profile of pathological and normal TMCs is critical to discover key regulatory molecules and pathways, which is the foundation for discovering the potential therapeutic targets. Simply reducing IOP by drugs, laser or surgery is not sufficient to guarantee a good prognosis in this disease. Therapies that focus on restoring TM cellularity and function could offer therapeutic benefits to POAG patients. The search for bioactive compounds with a protective effect on TM is of particular interest.

Acknowledgements

This work was supported in part by the projects (cstc2020jxjl130015, cstc2021jcyj-msxmX0767, and cstc2018jcyjAX0460) from the Natural Science Foundation of Chongqing.

Author details

Li Tang†, Chao Tang†, Ying Wang* and Xiaolong Shi*
Radiation and Cancer Biology Laboratory, Radiation Oncology Center, Chongqing Key Laboratory of Translational Research for Cancer Metastasis and Individualized Treatment, Chongqing University Cancer Hospital and Chongqing Cancer, Institute and Chongqing Cancer Hospital, Chongqing, China

*Address all correspondence to: 13996412826@163.com and xshi.bear@foxmail.com

† Both authors contributed equally to this work.

References

[1] He S, Stankowska DL, Ellis DZ, Krishnamoorthy RR, Yorio T. Targets of neuroprotection in glaucoma. Journal of Ocular Pharmacology and Therapeutics. 2018;**34**:85-106

[2] Kasetti RB, Patel PD, Maddineni P, Patil S, Kiehlbauch C, Millar JC, et al. ATF4 leads to glaucoma by promoting protein synthesis and ER client protein load. Nature Communications. 2020;**11**:5594

[3] Berrino E, Supuran CT. Rho-kinase inhibitors in the management of glaucoma. Expert Opinion on Therapeutic Patents. 2019;**29**:817-827

[4] Roy S, Villamarin A, Stergiopulos N, Mermoud A. MRI after successful eye Watch (TM) implantation. European Journal of Ophthalmology. 2020;**13**:1120672120973617

[5] Wang K, Read AT, Sulchek T, Ethier CR. Trabecular meshwork stiffness in glaucoma. Experimental Eye Research. 2017;**158**:3-12

[6] Izzotti A, Saccà SC, Longobardi M, Cartiglia C. Mitochondrial damage in the trabecular meshwork of patients with glaucoma. Archives of Ophthalmology. 2010;**128**:724-730

[7] Tamm ER, Braunger BM, Fuchshofer R. Intraocular pressure and the mechanisms involved in resistance of the aqueous humor flow in the trabecular meshwork outflow pathways. Progress in Molecular Biology and Translational Science. 2015;**134**:301-314

[8] Buffault J, Labbé A, Hamard P, Brignole-Baudouin F, Baudouin C. The trabecular meshwork: Structure, function and clinical implications. A review of the literature. Journal Français d'Ophtalmologie. 2020;**43**:e217-e230

[9] Patel G, Fury W, Yang H, Gomez-Caraballo M, Bai Y, Yang T, et al. Molecular taxonomy of human ocular outflow tissues defined by single-cell transcriptomics. Proceedings of the National Academy of Sciences of the United States of America. 2020;**117**:12856-12867

[10] van Zyl T, Yan W, McAdams A, Peng YR, Shekhar K, Regev A, et al. Cell atlas of aqueous humor outflow pathways in eyes of humans and four model species provides insight into glaucoma pathogenesis. Proceedings of the National Academy of Sciences of the United States of America. 2020;**117**:10339-10349

[11] Moazzeni H, Khani M, Elahi E. Insights into the regulatory molecules involved in glaucoma pathogenesis. American Journal of Medical Genetics. Part C, Seminars in Medical Genetics. 2020;**184**:782-827

[12] Wordinger RJ, Sharma T, Clark AF. The role of TGF-beta2 and bone morphogenetic proteins in the trabecular meshwork and glaucoma. Journal of Ocular Pharmacology and Therapeutics. 2014;**30**:154-162

[13] Saccà SC, Pulliero A, Izzotti A. The dysfunction of the trabecular meshwork during glaucoma course. Journal of Cellular Physiology. 2015;**230**:510-525

[14] Bollinger KE, Crabb JS, Yuan X, Putliwala T, Clark AF, Crabb JW. Quantitative proteomics: $TGF\beta_2$ signaling in trabecular meshwork cells. Investigative Ophthalmology & Visual Science. 2011;**52**:8287-8294

[15] Thomson J, Singh M, Eckersley A, Cain SA, Sherratt MJ, Baldock C. Fibrillin microfibrils and elastic fibre proteins: Functional interactions and extracellular regulation of growth factors. Seminars in Cell & Developmental Biology. 2019;**89**:109-117

[16] Faralli JA, Desikan H, Peotter J, Kanneganti N, Weinhaus B, Filla MS, et al. Genomic/proteomic analyses of dexamethasone-treated human trabecular meshwork cells reveal a role for GULP1 and ABR in phagocytosis. Molecular Vision. 2019;**25**:237-254

[17] Rao VR, Lautz JD, Kaja S, Foecking EM, Lukács E, Stubbs EB. Mitochondrial-targeted antioxidants attenuate TGF-β2 signaling in human trabecular meshwork cells. Investigative Ophthalmology & Visual Science. 2019;**60**:3613-3624

[18] Ahmad A, Ahsan H. Biomarkers of inflammation and oxidative stress in ophthalmic disorders. Journal of Immunoassay & Immunochemistry. 2020;**41**:257-271

[19] Nettesheim A, Shim MS, Hirt J, Liton PB. Transcriptome analysis reveals autophagy as regulator of TGFbeta/Smad-induced fibrogenesis in trabecular meshwork cells. Scientific Reports. 2019;**9**:16092

[20] Dismuke WM, Liang J, Overby DR, Stamer WD. Concentration-related effects of nitric oxide and endothelin-1 on human trabecular meshwork cell contractility. Experimental Eye Research. 2014;**120**:28-35

[21] Stamer WD, Lei Y, Boussommier-Calleja A, Overby DR, Ethier CR. eNOS, a pressure-dependent regulator of intraocular pressure. Investigative Ophthalmology & Visual Science. 2011;**52**:9438-9344

[22] Lei Y, Zhang X, Song M, Wu J, Sun X. Aqueous humor outflow physiology in NOS_3 knockout mice. Investigative Ophthalmology & Visual Science. 2015;**56**:4891-4898

[23] Patel PD, Chen YL, Kasetti RB, Maddineni P, Mayhew W, Millar JC, et al. Impaired TRPV4-eNOS signaling in trabecular meshwork elevates intraocular pressure in glaucoma. Proceedings of the National Academy of Sciences of the United States of America. 2021;**118**:e2022461118

[24] Salari N, Bokaee S, Farshchian N, Mohammadi M, Kazeminia M. The role of polymorphisms rs2070744 and rs1799983 eNOS gene in patients with POAG: A systematic review and meta-analysis. International Ophthalmology. 2021;**41**:2747-2763

[25] Saccà SC, Tirendi S, Scarfì S, Passalacqua M, Oddone F, Traverso CE, et al. An advanced in vitro model to assess glaucoma onset. ALTEX. 2020;**37**:265-274

[26] Wang M, Zheng Y. Oxidative stress and antioxidants in the trabecular meshwork. Peer Journal. 2019;**7**:e8121

[27] Gabelt BT, Kaufman PL. Changes in aqueous humor dynamics with age and glaucoma. Progress in Retinal and Eye Research. 2005;**24**:612-637

[28] Siegfried CJ, Shui YB. Intraocular oxygen and antioxidant status: New insights on the effect of vitrectomy and glaucoma pathogenesis. American Journal of Ophthalmology. 2019;**203**:12-25

[29] Tang B, Li S, Cao W, Sun X. The Association of oxidative stress status with open-angle glaucoma and exfoliation glaucoma: A systematic review and meta-analysis. Journal of Ophthalmology. 2019;**2019**:1803619

[30] Zhou L, Li Y, Yue BY. Oxidative stress affects cytoskeletal structure and cell-matrix interactions in cells from an ocular tissue: The trabecular meshwork. Journal of Cellular Physiology. 1999;**180**:182-189

[31] Pantalon A, Obadă O, Constantinescu D, Feraru C, Chiseliță D. Inflammatory model in patients with primary open angle glaucoma and diabetes. International Journal of Ophthalmology. 2019;**12**:795-801

[32] Avotri S, Eatman D, Russell-Randall K. Effects of resveratrol on inflammatory biomarkers in glaucomatous human trabecular meshwork cells. Nutrients. 2019;**11**:984

[33] Kaeslin MA, Killer HE, Fuhrer CA, Zeleny N, Huber AR, Neutzner A. Changes to the aqueous humor proteome during glaucoma. PLoS One. 2016;**11**: e0165314

[34] Oliveira MB, de Vasconcellos JPC, Ananina G, Costa VP, de Melo MB. Association between IL1A and IL1B polymorphisms and primary open angle glaucoma in a Brazilian population. Experimental Biology and Medicine (Maywood, N.J.). 2018;**243**:1083-1091

[35] Hill LJ, Mead B, Thomas CN, Foale S, Feinstein E, Berry M, et al. TGF-beta-induced IOP elevations are mediated by RhoA in the early but not the late fibrotic phase of open angle glaucoma. Molecular Vision. 2018;**24**:712-726

[36] Wang Y, Zhou H, Liu X, Han Y, Pan S, Wang Y. MiR-181a inhibits human trabecular meshwork cell apoptosis induced by H2O2 through the suppression of NF-kappaB and JNK pathways. Advances in Clinical and Experimental Medicine. 2018;**27**:577-582

[37] Weinreb RN, Toris CB, Gabelt BT, Lindsey JD, Kaufman PL. Effects of prostaglandins on the aqueous humor outflow pathways. Survey of Ophthalmology. 2002;**47**:53-64

[38] Weinreb RN, Kashiwagi K, Kashiwagi F, Tsukahara S, Lindsey JD. Prostaglandins increase matrix metalloproteinase release from human ciliary smooth muscle cells. Investigative Ophthalmology & Visual Science. 1997;**38**:2772-2780

[39] Grzybowski A, Och M, Kanclerz P, Leffler C, Moraes CG. Primary open angle glaucoma and vascular risk factors: A review of population based studies from 1990 to 2019. Journal of Clinical Medicine. 2020;**9**:761

[40] Pfahler NM, Barry JL, Bielskus IE, Kakouri A, Giovingo MC, Volpe NJ, et al. Nailfold capillary hemorrhages: Microvascular risk factors for primary open-angle glaucoma. Journal of Ophthalmology. 2020;**2020**:8324319

[41] Chou WY, Liu CJ, Chen MJ, Chiou SH, Chen WT, Ko YC. Effect of cold provocation on vessel density in eyes with primary open angle glaucoma: An optical coherence tomography angiography study. Scientific Reports. 2019;**9**:9384

[42] Pang JJ, Wu SM. Ocular pressure-volume relationship and ganglion cell death in glaucoma. OBM Neurobiology. 2021;**5**. DOI: 10.21926/obm.neurobiol.2102098

[43] Matlach J, Bender S, König J, Binder H, Pfeiffer N, Hoffmann EM. Investigation of intraocular pressure fluctuation as a risk factor of glaucoma progression. Clinical Ophthalmology. 2018;**18**(13):9-16

[44] McMonnies C. Reactive oxygen species, oxidative stress, glaucoma and hyperbaric oxygen therapy. Journal of Optometry. 2018;**11**:3-9

[45] Bouchemi M, Soualmia H, Midani F, El Afrit MA, El Asmi M, Feki M. Impaired nitric oxide production in patients with primary open-angle glaucoma. La Tunisie Médicale. 2020;**98**:144-149

[46] Rozpędek-Kamińska W, Wojtczak R, Szaflik JP, Szaflik J, Majsterek I. The genetic and endoplasmic reticulum-mediated molecular mechanisms of primary open-angle glaucoma. International Journal of Molecular Sciences. 2020;**21**:4171

[47] Moriguchi M, Watanabe T, Fujimuro M. Capsaicin induces ATF4 translation with upregulation of CHOP, GADD34 and PUMA. Biological & Pharmaceutical Bulletin. 2019;**42**:1428-1432

[48] Wu MZ, Fu T, Chen JX, Lin YY, Yang JE, Zhuang SM. LncRNA GOLGA2P10 is induced by PERK/ATF4/CHOP signaling and protects tumor cells from ER stress-induced apoptosis by regulating Bcl-2 family members. Cell Death & Disease. 2020;**11**:276

[49] Wu Z, Huang C, Xu C, Xie L, Liang JJ, Liu L, et al. Caveolin-1 regulates human trabecular meshwork cell adhesion, endocytosis, and autophagy. Journal of Cellular Biochemistry. 2019;**120**:13382-13391

[50] Sands WA, Page MM, Selman C. Proteostasis and ageing: Insights from long-lived mutant mice. Physiologie. 2017;**595**:6383-6390

[51] Lynch JM, Li B, Katoli P, Xiang C, Leehy B, Rangaswamy N, et al. Binding of a glaucoma-associated myocilin variant to the alpha B-crystallin chaperone impedes protein clearance in trabecular meshwork cells. The Journal of Biological Chemistry. 2018;**293**:20137-20156

[52] Huard DJE, Jonke AP, Torres MP, Lieberman RL. Different Grp94 components interact transiently with the myocilin olfactomedin domain in vitro to enhance or retard its amyloid aggregation. Scientific Reports. 2019;**9**:12769

[53] Yun HR, Jo YH, Kim J, Shin Y, Kim SS, Choi TG. Roles of autophagy in oxidative stress. International Journal of Molecular Sciences. 2020;**21**:3289

[54] Porter K, Nallathambi J, Lin Y, Liton PB. Lysosomal basification and decreased autophagic flux in oxidatively stressed trabecular meshwork cells: Implications for glaucoma pathogenesis. Autophagy. 2013;**9**:581-594

[55] Liton PB. The autophagic lysosomal system in outflow pathway physiology and pathophysiology. Experimental Eye Research. 2016;**144**:29-37

[56] Khalil AK, Kubota T, Tawara A, Inomata H. Ultrastructural age-related changes on the posterior iris surface: A possible relationship to the pathogenesis of exfoliation. Archives of Ophthalmology. 1996;**114**:721-725

[57] Izzotti A, Ceccaroli C, Longobardi MG, Micale RT, Pulliero A, Maestra SL, et al. Molecular damage in glaucoma: From anterior to posterior eye segment. The MicroRNA Role. Microrna. 2015;**4**:3-17

[58] Alvarado J, Murphy C, Polansky J, Juster R. Age-related changes in trabecular meshwork cellularity. Investigative Ophthalmology & Visual Science. 1981;**21**:714-727

[59] Tabak S, Schreiber-Avissar S, Beit-Yannai E. Influence of anti-glaucoma drugs on uptake of extracellular vesicles by trabecular meshwork cells. International Journal of Nanomedicine. 2021;**16**:1067-1081

[60] Dismuke WM, Challa P, Navarro I, Stamer WD, Liu Y. Human aqueous humor exosomes. Experimental Eye Research. 2015;**132**:73-77

[61] Schmidl D, Schmetterer L, Garhofer G, Popa-Cherecheanu A. Pharmacotherapy of glaucoma. Journal of Ocular Pharmacology and Therapeutics. 2015;**31**:63-77

[62] Lerner N, Avissar S, Beit-Yannai E, Katoh M. Extracellular vesicles mediate signaling between the aqueous humor producing and draining cells in the ocular system. PLoS One. 2017;**12**:e0171153

[63] Lerner N, Schreiber-Avissar S, Beit-Yannai E. Extracellular vesicle-mediated crosstalk between NPCE cells and TM cells result in modulation of Wnt signaling pathway and ECM remodeling. Journal of Cellular and Molecular Medicine. 2020;**24**:4646-4658

[64] Tabak S, Schreiber-Avissar S, Beit-Yannai E. Extracellular vesicles have variable dose-dependent effects on cultured draining cells in the eye. Journal of Cellular and Molecular Medicine. 2018;**22**:1992-2000

[65] Lerner N, Chen I, Schreiber-Avissar S, Beit-Yannai E. Extracellular vesicles mediate anti-oxidative response-in vitro study in the ocular drainage system. International Journal of Molecular Sciences. 2020;**21**:6105

[66] Choquet H, Wiggs JL, Khawaja AP. Clinical implications of recent advances in primary open-angle glaucoma genetics. Eye (London, England). 2020;**34**:29-39

[67] Liesenborghs I, Eijssen LMT, Kutmon M, Gorgels TGMF, Evelo CT, Beckers HJM, et al. Comprehensive bioinformatics analysis of trabecular meshwork gene expression data to unravel the molecular pathogenesis of primary open-angle glaucoma. Acta Ophthalmologica. 2020;**98**:48-57

[68] Liu T, Tang C, Shi XL. Analysis of variants in Chinese individuals with primary open-angle glaucoma using molecular inversion probe (MIP)-based panel sequencing. Molecular Vision. 2020;**26**:378-391

[69] Wang HW, Sun P, Chen Y, Jiang LP, Wu HP, Zhang W, et al. Research progress on human genes involved in the pathogenesis of glaucoma (Review). Molecular Medicine Reports. 2018;**18**:656-674

[70] Gharahkhani P, Jorgenson E, Hysi P, Khawaja AP, Pendergrass S, Han X, et al. Genome-wide meta-analysis identifies 127 open-angle glaucoma loci with consistent effect across ancestries. Nature Communications. 2021;**12**:1258

[71] Gould DB, Miceli-Libby L, Savinova OV, Torrado M, Tomarev SI, Smith RS, et al. Genetically increasing Myoc expression supports a necessary pathologic role of abnormal proteins in glaucoma. Molecular and Cellular Biology. 2004;**24**:9019-9125

[72] Kim BS, Savinova OV, Reedy MV, Martin J, Lun Y, Gan L, et al. Targeted disruption of the myocilin gene (Myoc) suggests that human glaucoma-causing mutations are gain of function. Molecular and Cellular Biology. 2001;**21**:7707-7713

[73] Yam GH, Gaplovska-Kysela K, Zuber C, Roth J. Aggregated myocilin induces russell bodies and causes apoptosis: Implications for the pathogenesis of myocilin-caused primary open-angle glaucoma. The American Journal of Pathology. 2007;**170**:100-109

[74] Liu Y, Vollrath D. Reversal of mutant myocilin non-secretion and cell killing:

Implications for glaucoma. Human Molecular Genetics. 2004;**13**:1193-1204

[75] Jetten AM. GLIS1-3 transcription factors: Critical roles in the regulation of multiple physiological processes and diseases. Cellular and Molecular Life Sciences. 2018;**75**:3473-3494

[76] Choquet H, Thai KK, Yin J, Hoffmann TJ, Kvale MN, Banda Y, et al. A large multi-ethnic genome-wide association study identifies novel genetic loci for intraocular pressure. Nature Communications. 2017;**8**:2108

[77] Khor CC, Do T, Jia H, Nakano M, George R, Abu-Amero K, et al. Genome-wide association study identifies five new susceptibility loci for primary angle closure glaucoma. Nature Genetics. 2016;**48**:556-562

[78] Khawaja AP, Cooke Bailey JN, Wareham NJ, Scott RA, Simcoe M, Igo RP Jr, et al. Genome-wide analyses identify 68 new loci associated with intraocular pressure and improve risk prediction for primary open-angle glaucoma. Nature Genetics. 2018;**50**:778-782

[79] Nair KS, Srivastava C, Brown RV, Koli S, Choquet H, Kang HS, et al. GLIS1 regulates trabecular meshwork function and intraocular pressure and is associated with glaucoma in humans. Nature Communications. 2021;**12**:4877

[80] Bailey JN, Loomis SJ, Kang JH, Allingham RR, Gharahkhani P, Khor CC, et al. Genome-wide association analysis identifies TXNRD2.; ATXN2 and FOXC1 as susceptibility loci for primary open-angle glaucoma. Nature Genetics. 2016;**48**:189-194

[81] Paylakhi SH, Moazzeni H, Yazdani S, Rassouli P, Arefian E, Jaberi E, et al. FOXC1 in human trabecular meshwork cells is involved in regulatory pathway that includes miR-204.; MEIS2.; and ITGβ1. Experimental Eye Research. 2013;**111**:112-121

[82] Berry FB, Skarie JM, Mirzayans F, Fortin Y, Hudson TJ, Raymond V, et al. FOXC1 is required for cell viability and resistance to oxidative stress in the eye through the transcriptional regulation of FOXO1A. Human Molecular Genetics. 2008;**17**:490-505

[83] Ito YA, Goping IS, Berry F, Walter MA. Dysfunction of the stress-responsive FOXC1 transcription factor contributes to the earlier-onset glaucoma observed in Axenfeld-Rieger syndrome patients. Cell Death & Disease. 2014;**5**:e1069

[84] Doucette LP, Footz T, Walter MA. FOXC1 regulates expression of prostaglandin receptors leading to an attenuated response to latanoprost. Investigative Ophthalmology & Visual Science. 2018;**59**:2548-2554

[85] Laffita-Mesa JM, Paucar M, Svenningsson P. Ataxin-2 gene: A powerful modulator of neurological disorders. Current Opinion in Neurology. 2021;**34**:578-588

[86] Lee J, Kim M, Itoh TQ, Lim C. Ataxin-2: A versatile posttranscriptional regulator and its implication in neural function. Wiley Interdisciplinary Review RNA. 2018;**9**:e1488

[87] Wolozin B, Ivanov P. Stress granules and neurodegeneration. Nature Reviews. Neuroscience. 2019;**20**:649-666

[88] Arimoto-Matsuzaki K, Saito H, Takekawa M. TIA1 oxidation inhibits stress granule assembly and sensitizes cells to stress-induced apoptosis. Nature Communications. 2016;**7**:10252

[89] Wardman JH, Henriksen EE, Marthaler AG, Nielsen JE, Nielsen TT. Enhancement of autophagy and solubilization of Ataxin-2 alleviate

apoptosis in spinocerebellar ataxia Type 2 patient cells. Cerebellum. 2020;**19**:165-181

[90] Lastres-Becker I, Nonis D, Eich F, Klinkenberg M, Gorospe M, Kotter P, et al. Mammalian ataxin-2 modulates translation control at the pre-initiation complex via PI3K/mTOR and is induced by starvation. Biochimica et Biophysica Acta. 2016;**1862**:1558-1569

[91] Kim YC, Guan KL. mTOR: A pharmacologic target for autophagy regulation. The Journal of Clinical Investigation. 2015;**125**:25-32

[92] Sundberg CA, Lakk M, Paul SP, Figueroa K, Scoles DR, Pulst SM, et al. The RNA-binding protein and stress granule component ATAXIN-2 is expressed in mouse and human tissues associated with glaucoma pathogenesis. The Journal of Comparative Neurology. 2022;**530**:537-552

[93] Stone EM, Lotery AJ, Munier FL, Héon E, Piguet B, Guymer RH, et al. A single EFEMP1 mutation associated with both Malattia Leventinese and Doyne honeycomb retinal dystrophy. Nature Genetics. 1999;**22**:199-202

[94] Narendran N, Guymer RH, Cain M, Baird PN. Analysis of the EFEMP1 gene in individuals and families with early onset drusen. Eye (London, England). 2005;**19**:11-15

[95] Meyer KJ, Davis LK, Schindler EI, Beck JS, Rudd DS, Grundstad AJ, et al. Genome-wide analysis of copy number vari- ants in age-related macular degeneration. Human Genetics. 2011;**129**:91-100

[96] Suriyapperuma SP, Child A, Desai T, Brice G, Kerr A, Crick RP, et al. A new locus (GLC1H) for adult-onset primary open-angle glaucoma maps to the 2p15-p16 region. Archives of Ophthalmology. 2007;**125**:86-92

[97] Liu T, Xie L, Ye J, Liu Y, He X. Screening of candidate genes for primary open angle glaucoma. Molecular Vision. 2012;**18**:2119-2126

[98] Lin Y, Liu T, Li J, Yang J, Du Q, Wang J, et al. A genome-wide scan maps a novel autosomal dominant juvenile-onset open- angle glaucoma locus to 2p15-16. Molecular Vision. 2008;**14**:739-744

[99] Mackay DS, Bennett TM, Shiels A. Exome sequencing identifies a missense variant in EFEMP1 co-segregating in a family with autosomal dominant primary open-angle glaucoma. PLoS One. 2015;**10**:e0132529

[100] Springelkamp H, Iglesias AI, Mishra A, Höhn R, Wojciechowski R, Khawaja AP, et al. New insights into the genetics of primary open-angle glaucoma based on meta-analyses of intraocular pressure and optic disc characteristics. Human Molecular Genetics. 2017;**26**:438-453

[101] Fuchshofer R, Stephan DA, Russell P, Tamm ER. Gene expression profiling of TGFbeta2- and/or BMP7-treated trabecular meshwork cells: Identification of Smad7 as a critical inhibitor of TGF-beta2 signaling. Experimental Eye Research. 2009;**88**:1020-1032

[102] Thorleifsson G, Magnusson KP, Sulem P, Walters GB, Gudbjartsson DF, Stefansson H, et al. Common sequence variants in the LOXL1 gene confer susceptibility to exfoliation glaucoma. Science. 2007;**317**:1397-1400

[103] Wu M, Zhu XY, Ye J. Associations of polymorphisms of LOXL1 gene with primary open-angle glaucoma:

A meta-analysis based on 5.;293 subjects. Molecular Vision. 2015;**21**:165-172

[104] Eliseeva N, Ponomarenko I, Reshetnikov E, Dvornyk V, Churnosov M. LOXL1 gene polymorphism candidates for exfoliation glaucoma are also associated with a risk for primary open-angle glaucoma in a Caucasian population from central Russia. Molecular Vision. 2021;**27**:262-269

[105] Shiga Y, Akiyama M, Nishiguchi KM, Sato K, Shimozawa N, Takahashi A, et al. Genome-wide association study identifies seven novel susceptibility loci for primary open-angle glaucoma. Human Molecular Genetics. 2018;**27**:1486-1496

[106] Debret R, Cenizo V, Aimond G, André V, Devillers M, Rouvet I, et al. Epigenetic silencing of lysyl oxidase-like-1 through DNA hypermethylation in an autosomal recessive cutis laxa case. The Journal of Investigative Dermatology. 2010;**130**:2594-2601

[107] Ye H, Jiang Y, Jing Q, et al. LOXL1 hypermethylation in pseudoexfoliation syndrome in the uighur population. Investigative Ophthalmology & Visual Science. 2015;**56**:5838-5843

[108] Wu G, Guo Z, Chang X, Kim MS, Nagpal JK, Liu J, et al. LOXL1 and LOXL4 are epigenetically silenced and can inhibit ras/extracellular signal-regulated kinase signaling pathway in human bladder cancer. Cancer Research. 2007;**67**:4123-4129

[109] Greene AG, Eivers SB, McDonnell F, Dervan EWJ, O'Brien CJ, Wallace DM. Differential Lysyl oxidase like 1 expression in pseudoexfoliation glaucoma is orchestrated via DNA methylation. Experimental Eye Research. 2020;**201**:108349

[110] Prum BE Jr, Rosenberg LF, Gedde SJ, Mansberger SL, Stein JD, Moroi SE, et al. Primary open-angle glaucoma preferred practice pattern(®) Guidelines. Ophthalmology. 2016;**123**:41-111

[111] Mathew DJ, McKay BR, Basilious A, Belkin A, Trope GE, Buys YM. Adherence to world glaucoma association guidelines for surgical trials in the era of microinvasive glaucoma surgeries. Ophthalmol Glaucoma. 2019;**2**:78-85

[112] Gan K, Liu Y, Stagg B, Rathi S, Pasquale LR, Damji K. Telemed J E Telemedicine for glaucoma: Guidelines and recommendations. Health. 2020;**26**:551-555

[113] European glaucoma society terminology and guidelines for glaucoma, 4th edn-Chapter 3: Treatment principles and options Supported by the EGS Foundation: Part 1: Foreword; Introduction; Glossary; Chapter 3 Treatment principles and options. The British Journal of Ophthalmology. 2017;**101**:130-195

[114] Perez CI, Singh K, Lin S. Relationship of lifestyle, exercise, and nutrition with glaucoma. Current Opinion in Ophthalmology. 2019;**30**:82-88

[115] Valero-Vello M, Peris-Martínez C, García-Medina JJ, Sanz-González SM, Ramírez AI, Fernández-Albarral JA, et al. Searching for the antioxidant, anti-inflammatory, and neuroprotective potential of natural food and nutritional supplements for ocular health in the mediterranean population. Food. 2021;**10**:1231

[116] Fan X, Bilir EK, Kingston OA, Oldershaw RA, Kearns VR, Willoughby CE, et al. Replacement of the trabecular meshwork cells: A way ahead in IOP control? Biomolecules. 2021;**11**:1371

[117] Weinreb RN, Aung T, Medeiros FA. The pathophysiology and treatment of glaucoma: A review. Journal of the American Medical Association. 2014;**311**:1901-1911

[118] Weinreb Robert N, Tee KP. Primary open-angle glaucoma. The Lancet. 2004;**363**:1711-1720

[119] Marshall LL, Hayslett RL, Stevens GA. Therapy for open-angle glaucoma. The Consultant Pharmacist. 2018;**33**:432-445

[120] Li G, Torrejon KY, Unser AM, Ahmed F, Navarro ID, Baumgartner RA, et al. Trabodenoson, an adenosine mimetic with A1 receptor selectivity lowers intraocular pressure by increasing conventional outflow facility in mice. Investigative Ophthalmology & Visual Science. 2018;**59**:383-392

[121] Myers JS, Sall KN, DuBiner H, Slomowitz N, McVicar W, Rich CC, et al. A dose-escalation study to evaluate the safety, tolerability, pharmacokinetics, and efficacy of 2 and 4 weeks of twice-daily ocular trabodenoson in adults with ocular hypertension or primary open-angle glaucoma. Journal of Ocular Pharmacology and Therapeutics. 2016;**32**:555-562

[122] Hoy SM. Netarsudil ophthalmic solution 0.02%: First global approval. Drugs. 2018;**78**:389-396

[123] Asrani S, Bacharach J, Holland E, McKee H, Sheng H, Lewis RA, et al. Fixed-Dose combination of netarsudil and latanoprost in ocular hypertension and open-angle glaucoma: Pooled efficacy/safety analysis of phase 3 mercury-1 and -2. Advances in Therapy. 2020;**37**:1620-1631

[124] Serle JB, Katz LJ, McLaurin E, Heah T, Ramirez-Davis N, Usner DW, et al. ROCKET-1 and ROCKET-2 study groups. Two phase 3 clinical trials comparing the safety and efficacy of netarsudil to timolol in patients with elevated intraocular pressure: Rho kinase elevated IOP treatment trial 1 and 2 (ROCKET-1 and ROCKET-2). American Journal of Ophthalmology. 2018;**186**:116-127

[125] Sit AJ, Gupta D, Kazemi A, McKee H, Challa P, Liu KC, et al. Netarsudil improves trabecular outflow facility in patients with primary open angle glaucoma or ocular hypertension: A phase 2 study. American Journal of Ophthalmology. 2021;**226**:262-269

[126] Mehran NA, Sinha S, Razeghinejad R. New glaucoma medications: Latanoprostene bunod, netarsudil, and fixed combination netarsudil-latanoprost. Eye (London, England). 2020;**34**:72-88

[127] Weinreb RN, Liebmann JM, Martin KR, Kaufman PL, Vittitow JL. Latanoprostene bunod 0.024% in subjects with open-angle glaucoma or ocular hypertension: Pooled phase 3 study findings. Journal of Glaucoma. 2018;**27**:7-15

[128] Fingeret M, Gaddie IB, Bloomenstein M. Latanoprostene bunod ophthalmic solution 0.024%: A new treatment option for open-angle glaucoma and ocular hypertension. Clinical & Experimental Optometry. 2019;**102**:541-550

[129] Addis VM, Miller-Ellis E. Latanoprostene bunod ophthalmic solution 0.024% in the treatment of open-angle glaucoma: Design, development, and place in therapy. Clinical Ophthalmology. 2018;**12**:2649-2657

[130] Miller Ellis E, Berlin MS, Ward CL, Sharpe JA, Jamil A, Harris A. Ocular hypotensive effect of the novel EP3/FP agonist ONO-9054 versus Xalatan: Results of a 28-day, double-masked,

randomised study. The British Journal of Ophthalmology. 2017;**101**:796-800

[131] Roy Chowdhury U, Dosa PI, Fautsch MP. ATP sensitive potassium channel openers: A new class of ocular hypotensive agents. Experimental Eye Research. 2017;**158**:85-93

[132] Chi SC, Kang YN, Hwang DK, Liu CJ. Selective laser trabeculoplasty versus medication for open-angle glaucoma: Systematic review and meta-analysis of randomised clinical trials. The British Journal of Ophthalmology. 2020;**104**:1500-1507

[133] Gazzard G, Konstantakopoulou E, Garway-Heath D, Garg A, Vickerstaff V, Hunter R, et al. Selective laser trabeculoplasty versus drops for newly diagnosed ocular hypertension and glaucoma: The LiGHT RCT. Health Technology Assessment. 2019;**23**:1-102

[134] Wang H, Xin C, Han Y, Shi Y, Ziaei S, Wang N. Intermediate outcomes of ab externo circumferential trabeculotomy and canaloplasty in POAG patients with prior incisional glaucoma surgery. BMC Ophthalmology. 2020;**20**:389

[135] Dickerson JE Jr, Brown RH. Circumferential canal surgery: A brief history. Current Opinion in Ophthalmology. 2020;**31**:139-146

[136] King AJ, Fernie G, Azuara-Blanco A, Burr JM, Garway-Heath T, Sparrow JM, et al. Treatment of advanced glaucoma study: A multicentre randomised controlled trial comparing primary medical treatment with primary trabeculectomy for people with newly diagnosed advanced glaucoma-study protocol. The British Journal of Ophthalmology. 2018;**102**:922-928

[137] Tian J, Liu Y, Chen K. Ginkgo biloba extract in vascular protection: Molecular mechanisms and clinical applications. Current Vascular Pharmacology. 2017;**15**:532-548

[138] Nguyen T, Alzahrani T, Biloba G. StatPearls [Internet]. Treasure Island (FL): StatPearls Publishing; 2021

[139] Horbowicz M, Wiczkowski W, Góraj-Koniarska J, Miyamoto K, Ueda J, Saniewski M. Effect of methyl jasmonate on the terpene trilactones, flavonoids, and phenolic acids in ginkgo biloba L. Leaves: Relevance to leaf senescence. Molecules. 2021;**26**:4682

[140] Tian J, Popal MS, Liu Y, Gao R, Lyu S, Chen K, et al. Erratum to "Ginkgo Biloba Leaf Extract Attenuates Atherosclerosis in Streptozotocin-Induced Diabetic ApoE−/−Mice by Inhibiting Endoplasmic Reticulum Stress via Restoration of Autophagy through the mTOR Signaling Pathway". Oxidative Medicine and Cellular Longevity. 2019;**2019**:3084083

[141] Loskutova E, O'Brien C, Loskutov I, Loughman J. Nutritional supplementation in the treatment of glaucoma: A systematic review. Survey of Ophthalmology. 2019;**64**:195-216

[142] Liu XW, Yang JL, Niu W, Jia WW, Olaleye OE, Wen Q, et al. Human pharmacokinetics of ginkgo terpene lactones and impact of carboxylation in blood on their platelet-activating factor antagonistic activity. Acta Pharmacologica Sinica. 2018;**39**:1935-1946

[143] Piazza S, Pacchetti B, Fumagalli M, Bonacina F, Dell'Agli M, Sangiovanni E. Comparison of two ginkgo biloba L. Extracts on oxidative stress and inflammation markers in human endothelial cells. Mediators of Inflammation. 2019;**2019**:6173893

[144] Wu TC, Chen JS, Wang CH, Huang PH, Lin FY, Lin LY, et al.

Activation of heme oxygenase-1 by Ginkgo biloba extract differentially modulates endothelial and smooth muscle-like progenitor cells for vascular repair. Scientific Reports. 2019;**9**:17316

[145] Kang JM, Lin S. Ginkgo biloba and its potential role in glaucoma. Current Opinion in Ophthalmology. 2018;**29**:116-120

[146] Cho HK, Kim S, Lee EJ, Kee C. Neuroprotective effect of ginkgo biloba extract against hypoxic retinal ganglion cell degeneration in vitro and in vivo. Journal of Medicinal Food. 2019;**22**:771-778

[147] Jia LY, Sun L, Fan D, Lam DSC, Pang CP, Yam G. Effect of topical ginkgo biloba extract on steroid-induced changes in the trabecular meshwork and intraocular pressure. Archives of Ophthalmology. 2008;**126**:1700-1706

[148] Ramdas WD. The relation between dietary intake and glaucoma: A systematic review. Acta Ophthalmologica. 2018;**96**:550-556

[149] Scuteri D, Rombolà L, Watanabe C, akurada S, Corasaniti MT, Bagetta G, et al. Impact of nutraceuticals on glaucoma: A systematic review. Progress in Brain Research. 2020;**257**:141-154

[150] Jabbehdari S, Chen JL, Vajaranant TS. Effect of dietary modification and antioxidant supplementation on intraocular pressure and open-angle glaucoma. European Journal of Ophthalmology. 2021;**31**:1588-1605

[151] Malik MA, Gupta V, Shukla S, Kaur J. Glutathione s-transferase (GSTM1, GSTT1) polymorphisms and JOAG susceptibility: A case control study and meta-analysis in glaucoma. Gene. 2017;**628**:246-252

[152] Ramdas WD, Schouten JSAG, Webers CAB. The effect of vitamins on glaucoma: A systematic review and meta-analysis. Nutrients. 2018;**10**:359

[153] Galanopoulos A, Smith JR. Vitamins for glaucoma. Clinical & Experimental Ophthalmology. 2020;**48**:877-878

[154] Williams PA, Harder JM, Foxworth NE, Cochran KE, Philip VM, Porciatti V, et al. Vitamin B(3) modulates mitochondrial vulnerability and prevents glaucoma in aged mice. Science. 2017;**355**:756-760

[155] Ulhaq ZS. Vitamin D and its receptor polymorphisms are associated with glaucoma. Journal Français d'Ophtalmologie. 2020;**43**:1009-1019

[156] Ahmad SS. Coenzyme Q and its role in glaucoma. Saudi Journal of Ophthalmology. 2020;**34**:45-49

[157] Lem DW, Gierhart DL, Davey PG. Carotenoids in the Management of Glaucoma: A systematic review of the evidence. Nutrients. 1949;**2021**:13

[158] Giannaccare G, Pellegrini M, Senni C, Bernabei F, Scorcia V, Cicero AFG. Clinical applications of astaxanthin in the treatment of ocular diseases: Emerging Insights. Marine Drugs. 2020;**18**:239

[159] Heitmar R, Brown J, Kyrou I. Saffron (*Crocus sativus* L.) in ocular diseases: A narrative review of the existing evidence from clinical studies. Nutrients. 2019;**11**:649

[160] Bungau S, Abdel-Daim MM, Tit DM, Ghanem E, Sato S, Maruyama-Inoue M, et al. Health benefits of polyphenols and carotenoids in age-related eye diseases. Oxidative Medicine and Cellular Longevity. 2019;**2019**:9783429

[161] Zhao L, Wang H, Du X. The therapeutic use of quercetin in

ophthalmology: Recent applications. Biomedicine & Pharmacotherapy. 2021;**137**:111371

[162] Liang W, Huang X, Chen W. The temp effects of baicalin and baicalein on cerebral Ischemia: A review. Aging and Disease. 2017;**8**:850-867

[163] Gong L, Zhu J. Baicalin alleviates oxidative stress damage in trabecular meshwork cells in vitro. Naunyn-Schmiedeberg's Archives of Pharmacology. 2018;**391**:51-58

[164] Radomska-Leśniewska DM, Osiecka-Iwan A, Hyc A, Góźdź A, Dąbrowska AM, Skopiński P. Therapeutic potential of curcumin in eye diseases. Central European Journal of Immunology. 2019;**44**:181-189

[165] Luo H, Zhuang J, Hu P, Ye W, Chen S, Pang Y, et al. Resveratrol delays retinal ganglion cell loss and attenuates gliosis-related inflammation from ischemia-reperfusion injury. Investigative Ophthalmology & Visual Science. 2018;**59**:3879-3888

[166] Means JC, Lopez AA, Koulen P. Resveratrol protects optic nerve head astrocytes from oxidative stress-induced cell death by preventing caspase-3 activation, tau dephosphorylation at ser(422) and formation of misfolded protein aggregates. Cellular and Molecular Neurobiology. 2020;**40**: 911-926

[167] Lu B, Wang X, Ren Z, Jiang H, Liu B. Anti-glaucoma potential of hesperidin in experimental glaucoma induced rats. AMB Express. 2020;**10**:94

[168] Wang J, Zhang D, Cao C, Yao J. Betalain exerts a protective effect against glaucoma is majorly through the association of inflammatory cytokines. AMB Express. 2020;**10**:125

[169] Cejka C, Kubinova S, Cejkova J. Trehalose in ophthalmology. Histology and Histopathology. 2019;**34**:611-618

[170] Fan Y, Guo L, Wei J, Chen J, Sun H, Guo T. Effects of salidroside on trabecular meshwork cell extracellular matrix expression and mouse intraocular pressure. Investigative Ophthalmology & Visual Science. 2019;**60**:2072-2082

[171] Song X, Tan L, Wang M, Ren C, Guo C, Yang B, et al. Myricetin: A review of the most recent research. Biomedicine & Pharmacotherapy. 2021;**134**:111017

[172] Yang Q, Li Y, Luo L. Effect of myricetin on primary open-angle glaucoma. Translational Neuroscience. 2018;**9**:132-141

[173] Rodríguez-Cruz M, Serna DS. Nutrigenomics of ω −3 fatty acids: Regulators of the master transcription factors. Nutrition. 2017;**41**:90-96

[174] Du Y, Taylor CG, Aukema HM, Zahradka P. Importance of extracellular matrix and growth state for the EA.hy926 endothelial cell response to polyunsaturated fatty acids. PLoS One. 2018;**13**:e0197613

[175] Ernst E. Effects of n-3 fatty acids on blood rheology. Journal of Internal Medicine. Supplement. 1989;**731**:129-132

[176] Saccà SC, Cutolo CA, Ferrari D, Corazza P, Traverso CE. The eye, oxidative damage and polyunsaturated fatty acids. Nutrients. 2018;**10**:668

[177] Wang YE, Tseng VL, Yu F, Caprioli J, Coleman AL. Association of dietary fatty acid intake with glaucoma in the united sates. JAMA Ophthalmol. 2018;**136**:141-147

[178] Downie LE, Vingrys AJ. Oral omega-3 supplementation lowers

intraocular pressure in normotensive adults. Translational Vision Science & Technology. 2018;7:1

[179] Villadoniga RS, Rodrıguez Garcıa E, Sagastagoia Epelde O, Dıaz MDA, Pedrol JCD. Effects of oral supplementation with docosahexaenoic acid (DHA) plus antioxidants in pseudoexfoliative glaucoma: A 6-month open-label randomized trial. Journal of Ophthalmology. 2018;**2018**:8259371

Chapter 3

Optic Nerve and Retinal Ganglion Cell Protection, Rejuvenation, and Regeneration as Glaucoma Treatment Strategies

Najam A. Sharif

Abstract

Once destroyed, neurons and their axons in the mammalian central nervous system, including retinal ganglion cells (RGCs) and their axons in the eye and neurons in the thalamic and cortical brain regions involved in visual perception, cannot automatically be replaced. Intrinsic inhibitory chemicals and structural components, suppressive transcription factors, scar formation, and the sheer long distances the RGC axons have to travel to the brain prevent or reduce regenerative capacity in the visual system damaged by aging and various diseases such as glaucoma. However, non-clinical and some clinical uses of transcorneal electrical stimulation, redlight therapy, gene-therapy, and cell replacement, among other novel technologies and techniques, appear promising to help overcome some of these hurdles. Early results indicate that indeed neuronal rejuvenation; potential regeneration and ultimate replacement of the lost RGCs and their axons, such as in glaucoma; and the reestablishment of the retina-optic nerve–brain connections may be possible. Improvement and/or partial restoration of eyesight due to ocular and neurological disease-induced visual impairment in humans may thus be possible in the near future. These aspects will be discussed in this chapter.

Keywords: glaucoma, optic neuropathy, degeneration, regeneration, retina, electroceuticals

1. Introduction

The process of visual perception is initiated when light enters the eye and is focused on the retina at the back of the eye (**Figure 1A**). Simplistically, photoreceptors convert the electromagnetic energy received into chemical signals that are transmitted to the bipolar cells, which communicate with the retinal ganglion cells (RGCs), of which there are many sub-types [1, 2]. The RGCs encode the integrated information received into electrical impulses that are then transmitted down their axons, which form the optic nerve. The optic nerves carrying RGC axons from each hemiretina cross over the optic chiasm, each half set innervates the relay station at the

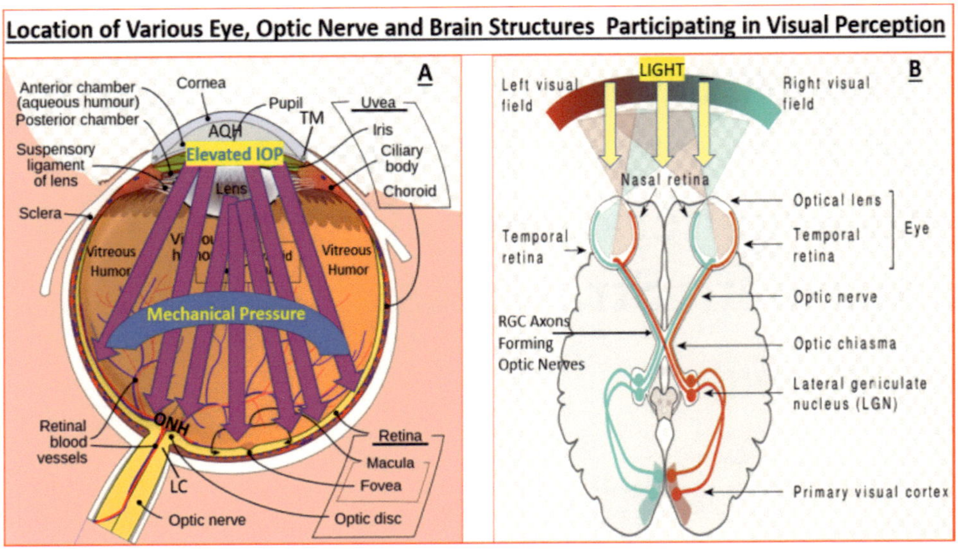

Figure 1.
*These schematics illustrate key anatomical elements of the human eye (A) and its connection, via the optic nerve, to the brain structures (B) involved in visual signal transmission and visual perception. (**A**) also depicts how elevated IOP damages the optic nerve head (ONH), lamina cribosa (LC), and ultimately the optic nerve through mechanical pressure such as in glaucoma. (**B**) shows the remarkable length of the optic nerves. AQH, aqueous humor; IOP, intraocular pressure; TM, trabecular meshwork. Adapted from Wikipedia; https://en.wikipedia.org/wiki/Eye; https://en.wikipedia.org/wiki/Visual_system (19Oct2022).*

lateral geniculate thalamic nuclei (and other nuclei), and from there, other neuronal axons connect to various parts of the visual cortex (**Figure 1B**). Successive integration and processing of the information finally emerge as visual images perceived by the person or animal. This whole simplified process happens in milliseconds, and binocular color vision is achieved under normal circumstances.

Loss of visual perception due to aging and pathological factors damaging the optic nerve and the RGCs are classic structural and functional deficits observed in patients with glaucoma [3–6]. Although there are many forms of glaucoma, the most prevalent types are open-angle glaucoma (OAG) and angle-closure glaucoma (ACG), followed by normotensive glaucoma (NTG) [3–9]. The two major disease-instigating and risk factors for OAG and ACG are advanced age and elevated intraocular pressure (IOP). Increased IOP results when the aqueous humor (AQH) accumulates in the anterior chamber of the eye due to blockage of the AQH drainage system, trabecular meshwork (TM), and Schlemm's canal (SC) (**Figure 1A**) [7–10]. Protracted IOP fluctuations and disc hemorrhage are additional risk factors of visual field deterioration and progression, especially in advanced glaucoma, even at low IOPs. Similarly, since NTG develops independent of high IOP, it is believed that local inflammation, tissue remodeling at the optic nerve head (ONH) and lamina cribosa (LC) in the retina (**Figures 1A** and **2**), and subsequent loss of RGCs and their axons that are supersensitive to injurious conditions are responsible for the pathogenesis of the disease. Many molecular and cellular elements conspire to cause this glaucomatous optic neuropathy (GON). Close to 80 million people worldwide suffer from OAG and ACG alone with projected numbers to increase to >112 million by 2040 [9]. Even though IOP-lowering drugs, devices, and surgical treatments slow down the disease progression [10–12],

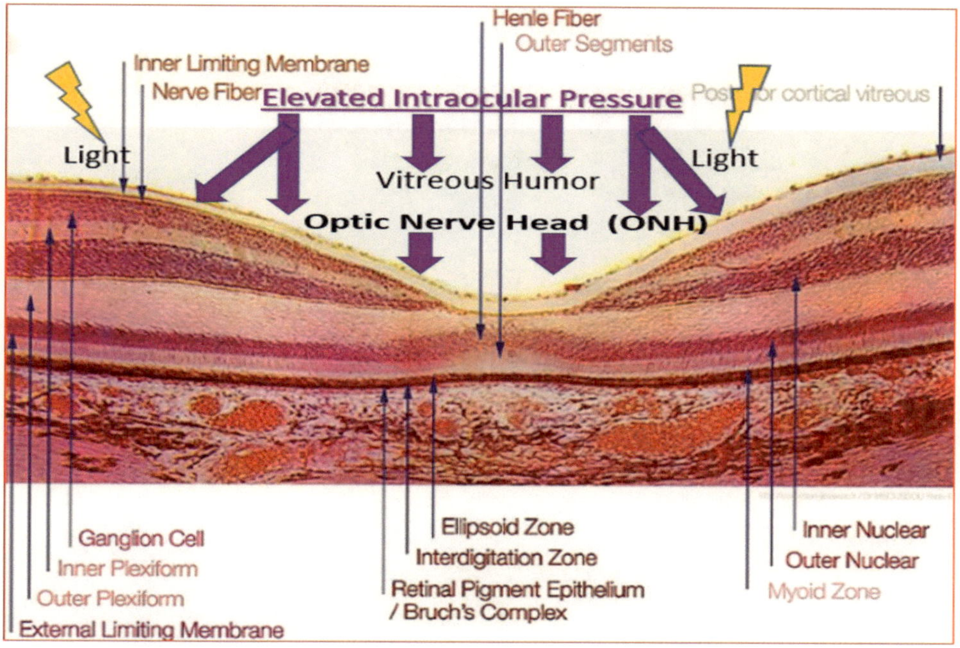

Figure 2.
Detailed view of the retinal architecture showing cross-sectional location of the cell types and their layering is depicted here. The physical/mechanical pressure exerted by elevated intraocular pressure in ocular hypertensive OAG glaucoma patients that damages the optic nerve head region, specially RGCs and their axons, is also illustrated. Adapted from Wikipedia; https://en.wikipedia.org/wiki/Retina (19Oct2022).

there remains a high unmet medical need to help protect, preserve, and restore visual field/visual perception in the OAG/ACG/NTG-afflicted patients and hence the need to discover and develop novel treatment modalities and technologies to mitigate these ocular diseases at various intervention points and through diverse receptor/enzyme/ion-channel targets [6, 11, 12].

2. Basic anatomy and pathology of GON

Multifaceted research into GON has revealed that one of the weakest structural components of the visual system is the retinal region known as the ONH and LC at the back of the eye (**Figures 1A-3**). The high IOP associated with OAG exerts physical compressive pressure and damages the latter tissues through mechanical forces [13, 14] and the ensuing microglial activation, infiltration of immune cells into the retina, aberrant activation of the complement system, and release of inflammatory cytokines (e.g., interleukins), vasoconstrictor (endothelin) and neurotoxic (glutamate; ATP) agents, and destructive proteases (matrix metalloproteinases [MMPs]) [15–24]. The most susceptible RGC axons and cell bodies are injured, and over time, their terminals retract away from the brain neurons, thereby reducing the delivery of mitochondria and neurotrophins to the RGC somas due to impaired retrograde axonal flow [19, 24]. The ischemia/hypoxia [25, 26] induced by vasoconstriction of retinal blood vessels that travel along with the RGC axons also causes immense oxidative stress on the whole visual system with resultant atrophic consequences [27–32].

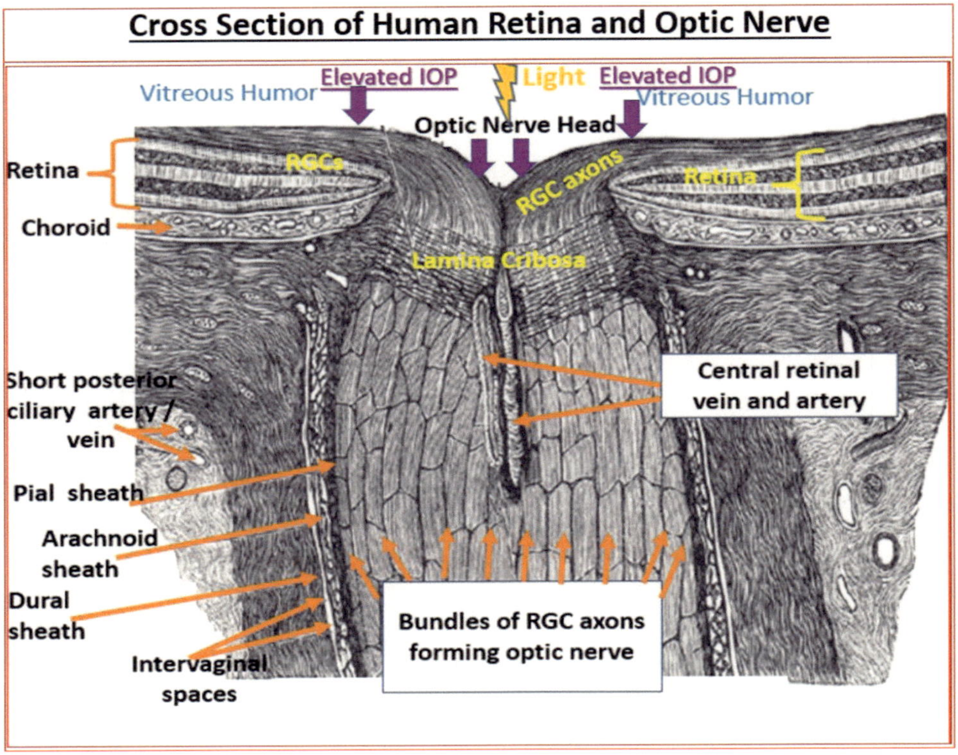

Figure 3.
The location of the optic nerve head, lamina cribosa, and the optic nerve structure and its blood supply (B) are shown in this figure. Additionally, the negative impact of elevated intraocular pressure (IOP) on these structures is also depicted. Adapted from Wikipedia; https://en.wikipedia.org/wiki/Optic_disc (19Oct2022).

Even though these events and this chronic disease progress slowly over decades, ultimately many RGCs and their axons wither and die, thus causing visual impairment, which, if it is not diagnosed and treatment administered, can lead to irreversible loss of eyesight. The asymptomatic nature of OAG and NTG means that the patients are totally oblivious to the damage being inflicted on their visual system and only notice vision defects when significant vision loss has occurred. Not only are the RGCs and the optic nerve damaged in OAG and NTG, but due to reduced retina–brain communication activity, many neurons in the thalamus, superior colliculus, suprachiasmatic nucleus, and visual cortex are also destroyed and cannot be replaced [27–32].

Due to the aging process, coupled with the pathological events described above, the autophagic clearance of dead or dying neurons and axonal debris in the retina and brain is impaired. The toxicity, oxidative insults, and glial proliferation caused by the pathological condition and milieu [2, 5, 6, 17–20] further slow down the intrinsic reparative mechanisms, and more cells and axons are destroyed. The patient now begins to notice blind-spots in the visual images, reduced contrast sensitivity, and an overall loss of visual acuity and loss of peripheral vision [14, 32]. At such time, it is imperative to lower and control the IOP in the patient's eyes and thus preserve the remaining RGCs and their axons and maintain good health of the brain's gray and white matter associated with vision. As mentioned above, lowering and controlling

IOP in glaucoma patients is no longer a huge issue [5, 6, 10], although patient compliance in administering prescribed eyedrops presents continued problems, and of course, more efficacious treatments with a longer duration of action and less side effects are still needed. However, what remains a major healthcare concern is the ways and means to directly protect the remaining visual infrastructure, to implement novel methods to rejuvenate and potentially regenerate or replace the lost RGCs and their axons, and to re-establish lost retina-optic nerve–brain connections, thereby restoring some lost visual function.

3. Concept and progress in neuroprotection for GON

Because GON is a multifactorial disease, it requires a multi-pronged therapeutic approach. Unfortunately, much of the reported research data published thus far has utilized a strategy involving a single insult (whether it is a neurotoxin, hypoxia, aglycemia, or neurotrophic factor deprivation or optic nerve crush) and a single test agent to protect the neurons and their axons. However, while not fully representing the *in vivo* GON condition, such cell-based or animal model(s) of glaucoma-based investigations have identified many classes of drug candidates capable of intervening and preventing RGC cell death *in vitro* and *in vivo* [11, 12]. These range from antioxidants; anti-inflammatory agents; peroxisome proliferator-activated receptor-γ agonists; vasodilators; nitric oxide synthase inhibitors; inhibitors of rho kinase, Janus kinase, and glycogen synthase kinase; statins; complement inhibitors; autophagy stimulators; endothelin receptor antagonists; glutamate receptor sub-type-selective antagonists; Krebs cycle activators/coenzymes to generate ATP (e.g., nicotinamide adenine dinucleotide [NAD^+] and vitamin B3); various neurotrophic factors; Nrf2 activators; Ca^{2+}-channel blocker; antibodies to NoGo (reticulon); a major neurite outgrowth inhibitory protein of CNS myelin; and even miRNAs (natural or synthetic) derived from specific cell or tissue exosomes/secretomes, extracellular vesicles, and so on [6, 10–12, 21, 30, 33–36]. The next challenge is to embark on a combinatorial approach and deploy assays and animal models where multiple chemical and/or metabolic or physical challenges can be subjected to determine the efficacy of potential neuroprotective agents. Drugs or other treatment modalities that can recruit and engage with several protective mechanisms would be deemed much more useful for combating GON than substances with a singular benefit. Ultimately, any efficacy findings from animal models of GON would need to be demonstrated in human subjects, and there is much hope that such translational goals will be achieved in the near future. Encouraging data on the benefits of vitamin B3 in ocular hypertensive/OAG patients appear promising [35, 36] and require clinical confirmation by other researchers.

4. Gene therapies for glaucoma treatment

With the success of gene therapy for a specific form of retinitis pigmentosa, Leber's congenital amaurosis [37], there has been a surge in genetic manipulation studies directed toward glaucoma treatment. Although such studies have so far been pre-clinical using animal models of disease, there is hope that some will enter clinical trials soon. Early studies focused on the use of adeno-associated viral (AAV) vectors delivering genes to the ANC cells and were aimed at opening up the TM drainage system to promote AQH outflow to lower IOP and thus reduce the mechanical pressure on the ONH/LC and thus indirectly protect the optic nerve. Indeed, insertion of AAV-mediated genes enhancing expression of MMP-1 in sheep [38] and MMP-3 in mice [39], to remodel the TM tissue, resulted in reduction of IOP. In a different way, genetic manipulation of the mouse ciliary body aquaporin-1 [40] and the silencing of the β-adrenoceptors in the same tissue [41], to reduce AQH production, also yielded significant IOP decreases. In an effort to promote AQH outflow via the uveoscleral pathway to decrease feline IOP, cells of the ANC were transduced with the gene for cyclooxygenase-2 (in order to produce endogenous prostaglandins) and a gene for an optimized FP-receptor protein [42].

Gene therapies specifically directed at protecting RGCs and other retinal neurons have also found some success in pre-clinical studies. Thus, transduction of gene encoding a form of erythropoietin in the eyes of mice with pigmentary glaucoma (DBA/2 J) suppressed infiltration of peripheral immune cells into their retinas, modulated microglial reactivity, reduced oxidative stress, and preserved their visual perception [43]. RGCs and their axons in DBA/2 J mice and other mice with microbead-induced ocular hypertension (OHT) could be protected by genetic expression of the anti-apoptotic soluble Fas-ligand [44], by over-expression of the complement C3 inhibitor CR2-Crry [45], and by retinal expression of scAAV2-C3 (exoenzyme C3 transferase), which significantly reduced the number of apoptotic RGCs and decreased cell loss in the ganglion cell layer after ischemia/reperfusion injury [46]. Additional examples of gene therapies for RGC preservation in the face of death signals after GON induction in various animal models have involved delivering X-linked inhibitor of apoptosis (XIAP; potent caspase inhibitor) [47], transduction of RGCs with the protective transcription factors BCL2L1 [48], and Myc-associated protein X (MAX) [49] and over-expression of NMNAT1, the key enzyme in the NAD^+ biosynthetic pathway to enhance RGC rejuvenation through increased intrinsic energy production [50]. A most advanced form of gene therapy that proved successful in animals has been the co-delivery of the neurotrophin BDNF and its receptor to impart neuroprotection to RGCs [51]. However, despite such non-clinical successes, the multifactorial nature of GON will most likely still require use of a combination of gene therapies to achieve clinically relevant efficacy. Furthermore, translation to the clinical management of various forms of glaucoma will remain rather challenging, but hopefully, this will become a reality in the near future.

5. Cell-replacement therapies for glaucoma treatment

Delivering missing genes or modifying genetic expression of certain gene products has its complexities and difficulties. However, replacing injured or dead cells as a form of treatment for ocular hypertension and GON is an even more daunting task. Nevertheless, several pre-clinical studies have demonstrated the effectiveness of such an approach. Due to cell senescence caused by aging or pathological conditions as in glaucoma, the TM region could benefit from enhanced cellularity to filter and drain AQH and maintain IOP within normal ranges. Hence, stem cells isolated from human TM and expanded *in vitro* homed to TM tissue and remained active for at least 4 months after injection in normal mice [52]. Abu-Hassan et al. [53] created an *in vitro* model of glaucoma by inducing a controlled loss of TM cellularity in perfused postmortem human eye anterior eye segments using saponin. Transplanting isolated human TM cells or induced pluripotent stems cells (iPSCs) that resemble

TM characteristics into these eye segments allowed the cells to intercalate into the TM, and over time, this procedure restored IOP to a large extent [54–56]. In another study, transplanted TM-like cells derived from induced pluripotent stem cells into the anterior chamber of a transgenic mouse model of glaucoma involving over-expression of myocilin led to significantly reduced IOP and improved aqueous humor outflow facility, which was maintained for >8 weeks [54]. These and other studies [57–60] clearly show the potential use of cell-replacement therapy to overcome glaucoma-induced loss of TM cells and recover their function in the future, perhaps in human subjects. Such cell replacement ventures would take advantage of autologous or allogenic approaches and utilize TM progenitor cells, iPSCs, or even mesenchymal stem cells (MSCs) or their combinations. However, in view of the gross heterogeneity of TM cells [61], the choice of cells for transplantation should account for demonstratable phagocytic activity and contractile properties to ensure maximum longevity of the cells and their function *in vivo*.

Unlike the TM cell replacement, the challenge of replacing lost RGCs in the retina of glaucomatous animals (and humans), due to physical barriers such as the inner and outer limiting membranes, fibrotic scarring, and the growth-inhibitory microenvironment, is much greater. However, some successes, at least in animals, are noteworthy. Firstly, a multitude of cell sources have been identified for potential in vitro differentiation, proliferation, and characterization before being considered for transplantation purposes. Additionally, techniques have been developed that permit re-programming [62, 63] or conversion of cells to specific desired cell types. Sources of cells include the following: allogenic cadaveric human cells, human fetal retinal stem cells, human CNS stem cells, adult hippocampal neural stem cells, ciliary pigmented epithelial cells, limbal stem cells, retinal progenitor cells (RPCs), mesenchymal stem cells (MSCs), human pluripotent stem cells (PSCs) [including both human embryonic stem cells (ESCs) and human-induced pluripotent stem cells (iPSCs)], and retinal organoids themselves. Regarding glaucoma treatment via cell replacement technologies, successful transfer of embryonic retinal progenitor cells labeled with green fluorescent protein into mouse eyes depleted of RGCs and their movement to the RGC layer and establishment of appropriate connections was demonstrated [64]. The transplanted cells began to express key RGC-related genes and extended bundled axons, although their numbers were not so high [64]. Subsequently, chemically induced conversion of human embryonic stem cells and iPSCs into functional RGCs was achieved using a Notch inhibitor [65], where >30% of the cells expressed key RGC markers, which generated action potentials. Such techniques have been further refined that included reprograming fibroblasts into RGC-like neurons via transcription factors *Asc11, Brn3b,* and *Is11* [66] and converting mature mouse Muller cells into RGCs using other transcription factors/genes such as *Math5* and *Brn3b* [67]. The newly created RGCs exhibited neuronal electrophysiological characteristics and extended axons to make connections to the appropriate visual centers when transplanted into mouse eyes lacking original RGCs and improved functional vision in the host animals [67]. Furthermore, a combination of stem cell therapy and optogenetics has paved the way for restoring vision in animals deficient in or with defective retinal architecture [68]. While promising, there are still many hurdles in terms of the duration of survival of the transplanted cells and the durability of their function in terms of vision restoration and the quality of the latter. Nevertheless, there is hope that further progress will be made such that translation of these laboratory findings to the glaucoma patients clinically can be achieved in the near future [69–71].

6. Electroceutical technologies for improving vision

Activity-dependent maturation and maintenance of synaptic connectivity, long-term potentiation for memory consolidation, and axonal regrowth and connectivity are essential for CNS homeostasis and normal functions of neural networks [72]. Action potential transmission keeps neural circuits healthy and functioning [73]. Based on these findings, electrotherapies have been shown to promote tissue and bone healing whether administered via acupuncture, electroacupuncture, or electrical stimulation via electrodes. Indeed, electroshock treatment for anxiety and depression is well known as is deep brain stimulation to help deal with motor dysfunctions as in Parkinson's disease and as beneficial paradigms for other neurological diseases.

As a continuum of the above application, electrical stimulation (ES) and trans-corneal electrical stimulation (TCES) have been utilized for visual perception improvement. Indeed, ES and TCES protected and preserved RGCs of rats in which optic nerve lesions had been introduced and where endogenously secreted insulin-like growth factor-1 (IGF-1) was demonstrated to be the neuroprotective agent [74, 75]. Interestingly, repetitive ES promoted axonal regeneration in a rat optic nerve crush model of glaucoma [76] and afforded retinal neuroprotection in a retinal ischemia injury model [77, 78]. Inhibition of inflammatory cell migration and release of their inflammatory cytokines coupled with concomitant release of endogenous neuro-trophic factors were observed following ES procedures [77–79]. Furthermore, TCES helped preserve and aided the recovery of retinal cells and their function following various external insults through reductions in microglial activation and suppression of cytokine secretion in the retina [80–82]. Similarly, in an animal model of pigmentary glaucoma (DBA2/J mice), TCES treatment suppressed infiltration and activation of inflammatory cells and microglia through improved energy utilization/homeostasis and by reducing cellular apoptosis [81]. The theme of neurotrophins release and suppression of inflammation, among other beneficial elements, induced by TCES in promoting RGC neuroprotection and their axonal growth is illustrated in **Figure 4**.

ES *in vivo* caused RGC neurite and/or axon elongation principally through brain-derived growth factor (BDNF) release and modulation of signal transduction pathways involving phosphoinositide-3-kinase (PI3K)/AKT, mitogen-activated kinase kinases (MEKs), and Ca^{2+}-calmodulin-kinases and by down-regulation of nuclear factor-κB and inhibition of PTEN phosphatase [82–84]. The stimulation of intracellular cAMP production and the down-stream effects involving cAMP response element-binding protein (CREB) in the nucleus induced by ES appeared important for RGC preservation and RGC axonal growth. Additional investigations in a rat optic nerve crush model of glaucoma revealed that RGC axonal growth and elongation could be induced if the rats received high contrast image stimulation (equivalent to ES or RGC axonal action potential activity) and that the axonal length could be further increased if the latter procedure was combined with knockout of the mammalian target of rapamycin [76]. Partial restoration of a subset of rat behaviors reliant on improved vision was observed, and this correlated well with re-establishment of many connections of the RGC axons with the thalamic brain nuclei, which in turn promoted reinnervation of the thalamic-visual cortical connections [76]. The elucidation of the mechanism(s) of action of TCES has been studied in animals and also *in vitro* by electrical stimulation techniques. The collective conclusions are that these procedures up-regulate protective transcriptional factors (e.g., Bcl-2) and concomitantly down-regulate the damaging ones (e.g., Bax) (**Figure 5**). Additionally, protective proteins are synthesized and/or activated intracellularly to promote

DOI: http://dx.doi.org/10.5772/intechopen.108914

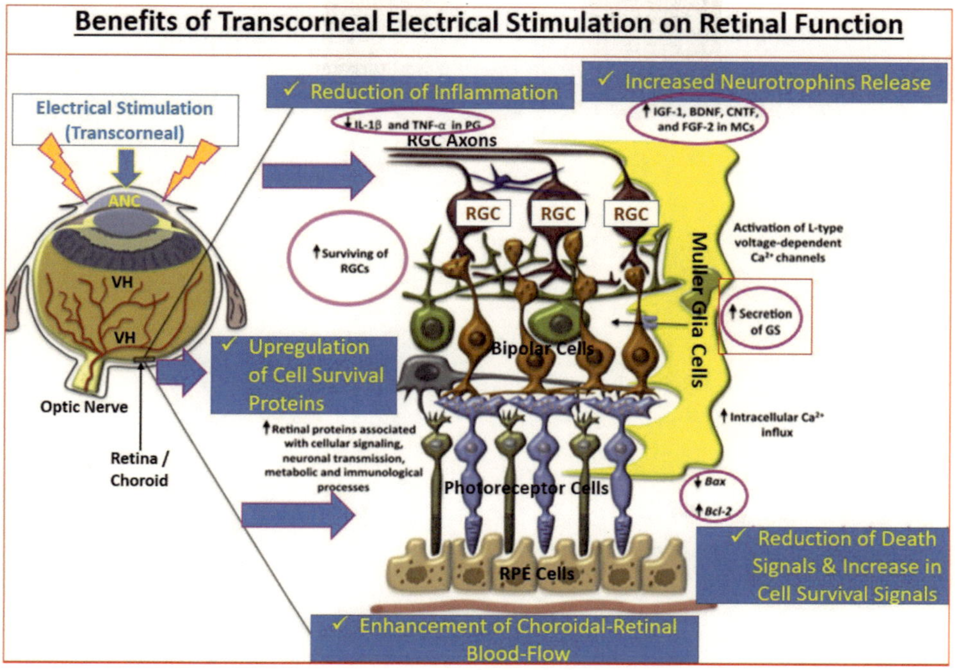

Figure 4.
The schematic illustrates the beneficial effects of transcorneal electrical stimulation (TCES) on the structure and function of the retina. Adapted from Ref. [77].

neuroprotection/cytoprotection of the retinal cells, especially RGCs. These beneficial effects are augmented by release of growth factors such as IGF-1/2, BDNF, and ciliary neurotrophic factor [74–79]. Simultaneous or consequential reductions in production and secretion of inflammatory cytokines also aid in preserving RGCs and their axons (**Figure 5**). Ultimately, initiation of axonogenesis and re-connectivity of the RGC axons to the visual centers within the brain lead to visual improvements. Additional studies have shown that electrical stimulation can induce retinal progenitor cell differentiation and Muller cell proliferation, which has positive feedback actions on structure and function (**Figure 5**) [84].

Even though ethical considerations and regulatory issues have thus far hampered translation of such studies to the glaucoma patients or to others afflicted with major retinal dystrophies, a few encouraging studies have been reported. Some improvement in vision was observed in patients with nonarteritic ischemic optic neuropathy and traumatic optic neuropathy administered TCES [85]. Likewise, patients with optic nerve lesions subjected to transorbital stimulation experienced improvement in their visual field size and visual acuity or increased detection ability within the visual field [86, 87]. Furthermore, transorbital alternating current stimulation of patients with optic neuropathy yielded increased thresholds in static perimetry tests and led to improved visual fields [87]. Investigations dealing with use of electrical stimulation to improve retinal circulation or to combat retinal vein occlusion issues demonstrated positive findings [88–90] and an improvement in retinal function after such treatment in patients who had retinal artery occlusions [90]. Transpalpebral stimulation using 10 Hz nonrectangular current pulses (100 μA) constant current in primary OAG (POAG) patients reduced their IOP down to 14.41–15.29 mmHg starting with

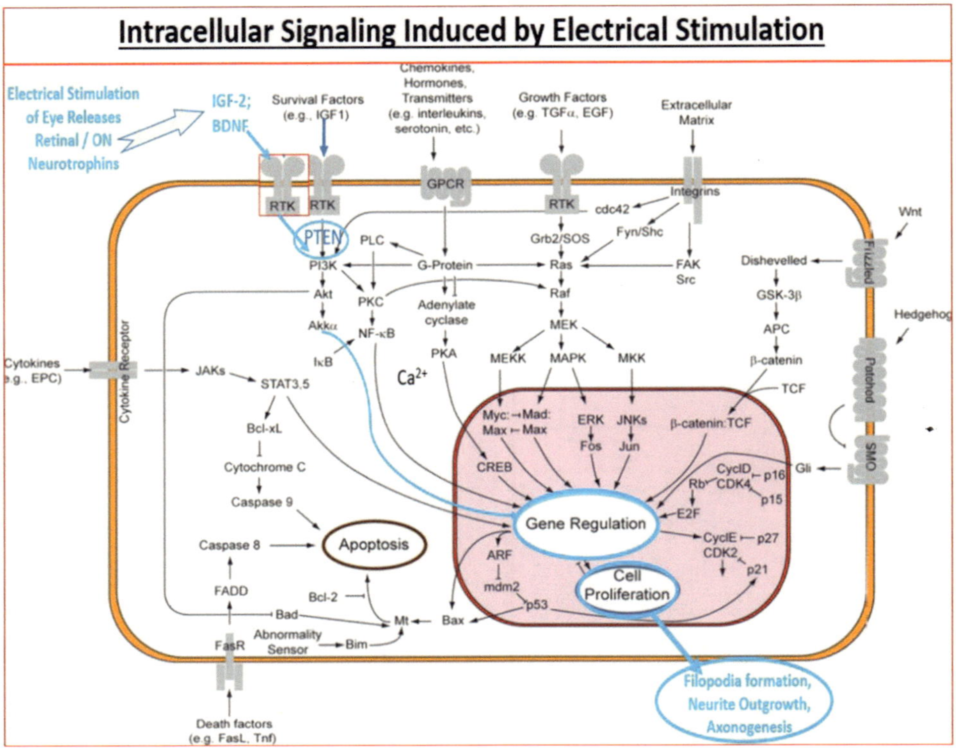

Figure 5.
This pictorial depicts the mechanism(s) of action of transcorneal electrical stimulation on neurotrophin release and the ensuing intracellular signal transduction pathway(s) activation, in particular the pathway shown in light blue. Adapted from Wikipedia; https://en.wikipedia.org/wiki/Signal_transduction (19Oct2022).

baseline IOPs of 19.25–20.38 mmHg [91]. Similarly, transorbital AC current (30 min/day for 10 days at 10 Hz) given to patients with visual field defects resulted in significant improvement in their visual fields due to local activation of their visual cortex and increased retinal blood flow [88–90]. Furthermore, a very recent study employing optic nerve stimulation (ONS) demonstrated highly significant improvements in visual fields (2 weeks to 1 year of daily treatment) in 101 eyes of 70 patients (composed of mainly POAG and NTG) and decreased the mean defects in their retinas (**Figures 6** and 7) [92]. An Eyetronic® device (Neuromodtronic GmbH, Potsdam, Germany) that applied electrical stimulation via goggles with embedded supraorbital and infraorbital electrodes and recorded EEG signals via an electrode cap was used to deliver the stimulation. All four electrodes, two on each side, in the stimulation goggles were controlled by four separate constant-current stimulators with the following stimulation parameters: Pulse shape: biphasic, symmetric rectangular; pulse amplitude: up to 1.2 mA; pulse duration: 14 to 20 ms; and repetition frequency in pulse trains: 5 to 34 Hz. The daily duration of the stimulation treatment was less than 40 min but varied slightly from one treatment day to another. While the results are impressive, we await confirmation of these types of studies in the near future.

Despite some successes described above, the use of electrical stimulation to tackle ocular diseases is still being refined, and many challenges remain. For instance, the choice of type of electrical stimulator, the type of electrical current to use (AC or

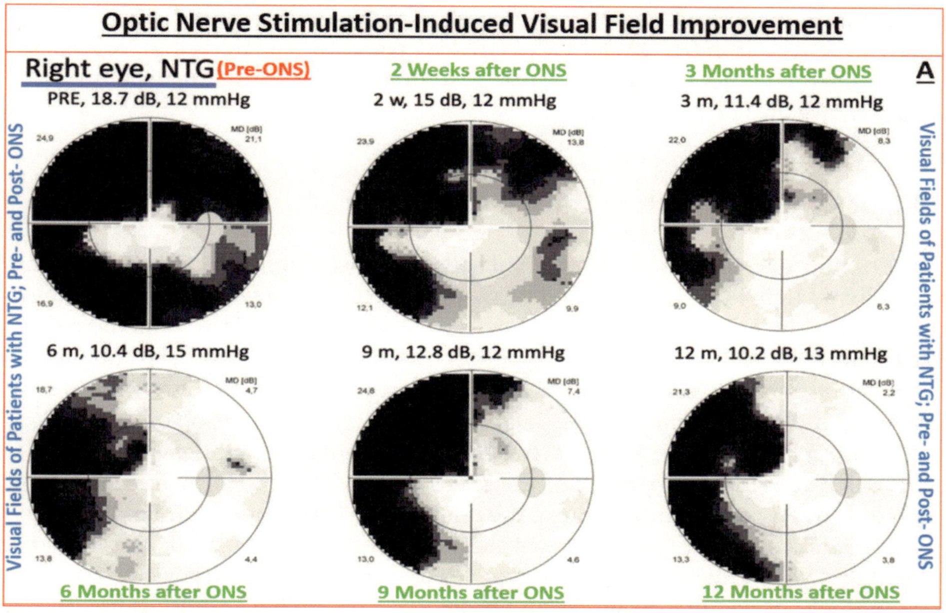

Figure 6.
Improvements in visual fields of NTG patients following optic nerve stimulation (ONS). Note the increase in white areas in the circles. Adapted from Ref. [92].

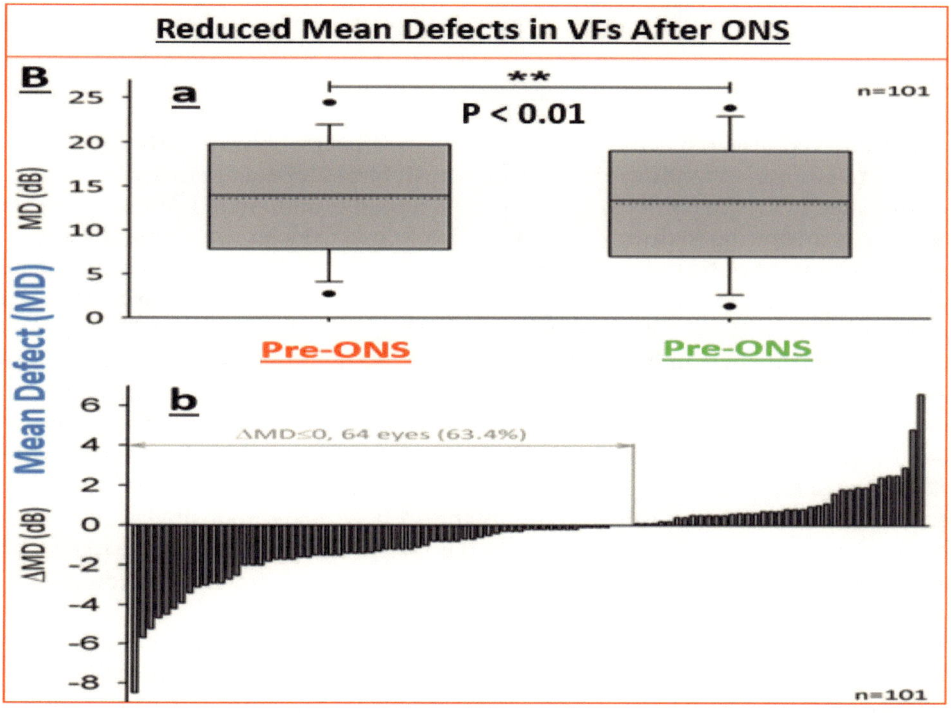

Figure 7.
Reduction of mean defects in NTG patients after ONS. Adapted from Ref. [92].

DC), the strength of the current (50–800 μA), and the frequency and duration of each treatment session for OAG, ACG, and NTG patients need defining. Nevertheless, the electroceutical therapeutics may prove useful in the future and may be adopted for clinical use on a routine basis.

7. Photobiomodulation for glaucoma treatment

Use of nonthermal, non-ionizing light sources (lasers, light emitting diodes, and/or broadband light) using visible and near-infrared light is now recognized as helpful treatment modalities to aid healing (muscles and joints) and for reducing pain. Furthermore, by generating CO, redlight (650 nm wavelength) has been shown to destroy certain viruses, to activate neurite outgrowth after blue-light-induced retraction, and to aid corneal epithelial healing through rejuvenation of cellular mitochondria [93, 94]. The principal MOA of photo biomodulation involves the activation of the respiratory chain of the Krebs cycle within the mitochondria of cells to enhance ATP production and cause the release of NO and free radicals. The beneficial effects of redlight resulting from these activities help increase local circulation and metabolism. Whilst blue light damaged retina cell mitochondria via oxidative stress, redlight prevented the injury and protected Muller glial and RGCs [94, 95]. Mice with autosomal optic atrophy subjected to redlight exposure for 5 days exhibited less RGC dendritic atrophy than control mice that did not receive redlight [96–98]. Thus, benefits of redlight exposure may benefit OAG/ACG/NTG patients and need to be investigated in the future.

8. Conclusions

Multifaceted research in ophthalmology and neuroscience has greatly contributed to our understanding of the pathogenesis of neurodegenerative diseases. Accumulated evidence points to several local microenvironmental deleterious events and factors conspiring to cause death of RGCs and brain nuclei neurons and axonal damage within the optic nerve. Inflammation and reduced ocular perfusion at the ONH/LC retinal region caused by elevated IOP appears to trigger the initial damage in the eyes of glaucoma patients, leading to weakening of the LC structure. The contusion, bending, and overall increased tortuosity of the injured RGCs axons and retinal blood vessels then cause oxidative damage, reduced axonal flow of neurotrophins and mitochondria to the RGC cell somas, and retraction of the axonal terminals in the thalamic and other parts of the brain. Decreased overall input from RGCs eventually leads to the death of brain neurons involved in visual image processing and loss of peripheral vision. Such detrimental events appear to be also responsible for decreased visual acuity, contrast sensitivity, and visual impairment in patients where the IOPs are within normal ranges (NTG), indicating involvement of genetic, environmental, and other factors in their RGC, axonal, and CNS atrophy.

While lowering and controlling IOP by pharmaceutical, surgical, and micro-shunt implantation procedures slows down the progression of GON, other direct and indirect means are needed to protect and preserve the retinal and visual center architecture and functions. The neuroprotective paradigm is now well accepted, and many drugs and food-derived agents have shown efficacy in cell-based and animal model-based systems. Likewise, gene- [51, 99] and cell-therapy [70, 100–102] and controlled electrical stimulation [92] and photobiomodulation [97, 102] have beneficial effects and a place in tackling degenerative maladies. The latter alone, or coupled with optogenetic [102], photoswitch [103], electromagnetic, and ultrasound-based technologies [104, 105], is also beginning to show promise in promoting cytoprotection and even potential axonal regeneration. Though many challenges remain, we look forward to further progress in translating these to help patients with GON and other related neurodegenerative eye and brain diseases in the near future.

Acknowledgements

The inspiration to compile literature information and to write this book chapter was provided by my family members and many colleagues and collaborators who are working tirelessly to find suitable remedial solutions for glaucoma patients. My appointments to several universities and interactions with faculty and students at these research institutions and at the Glaucoma Foundation have further infused energy and enthusiasm toward this goal. I am also grateful to Santen for allowing me to pursue such scholarly activities.

Conflict of interest

The author declares no conflict of interest and simply wishes to advance sharing of knowledge to help in the discovery and development of methods and compositions to help patients suffering from neurodegenerative eye and brain disorders.

Author details

Najam A. Sharif[1,2,3,4,5,6,7,8]

1 Eye ECP Duke-NUS Ophthalmology and Visual Sciences Academic Clinical Programme, Duke-National University of Singapore Medical School, Singapore, Singapore

2 Department of Surgery and Cancer, Imperial College of Science and Technology, London, UK

3 Singapore Eye Research Institute (SERI), Singapore, Singapore

4 Department of Pharmaceutical Sciences, College of Pharmacy and Health Sciences, Texas Southern University, Houston, USA

5 Department of Pharmacy Sciences, Creighton University, Omaha, USA

6 Department of Pharmacology and Neuroscience, University of North Texas Health Sciences Center, Fort Worth, USA

7 University College London, Institute of Ophthalmology, London, UK

8 Global Alliances and External Research, Ophthalmology Innovation Center, Santen Inc, Emeryville, California, USA

*Address all correspondence to: najam.sharif@santen.com

References

[1] Grünert U, Martin PR. Cell types and cell circuits in human and non-human primate retina. Progress in Retinal and Eye Research. 2020;**5**:100844

[2] Ou Y, Jo RE, Ullian EM, et al. Selective vulnerability of specific retinal ganglion cell types and synapses after transient ocular hypertension. The Journal of Neuroscience. 2016;**36**(35):9240-9252

[3] Weinreb RN, Aung T, Medeiros FA. The pathophysiology and treatment of glaucoma: A review. JAMA. 2014;**311**:1901-1911

[4] Jonas JB, Aung T, Bourne RR, et al. Glaucoma. Lancet. 2017;**390**:2183-2193

[5] Sharif NA. Ocular hypertension and glaucoma: A review and current perspectives. International Journal of Ophthalmology & Visual Science. 2017;**2**(3):22-36

[6] Sharif NA. Therapeutic drugs and devices for tackling ocular hypertension and glaucoma, and need for neuroprotection and cytoprotective therapies. Frontiers in Pharmacology. 2021;**12**:729249

[7] Abu-Hassan DW, Acott TS, Kelley MJ. The trabecular meshwork: A basic review of form and function. Journal of Ocular Biology. 2014;**2**(1):9

[8] Acott TS, Vranka JA, Keller KE, et al. Normal and glaucomatous outflow regulation. Progress in Retinal and Eye Research. 2020;**11**:100897

[9] Tham Y-C, Li X, Wong TY, et al. Global prevalence of glaucoma and projections of glaucoma burden through 2040. Ophthalmology. 2014;**121**:2081-2090

[10] Bucolo C, Salomone S, Drago F, et al. Pharmacological management of ocular hypertension: Current approaches and future prospectives. Current Opinion in Pharmacology. 2013;**13**:50-55

[11] He S, Stankowska DL, Ellis DZ, Krishnamoorthy RR, Yorio T. Targets of neuroprotection in glaucoma. Journal of Ocular Pharmacology and Therapeutics. 2018;**34**(1-2):85-106

[12] Sharif NA. iDrugs and iDevices discovery and development - preclinical assays, techniques and animal model studies for ocular hypotensives and neuroprotectants. Journal of Ocular Pharmacology and Therapeutics. 2018;**34**:7-39

[13] Burgoyne CF, Downs JC, Bellezza AJ, et al. The optic nerve head as a biomechanical structure; a new paradigm for understanding the role of IOP-related stress and strain in the pathophysiology of glaucomatous optic nerve head damage. Progress in Retinal and Eye Research. 2005;**24**:39-73

[14] Downs JC, Roberts MD, Sigal IA. Glaucomatous cupping of the lamina cribrosa: A review of the evidence for active progressive remodeling as a mechanism. Experimental Eye Research. 2011;**93**:133-140

[15] Chintala SK, Putris N, Geno M. Activation of TLR3 promotes the degeneration of retinal ganglion cells by upregulating the protein levels of JNK3. Investigative Ophthalmology & Visual Science. 2015;**56**:505-514

[16] Sanderson J, Dartt DA, Trinkaus-Randall V, et al. Purines in the eye: Recent evidence for the physiological and pathological role of purines in the

RPE, retinal neurons, astrocytes, Müller cells, lens, trabecular meshwork, cornea and lacrimal gland. Experimental Eye Research. 2014;**127**:270-279

[17] Tezel G, Yang X, Luo C, et al. Oxidative stress and the regulation of complement activation in human glaucoma. Investigative Ophthalmology & Visual Science. 2010;**51**:5071-5082

[18] Harder JM, Williams PA, Braine CE, et al. Complement peptide C3a receptor 1 promotes optic nerve degeneration in DBA/2J mice. Journal of Neuroinflammation. 2020;**17**(1):336

[19] Howell GR, Libby RT, Jakobs TC, et al. Axons of retinal ganglion cells are insulted in the optic nerve early in DBA/2J glaucoma. The Journal of Cell Biology. 2011;**179**(7):1523-1537

[20] Bosco A, Steele MR, Vetter ML. Early microglia activation in a mouse model of chronic glaucoma. The Journal of Comparative Neurology. 2011;**519**:599-620

[21] Calkins DJ, Horner PJ. The cell and molecular biology of glaucoma: Axonopathy and the brain. Investigative Ophthalmology & Visual Science. 2012;**53**:2482-2484

[22] Inman DM, Horner PJ. Reactive nonproliferative gliosis predominates in a chronic mouse model of glaucoma. Glia. 2007;**55**:942-953

[23] Prassana G, Krishnamoorthy R, Yorio T. Endothelin, astrocytes and glaucoma. Experimental Eye Research. 2011;**93**:170-177

[24] Maddineni P, Kasetti RB, Patel PD, et al. CNS axonal degeneration and transport deficits at the optic nerve head precede structural and functional loss of retinal ganglion cells in a mouse model of glaucoma. Molecular Neurodegeneration. 2020;**15**(1):48

[25] Flammer J, Orgül S, Costa VP, et al. The impact of ocular blood flow in glaucoma. Progress in Retinal and Eye Research. 2002;**21**(4):359-393

[26] Mozaffarieh M, Grieshaber MC, Flammer J. Oxygen and blood flow: Players in the pathogenesis of glaucoma. Molecular Vision. 2008;**14**:224-233

[27] Gupta N, Ly T, Zhang Q, et al. Chronic ocular hypertension induces dendrite pathology in the lateral geniculate nucleus of the brain. Experimental Eye Research. 2007;**84**:176-184

[28] Sasaoka M, Nakamura K, Shimazawa M, et al. Changes in visual fields and lateral geniculate nucleus in monkey laser-induced high intraocular pressure model. Experimental Eye Research. 2005;**86**:770-782

[29] Sponsel WE, Growth SL, Satangi N, et al. Refined data analysis provides clinical evidence for central nervous system control of chronic glaucomatous neurodegeneration. Translational Vision Science & Technology. 2014;**3**:1-13

[30] Adornetto A, Parisi V, Morrone LA, et al. The role of autophagy in glaucomatous optic neuropathy. Frontiers in Cell and Development Biology. 2020;**8**:121

[31] Yu L, Xie L, Dai C, et al. Progressive thinning of visual cortex in primary open-angle glaucoma of varying severity. PLoS One. 2015;**10**:e0121960

[32] Crabb DP. A view on glaucoma— Are we seeing it clearly? Eye. 2016;**30**:304-313

[33] Fitzner D, Schnaars M, van Rossum D, et al. Selective transfer of

exosomes from oligodendrocytes to microglia by macropinocytosis. Journal of Cell Science. 2011;**124**:447-458

[34] Eastlake K, Lamb WDB, Luis J, et al. Prospects for the application of Müller glia and their derivatives in retinal regenerative therapies. Progress in Retinal and Eye Research. 2021;**85**:100970

[35] Williams PA, Harder JM, John SWM. Glaucoma as a metabolic optic neuropathy: Making the case for nicotinamide treatment in glaucoma. Journal of Glaucoma. 2017;**26**(12):1161-1168

[36] Hui F, Tang J, Williams PA, et al. Improvement in inner retinal function in glaucoma with nicotinamide (vitamin B3) supplementation: A crossover randomized clinical trial. Clinical & Experimental Ophthalmology. 2020;**48**(7):903-914

[37] Nuzbrokh Y, Ragi SD, Tsang SH. Gene therapy for inherited retinal diseases. Annals of Translational Medicine. 2021;**9**(15):1278

[38] Gerometta R, Spiga MG, Borrás T, Candia OA. Treatment of sheep steroid-induced ocular hypertension with a glucocorticoid-inducible MMP1 gene therapy virus. Investigative Ophthalmology & Visual Science. 2010;**51**(6):3042-3048

[39] O'Callaghan J, Crosbie DE, Cassidy PS, et al. Therapeutic potential of AAV-mediated MMP-3 secretion from corneal endothelium in treating glaucoma. Human Molecular Genetics. 2017;**26**(7):1230-1246

[40] Wu J, Bell OH, Copland DA, et al. Gene therapy for glaucoma by ciliary body aquaporin 1 disruption using CRISPR-Cas9. Molecular Therapy. 2020;**28**(3):820-829

[41] Martínez T, González MV, Roehl I, et al. In vitro and in vivo efficacy of SYL040012, a novel siRNA compound for treatment of glaucoma. Molecular Therapy. 2014;**22**(1):81-91

[42] Barraza RA, McLaren JW, Poeschla EM. Prostaglandin pathway gene therapy for sustained reduction of intraocular pressure. Molecular Therapy. 2010;**18**(3):491-501

[43] Hines-Beard J, Wesley S, Bond WS, et al. Virus-mediated EpoR76E gene therapy preserves vision in a glaucoma model by modulating neuroinflammation and decreasing oxidative stress. Journal of Neuroinflammation. 2016;**13**:39

[44] Krishnan A, Kocab AJ, Zacks DN, et al. A small peptide antagonist of the Fas receptor inhibits neuroinflammation and prevents axon degeneration and retinal ganglion cell death in an inducible mouse model of glaucoma. Journal of Neuroinflammation. 2019;**16**(1):184

[45] Bosco A, Anderson SR, Breen KT, et al. Complement C3-targeted gene therapy restricts onset and progression of neurodegeneration in chronic mouse glaucoma. Molecular Therapy. 2018;**26**:2379-2396

[46] Tan J, Liu G, Lan C, et al. Lentiviral vector-mediated expression of C3 transferase attenuates retinal ischemia and reperfusion injury in rats. Life Sciences. 2021;**272**:119269

[47] Visuvanathan S, Baker AN, Lagali PS, et al. XIAP gene therapy effects on retinal ganglion cell structure and function in a mouse model of glaucoma. Gene Therapy. 2022;**29**(3-4):147-156

[48] Donahue RJ, Fehrman RL, Gustafson JR, Nickells RW. BCLXL gene therapy moderates neuropathology in the DBA/2J mouse model of inherited

glaucoma. Cell Death & Disease. 2021;**12**(8):781

[49] Lani-Louzada R, Marra C, Dias MS, et al. Neuroprotective gene therapy by overexpression of the transcription factor MAX in rat models of glaucomatous neurodegeneration. Investigative Ophthalmology & Visual Science. 2022;**63**(2):5

[50] Fang F, Zhuang P, Feng X, et al. NMNAT2 is downregulated in glaucomatous RGCs, and RGC-specific gene therapy rescues neurodegeneration and visual function. Molecular Therapy. 2022;**30**(4):1421-1431

[51] Khatib TZ, Osborne A, Yang S, et al. Receptor-ligand supplementation via a self-cleaving 2A peptide-based gene therapy promotes CNS axonal transport with functional recovery. Science Advances. 2021;**7**(14):eabd2590

[52] Du Y, Yun H, Yang E, Schuman JS. Stem cells from trabecular meshwork home to TM tissue in vivo. Investigative Ophthalmology & Visual Science. 2013;**54**(2):1450-1459

[53] Abu-Hassan DW, Li X, Ryan EI, Acott TS, Kelley MJ. Induced pluripotent stem cells restore function in a human cell loss model of open-angle glaucoma. Stem Cells. 2015;**33**(3):751-761

[54] Zhu W, Gramlich OW, Laboissonniere L, et al. Transplantation of iPSC-derived TM cells rescues glaucoma phenotypes in vivo. Proceedings of the National Academy of Sciences of the United States of America. 2016;**113**(25):E3492-E3500

[55] Zhu Q, Zhang Y, Tighe S, et al. Human trabecular meshwork progenitors. International Journal of Medical Sciences. 2019;**16**(5):704-710

[56] Sharif NA. Neuropathology and therapeutics addressing glaucoma, a prevalent sight threatening retina-optic nerve-brain disease. OBM Neurobiology. 2022;**6**(1):42

[57] Ding QJ, Zhu W, Cook AC, et al. Induction of trabecular meshwork cells from induced pluripotent stem cells. Investigative Ophthalmology & Visual Science. 2014;**55**(11):7065-7072

[58] Sun H, Zhu Q, Guo P, et al. Trabecular meshwork cells are a valuable resource for cellular therapy of glaucoma. Journal of Cellular and Molecular Medicine. 2019;**23**(3):1678-1686

[59] Mallick S, Sharma M, Kumar A, Du Y. Cell-based therapies for trabecular meshwork regeneration to treat glaucoma. Biomolecules. 2021;**11**(9):1258

[60] Nicoară SD, Brie I, Jurj A, Sorițău O. The future of stem cells and their derivates in the treatment of glaucoma. A critical point of view. International Journal of Molecular Sciences. 2021;**22**(20):11077

[61] Patel G, Fury W, Yang H, et al. Molecular taxonomy of human ocular outflow tissues defined by single-cell transcriptomics. Proceedings of the National Academy of Sciences of the United States of America. 2020;**117**(23):12856-12867

[62] Karl MO. The potential of stem cell research for the treatment of neuronal damage in glaucoma. Cell and Tissue Research. 2013;**353**(2):311-325

[63] Lu Y, Brommer B, Tian X, et al. Reprogramming to recover youthful epigenetic information and restore vision. Nature. 2020;**588**(7836):124-129

[64] Cho JH, Mao CA, Klein WH. Adult mice transplanted with embryonic

retinal progenitor cells: New approach for repairing damaged optic nerves. Molecular Vision. 2012;**18**:2658-2672

[65] Riazifar H, Jia Y, Chen J, Lynch G, Huang T. Chemically induced specification of retinal ganglion cells from human embryonic and induced pluripotent stem cells. Stem Cells Translational Medicine. 2014;**3**(4):424-432

[66] Wang J, He Q, Zhang K, et al. Quick commitment and efficient reprogramming route of direct induction of retinal ganglion cell-like neurons. Stem Cell Reports. 2020;**15**(5):1095-1110

[67] Xiao D, Jin K, Qiu S, et al. In vivo Regeneration of Ganglion Cells for Vision Restoration in Mammalian Retinas. Frontiers in Cell and Development Biology. 2021;**9**:755544

[68] Garita-Hernandez M, Lampič M, Chaffiol A, et al. Restoration of visual function by transplantation of optogenetically engineered photoreceptors. Nature Communications. 2019;**10**(1):4524

[69] Behtaj S, Öchsner A, Anissimov YG, Rybachuk M. Retinal tissue bioengineering, materials and methods for the treatment of glaucoma. Tissue Engineering and Regenerative Medicine. 2020;**17**(3):253-269

[70] Zhang J, Wu S, Jin ZB, Wang N. Stem cell-based regeneration and restoration for retinal ganglion cell: Recent advancements and current challenges. Biomolecules. 2021;**11**(7):987

[71] Coco-Martin RM, Pastor-Idoate S, Pastor JC. Cell replacement therapy for retinal and optic nerve diseases: Cell sources, clinical trials and challenges. Pharmaceutics. 2021;**13**(6):865

[72] de Faria O, Jr GDG, Nicholson M, Xiao J. Activity-dependent central nervous system myelination throughout life. Journal of Neurochemistry. 2019;**148**:447-461

[73] Wake H, Lee PR, Fields RD. Control of local protein synthesis and initial events in myelination by action potentials. Science. 2011;**333**:1647-1651

[74] Morimoto T, Miyoshi T, Fujikado T, Tano Y, Fukuda Y. Electrical stimulation enhances the survival of axotomized retinal ganglion cells in vivo. Neuroreport. 2002;**13**(2):227-230

[75] Morimoto T, Miyoshi T, Matsuda S, Tano Y, et al. Transcorneal electrical stimulation rescues axotomized retinal ganglion cells by activating endogenous retinal IGF-1 system. Investigative Ophthalmology & Visual Science. 2005;**46**(6):2147-2155

[76] Lim JH, Stafford BK, Nguyen PL, et al. Neural activity promotes long-distance, target-specific regeneration of adult retinal axons. Nature Neuroscience. 2016;**19**(8):1073-1084

[77] Pardue MT, Ciavatta VT, Hetling JR, et al. Neuroprotective effects of low-level electrical stimulation therapy on retinal degeneration. Advances in Experimental Medicine and Biology. 2014;**801**:845-851

[78] Pardue MT, Allen RS. Neuroprotective strategies for retinal disease. Progress in Retinal and Eye Research. 2018;**65**:50-76

[79] Sato T, Fujikado T, Lee TS, Tano Y. Direct effect of electrical stimulation on induction of brain-derived neurotrophic factor from cultured retinal Müller cells. Investigative Ophthalmology & Visual Science. 2008;**49**(10):4641-4646

[80] Zhou WT, Ni YQ, Jin ZB, Zhang M, et al. Electrical stimulation

ameliorates light-induced photoreceptor degeneration in vitro via suppressing the proinflammatory effect of microglia and enhancing the neurotrophic potential of Müller cells. Experimental Neurology. 2012;**238**(2):192-208

[81] Jassim AH, Cavanaugh M, Shah JS, et al. Transcorneal electrical stimulation reduces neurodegenerative process in a mouse model of glaucoma. Annals of Biomedical Engineering. 2021;**49**(2):858-870

[82] Yin Y, De Lima S, Gilbert HY, et al. Optic nerve regeneration: A long view. Restorative Neurology and Neuroscience. 2019;**37**(6):525-544

[83] Yang S-G, Li C-P, Peng X-Q, et al. Strategies to promote long-distance optic nerve regeneration. Frontiers in Cellular Neuroscience. 2020;**14**:119

[84] Enayati S, Chang K, Achour H, Cho KS, et al. Electrical stimulation induces retinal Müller cell proliferation and their progenitor cell potential. Cell. 2020;**9**(3):781

[85] Fujikado T, Morimoto T, Matsushita K, et al. Effect of transcorneal electrical stimulation in patients with nonarteritic ischemic optic neuropathy or traumatic optic neuropathy. Japanese Journal of Ophthalmology. 2006;**50**:266-273

[86] Sabel BA, Fedorov AB, Naue N, et al. Non-invasive alternating current stimulation improves vision in optic neuropathy. Restorative Neurology and Neuroscience. 2011;**29**:493-505

[87] Gall C, Schmidt S, Schittkowski MP, et al. Alternating current stimulation for vision restoration after optic nerve damage: A randomized clinical trial. PLoS One. 2016;**11**:e0156134

[88] Inomata K, Shinoda K, Ohde H, Tsunoda K, et al. Transcorneal electrical stimulation of retina to treat longstanding retinal artery occlusion. Graefe's Archive for Clinical and Experimental Ophthalmology. 2007;**245**:1773-1780

[89] Naycheva L, Schatz A, Willmann G, et al. Transcorneal electrical stimulation in patients with retinal artery occlusion: A prospective, randomized, sham-controlled pilot study. Ophthalmology and Therapy. 2013;**2**:25-39

[90] Oono S, Kurimoto T, Kashimoto R, et al. Transcorneal electrical stimulation improves visual function in eyes with branch retinal artery occlusion. Clinical Ophthalmology. 2011;**5**:397-402

[91] Gil-Carrasco F, Ochoa-Contreras D, Torres MA, et al. Transpalpebral electrical stimulation as a novel therapeutic approach to decrease intraocular pressure for open-angle glaucoma: A pilot study. Journal of Ophthalmology. 2018;**2018**:2930519

[92] Erb C, Eckert S, Gindorf P, et al. Electrical neurostimulation in glaucoma with progressive vision loss. Bioelectronic Medicine. 2022;**8**:6

[93] Kao YC, Liao YC, Cheng PL, Lee CH. Neurite regrowth stimulation by a red-light spot focused on the neuronal cell soma following blue light-induced retraction. Scientific Reports. 2019;**9**(1):18210

[94] Núñez-Álvarez C, Osborne NN. Blue light exacerbates and red light counteracts negative insults to retinal ganglion cells in situ and R28 cells in vitro. Neurochemistry International. 2019;**125**:187-196

[95] Osborne NN, Núñez-Álvarez C, Del Olmo-Aguado S, Merrayo-Lloves J.

Visual light effects on mitochondria: The potential implications in relation to glaucoma. Mitochondrion. 2017;**36**:29-35

[96] Beirne K, Freeman TJ, Rozanowska M, Votruba M. Red light irradiation in vivo upregulates DJ-1 in the retinal ganglion cell layer and protects against axotomy-related dendritic pruning. International Journal of Molecular Sciences. 2021;**22**(16):8380

[97] Del Olmo-Aguado1 S, Núñez-Álvarez C, Osborne NN. Red light of the visual spectrum attenuates cell death in culture and retinal ganglion cell death in situ. Acta Ophthalmologica. 2016;**94**(6):e481-e491

[98] Albarracin R, Valter K. 670 nm red light preconditioning supports Müller cell function: Evidence from the white light-induced damage model in the rat retina. Photochemistry and Photobiology. 2012;**88**(6):1418-1427

[99] Komáromy AM, Koehl KL, Park SA. Looking into the future: Gene and cell therapies for glaucoma. Veterinary Ophthalmology. 2021;**24**(Suppl. 1):16-33

[100] Johnson TV, Martin KR. Cell transplantation approaches to retinal ganglion cell neuroprotection in glaucoma. Current Opinion in Pharmacology. 2013;**13**:78-82

[101] Chamling X, Sluch SM, Zack DJ. The potential of human stem cells for the study and treatment of glaucoma. Investigative Ophthalmology & Visual Science. 2016;**57**:ORSFi1-ORSFi6

[102] Duebel J, Marazova K, Sahel JA. Optogenetics. Current Opinion in Ophthalmology. 2015;**26**(3):226-232

[103] Marc R, Pfeiffer R, Jones B. Retinal prosthetics, optogenetics, and chemical photoswitches. ACS Chemical Neuroscience. 2014;**5**(10):895-901

[104] Daeschler SC, Harhaus L, Schoenle P, et al. Ultrasound and shock-wave stimulation to promote axonal regeneration following nerve surgery: A systematic review and meta-analysis of preclinical studies. Scientific Reports. 2018;**8**(1):3168

[105] Haffey PR, Bansal N, Kaye E, et al. The regenerative potential of therapeutic ultrasound on neural tissue: A pragmatic review. Pain Medicine. 2020;**21**(7):1494-1506

Section 3

Diagnostics and Glaucoma

Chapter 4

Factors Affecting Intraocular Pressure Measurement and New Methods for Improving Accuracy: What Can IOP Tell Us about Glaucoma? How Can Practitioners Improve IOP Utility and Glaucoma Outcomes?

Sean J. McCafferty, Khin P. Kilgore and Jason M. Levine

Abstract

An increased awareness of how central corneal thickness (CCT) and corneal material properties such as corneal hysteresis has changed both tonometry accuracy and the resultant understanding of glaucoma risk. New research findings and methods of tonometry provide differing information on the diagnosis and treatment of ocular conditions which should be understood to appropriately incorporate this information into individual patient care. Additionally, a useful re-examination of what IOP can tell us about glaucoma empowers practitioners to improve glaucoma outcomes. All clinically utilized tonometry methods are estimates of true IOP, which is only assessed using direct intracameral techniques. Different described tonometry techniques are associated with their own overall bias and interpatient variability, due most typically to tissue biomechanics.

Keywords: intraocular pressure, glaucoma, IOP, tonometer, tonometry, Goldmann, corneal biomechanics, corneal hysteresis, correcting applanation tonometry, central corneal thickness

1. Introduction

Intraocular pressure (IOP) is mostly associated with the disease of Glaucoma, but it is arguably the second-most critical metric for assessing the overall ocular health of an individual next to visual acuity. Therefore, accurate and repeatable IOP measurements are necessary for the screening exams and adequate treatment of ocular disease. Accurate IOP measurement is not only essential to the accurate diagnoses, but it is also a necessary guide to effective treatment strategies. Glaucoma is a chronic and progressively debilitating disease requiring life-long monitoring and treatment.

This disease affects approximately 3.3 million Americans [1]. Glaucoma is now the leading cause of blindness in the aging Hispanic and African American populations, and several-fold more common in African Americans as in Caucasian Americans [2]. World-wide, there were an estimated 69 million people with glaucoma in 2020 [1]. Patients still go blind and suffer debilitating glaucomatous vision loss due to its mismanagement and misdiagnosis [3].

For more than 65 years, the clinical standard for IOP measurement has been Goldmann Applanation Tonometry (GAT) [4]. Several significant patient specific errors in the GAT IOP measurement have been identified and include: Corneal rigidity (±8 mmHg), corneal thickness (±7 mmHg), corneal curvature (±3 mmHg), and corneal tear film (±5 mmHg) [5–7]. The combination of these patient-variable errors may lead to an erroneous low IOP measurement and can be sight-threatening to a large population of patients.. The at-risk population includes glaucoma or undiagnosed ocular hypertension. Despite these known errors, currently GAT remains the standard-of-care. Despite GAT's numerous shortcomings, nothing had improved upon its inexpensive utility and accuracy. Limitations to GAT IOP were highlighted in the Ocular Hypertension Treatment Study (OHTS), which demonstrated that thicker cornea stand to be overestimate IOP, and thin corneas tend to be underestimated. This leads to a misdiagnosis of glaucoma [8]. Based upon the OHTS findings, the standard of practice has been modified to include a measurement of central corneal thickness (CCT) and many use a nomogram to correct the pressure for the CCT. Additionally, it is well-recognized that the effects of laser-assisted *in situ* keratomileusis (LASIK) surgery render accurate IOP measurement by the GAT inaccurate [9]. Attempts have been made to quantify the numerous GAT IOP errors and produce a corrected standard GAT measurement comparable between patients [10]. However, the corrections are cumbersome and prone their own error, leading to minimal clinical adoption, with the exception of CCT.

The Imbert-Fick principle assumes the cornea is an infinitely thin membrane which, by definition, has no rigidity, only strength in tension [5, 6]. CCT or corneal thickness in general, however, is a geometric quantity affecting the rigidity of the cornea [6]. The rigidity of the cornea is also affected by the corneal curvature. A steeply curved cornea must be bent more when applanated by the tonometer prism (**Figure 1**). The intrinsic material property of the cornea (the modulus of elasticity - both Young's and shear) also greatly affect the rigidity of the cornea [11, 12]. All of these rigidity-affecting components increase the force on the tonometer prism, which is erroneously attributed to intraocular pressure despite having no direct relation to IOP. Finally, the hydrostatic attraction created by the tear film was theorized to negate much of the rigidity error, but tear films are also highly variable among patients [13–15]. Intraocular pressure, with all presently utilized clinical methods of tonometry, is thus just an approximation of IOP with associated inter-patient biases due to biomechanical variability. Yet IOP is the leading risk factor for glaucomatous optic neuropathy (GON) progression and the only modifiable treatment parameter [16].

Given the numerous patient-dependent variables affecting GAT IOP, there is a common perception that IOP gives little information on glaucoma diagnosis and progression of GON. IOP has therefore been relegated to more of a supportive role in glaucoma diagnosis and treatment. We now rely more on optic nerve visualization, optical coherence tomography (OCT) and visual fields (VF) to diagnose glaucoma after the glaucomatous optic neuropathy (GON) has begun and adjust the IOP medically or surgically to prevent further GON. This process may take years to stabilize with IOP adjustments. Unfortunately, a significant minority continue to progress, which may be prevented with earlier treatment.

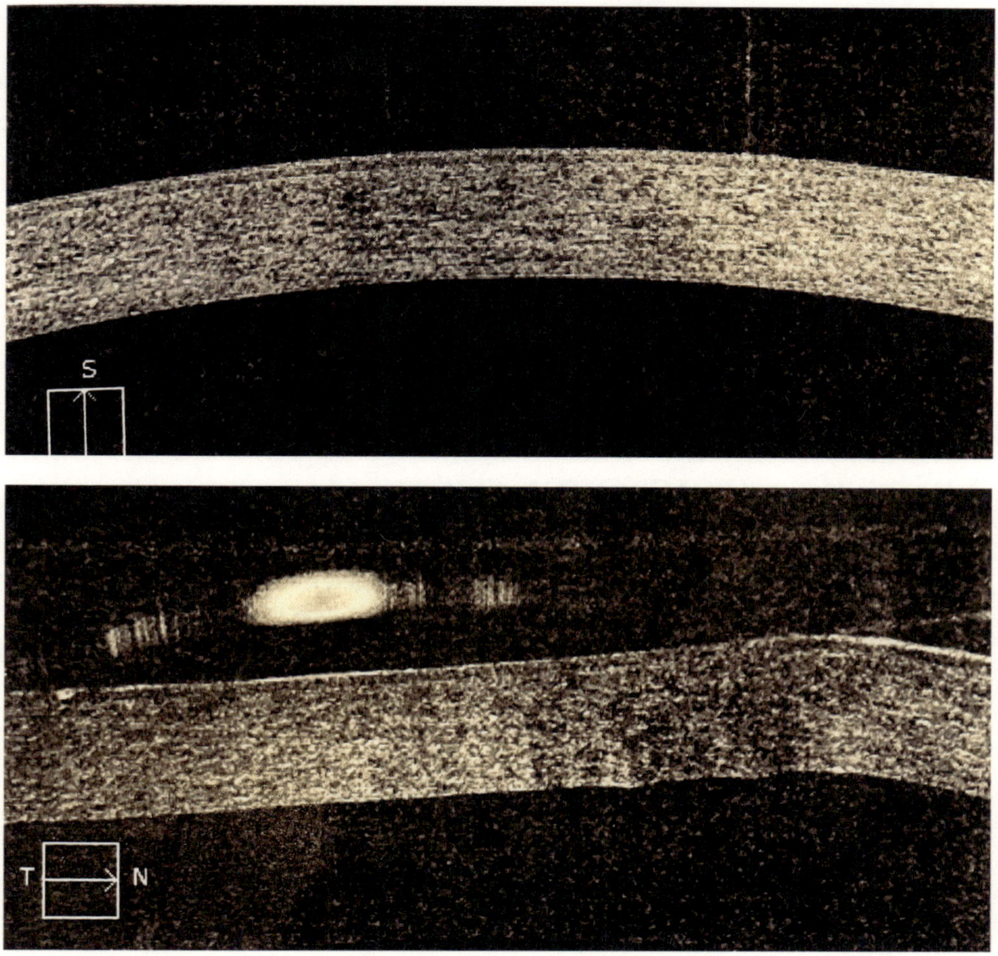

Figure 1.
Corneal OCT imaging before and during applanation demonstrating posterior lamellar corneal buckling.

So can IOP help us catch patients before they develop noticeable GON? The answer depends upon the question you ask.

2. Does my patient have ocular hypertension?

IOP is the only leading indicator of GON and is of primary importance in preventing GON before loss of the retinal nerve fiber layer (RNFL), as highlighted in the OHT study. Based on OHTS, most clinicians treat an IOP ≥26 mmHg as glaucoma even without evidence of GON due to the high probability of progression (2–36% progression depending upon CCT) [17]. This translates to a 1.2–8.1% chance of eventual functional vision loss with ocular hypertension (OHT) [16], leaving a significant portion of OHT patients who will never suffer vision loss from glaucoma (3–6 million in the US with OHT). An IOP cut-off alone may be a sensitive, but not a specific, early-detection system for GON, but designating an IOP = 26 mmHg to detect OHT produces a sensitivity and specificity which are by definition both 100% because the binary metric of disease presence (OHT) is an IOP value.

3. Does my patient have primary open angle or Normal tension Glaucoma?

Open angle glaucoma (OAG) includes primary open angle glaucoma (POAG) and normal tension glaucoma (NTG). POAG includes evidence of progressive GON with an untreated IOP ≥ 22 mmHg, while NTG requires IOP <22 mmHg untreated). Among NTG patients, IOP has been a fairly unreliable metric for predicting progressive GON, so we also examine OCT, VF, and visual optic nerve exam. In a recent study, currently pending publication, IOP sensitivity and specificity to progressive retinal nerve fiber layer (RNFL) loss was examined using the Receiver Operator Curve (ROC, **Figure 2**). The GAT prism IOP at 22 mmHg had a relatively low 70% sensitivity and 86% specificity.

4. Does my treated POAG or NTG patient require more aggressive treatment?

This is where the Goldmann IOP metric has traditionally done a poor job. Hence when a treated glaucoma patient asks, "How low does my pressure need to be?", the answer typically is, "Low enough so that the glaucoma doesn't progress". IOP's diagnostic

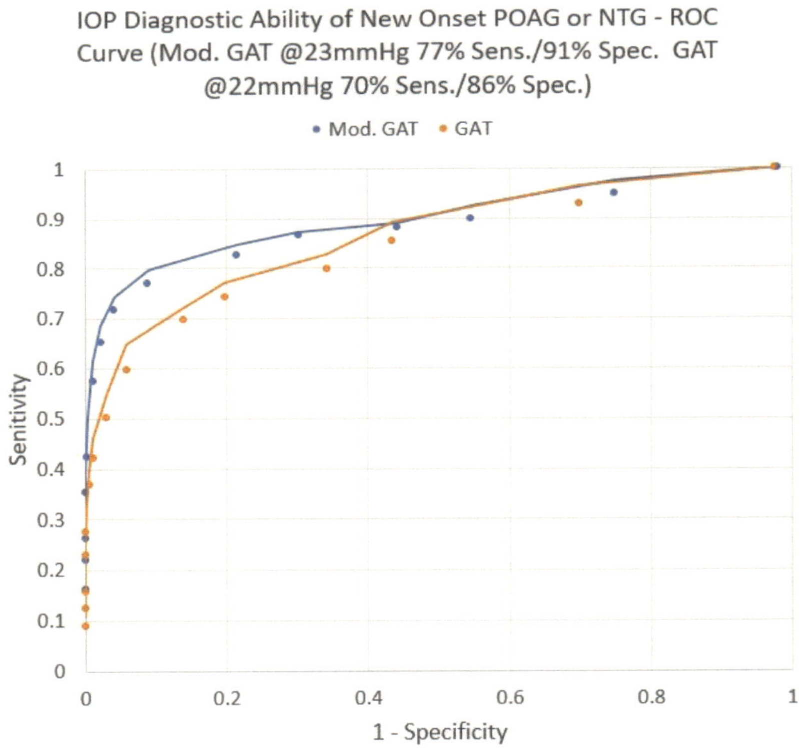

Figure 2.
Increased IOP sensitivity and specificity to RNFL loss progression in treated OAG eyes using a modified surface (mod.) GAT compared to GAT.

ability is illustrated by a near-linear ROC curve where there is an almost linear relationship between GAT IOP and progressive GON measured by RNFL loss. This means that there is no specific IOP where we could see a significant increase in the diagnostic ability of IOP, just that lower IOP is less likely to be associated with GON progression.

5. Tonometry affected by central corneal thickness, and corneal biomechanics

Studies have illustrated the effects of CCT on GAT in comparing trans-corneal applanation tonometry to intracameral transducer pressure, *in vivo*, in eyes undergoing cataract surgery [18, 19]. Both studies found the GAT IOP sensitivity to CCT was between ±4 and ± 7 mmHg per 100 μm deviation in CCT. It should be noted that typically older patients, who are more likely to undergo cataract surgery, have stiffer corneas than younger individuals. Stiffer corneas have been shown to have a significant correlation between CCT and GAT IOP error [5]. Nevertheless, CCT variations may lead to mischaracterization of patients in both ocular hypertension and normal-tension glaucoma [20, 21].

The Ocular Hypertension Treatment Study (OHTS) has illustrated the importance of CCT in glaucoma management. In the study, thinner corneas were noted in African-American patients [16, 22]. The European Glaucoma Prevention Study (EGPS) has confirmed these findings and both studies describe CCT as a major risk factor for glaucoma [23, 24]. However, the application of correction factors to GAT measured IOP did not improve its prediction of GON [25]. These findings indicate that patients may have a glaucoma risk mischaracterization due to GAT IOP error. However, CCT alone is insufficient to quantify a corrected IOP due to its dependence on several other corneal biomechanical factors such as corneal rigidity, which eclipse the effect of corneal thickness.

The lamellar cornea is bio-mechanically complex behaving unlike a simple plastic material. The modulus of elasticity of the cornea is an intrinsic measure of corneal rigidity, likely having a greater effect in GAT IOP measurement error than the geometric factor of CCT [5]. The values of the modulus of elasticity for the cornea vary considerably from 0.01 to 10 MPa [26, 27]. Generally, the cornea stiffens as it ages, with the presence of corneal disease, corneal surgery and glaucoma treatment.

With corneal hysteresis (CH), it is important to distinguish viscoelasticity from simply elasticity. The spring constant elastic response of the cornea is a static component, whereas hysteresis measuring the viscoelastic component is time-dependent. Presently, there is no commercially available technology to measure corneal elasticity in the clinic although a corneal indentation device (CID) may soon be in the market [28].

Differential tonometry is the use of sequential IOP measurement of an eye using of two different tonometers. This method has been described in studies to measure changes in corneal elasticity [28–30]. Recently, pre-approval studies using the corneal indentation device (CID) demonstrated measurement of a corneal tangent modulus by determining the slope of the force displacement curve [31, 32]. Studies, including intracameral pressure comparisons, have shown a modified Goldmann prism (CATS prism) to have a significantly decreased sensitivity to corneal biomechanical properties compared to the GAT prism [13, 19, 33–36]. IOP differences between CATS and GAT IOP measurements were strongly correlated with variations in CCT and CH [33–35]. Both prisms measure the same IOP in corneas with average properties, therefore, the difference in CATS and GAT IOP ($IOP_{CATS\text{-}GAT}$) measures those combined corneal biomechanical properties resisting its applanation [33, 34]. Significantly increased and sustained differential IOP was demonstrated following corneal cross linking (CXL) for early progressive keratoconus [37]. $IOP_{CATS-GAT}$ measures corneal biomechanical changes due to procedures similar to CXL. Likewise, differential tonometry demonstrated increased $IOP_{CATS-GAT}$ when using a prostaglandin analog glaucoma treatment, latanoprost 0.005% [38]. Prostaglandin analogs were shown to decrease corneal elasticity (**Figure 3**). No differential IOP changes were demonstrated with the use of timolol 0.5%, indicating that timolol does not affect corneal biomechanics [38].

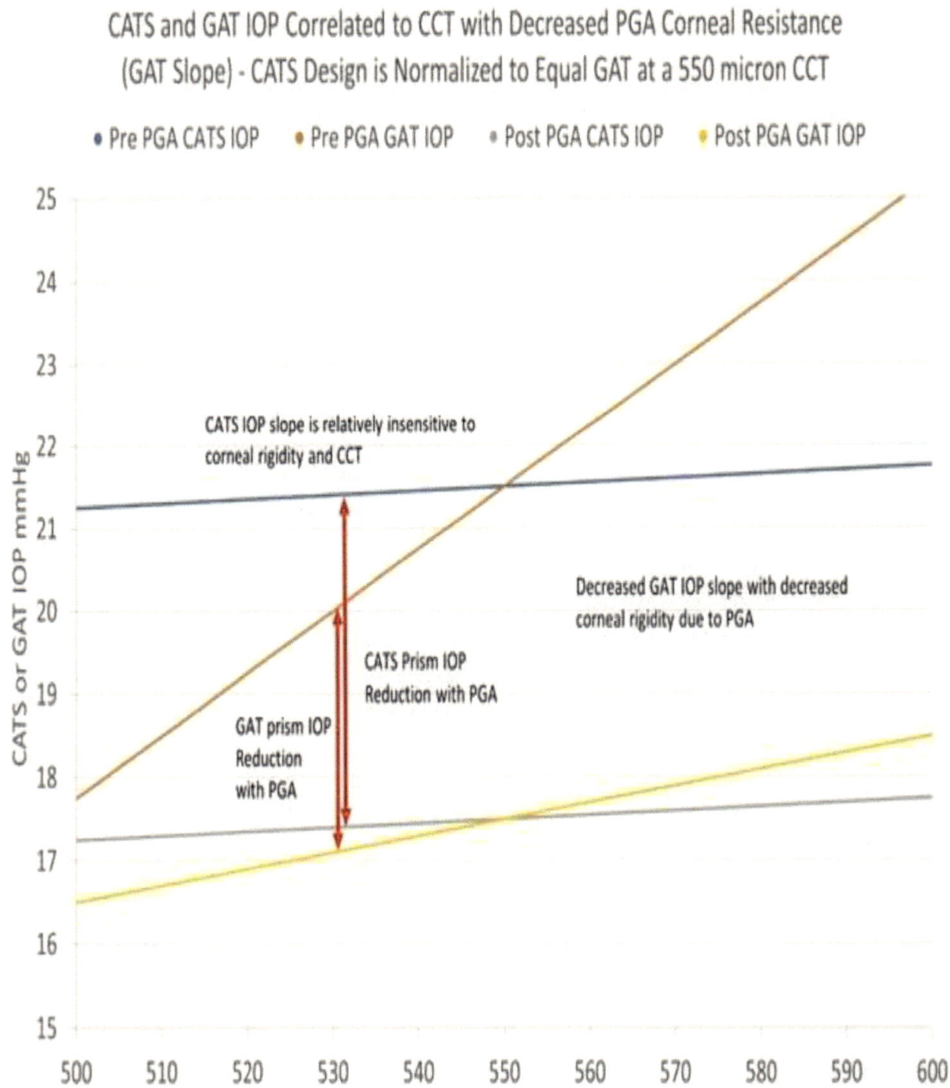

Figure 3.
Applanation IOP vs. CCT for variations in corneal rigidity before and after institution of PGA use.

The Ocular Response Analyzer (ORA) is able to measure corneal viscoelasticity. The ORA outputs the parameters Goldmann correlated IOPg, corneal hysteresis (CH), and a corneal corrected IOPcc. The CH and IOPcc parameters are viscoelastic and can be interpreted as strict elasticity only under very narrow critically damped dynamic applanating circumstances. Therefore, a cornea with a low hysteresis will generally have a lower elasticity, but the opposite may also be true. A pediatric cornea is a clinically relevant counter intuitive example in which it has a higher hysteresis but is obviously less rigid than an adult cornea. Therefore, it is inaccurate to always interpret low hysteresis as low elasticity.

6. Refractive and corneal surgery effect of tonometry

Intraocular pressure accuracy is a common concern to the practitioner following corneal refractive procedures and keratoplasty. Corneal refractive procedures adjust the CCT, CH, and modulus of elasticity, which may have a significant effect on IOP error. Studies have shown a GAT-measured IOP reduction following myopic LASIK or other corneal refractive surgery [4–41]. However, other refractive procedures and other methods of IOP measurement have indicated a large variation in IOP measurement, even some with an increase in GAT-measured IOP. Other corneal procedures such as radial keratotomy, small incision lenticule extraction (SMILE), and keratoplasty (endothelial, lamellar, or full-thickness) can also make the assessment of IOP very difficult. In the case of myopic LASIK, the IOP reduction can be explained using current models (**Figure 4**) as the reduction in GAT-measured IOP is a function of reduced CCT and a decreased corneal elastic modulus. The present model described below would predict a lower post-LASIK GAT IOP by a leftward shift in **Figure 4**

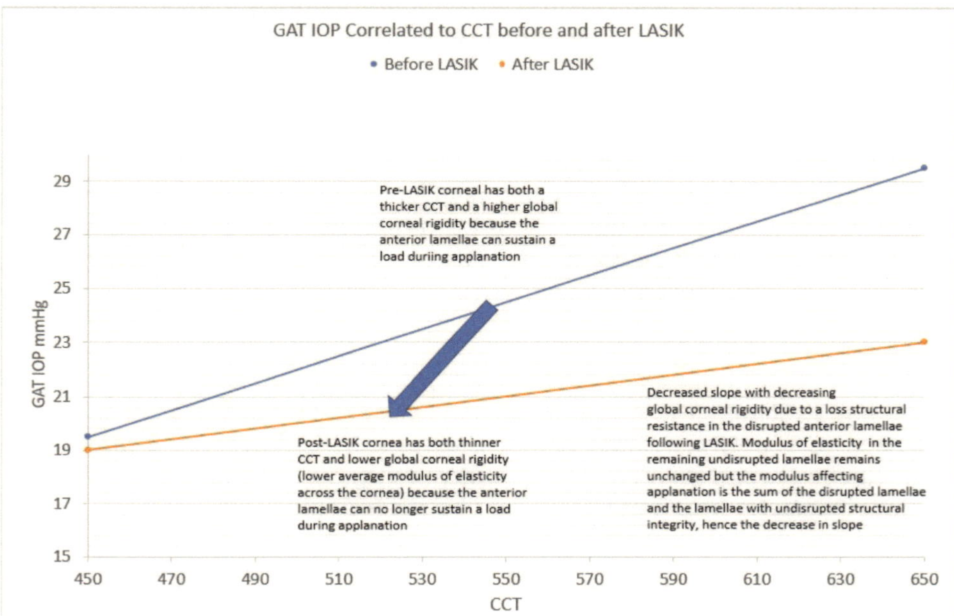

Figure 4.
GAT IOP curves before and after myopic LASIK, correlated to CCT and corneal elasticity.

with reduced CCT and flatter elastic modulus curve. The LASIK corneal flap makes negligible contribution to the corneal resistance during applanation in the post-LASIK cornea [40]. However, procedures such as radial keratotomy and keratoplasty may behave in a very different manner. The relationship of corneal elasticity and CCT generally obeys the model, but the level to which the factors contribute to IOP error is largely unknown and will require more study to understand.

7. IOP measurement comparison to true intracameral pressure

All presently utilized clinical methods of measuring IOP are compared and tested against Goldmann (GAT). Therefore, any inherent bias in IOP from intracameral pressure will be carried through all present clinical measurement techniques. Goldmann applanation tonometry underestimates true intracameral IOP by about 5 mmHg [18, 42]. Any IOP measurement technique which is calibrated to true intracameral pressure must then contend with the clinician adoption problem resetting long historic benchmarks of IOP such as 21 mmHg being the upper end of normal [42].

7.1 New methods to clinically measure IOP

The scope of this chapter includes a review of major new tonometry techniques, including GAT. The only innovation to the Goldmann tonometer design is the Correcting Applanation Tonometry Surface (CATS) prism modification, which incorporates an applanating surface conforming to the cornea. The CATS modified prism has demonstrated decreased sensitivity to variation in CCT and has shown decreased sensitivity to corneal rigidity and tear-film errors seen with GAT [36]. The TonoPen and noncontact tonometry (NCT) such as ORA both applanate the central cornea to estimate IOP. A rebound tonometer measures IOP based upon the velocity of a probe rebounding off of the cornea and a home version of it has the advantage of measuring daily variations in IOP. A Corvis ST non-contact high speed Scheimpflug camera visualizes corneal deformation during air-pulse deformation. Both surface continuous contact lens and implanted tonometers have the advantage of continuous IOP monitoring and diurnal variation. Other tools include transpalpebral IOP measurement and an older method, pneumotonometry. Each of these IOP measurement techniques has its advantages and disadvantages in terms of usability, complexity, patient acceptance, and accuracy. All are affected, to some degree, by variations in corneal biomechanical properties, including CCT.

7.2 Goldmann GAT/CATS

The gold standard for IOP measurement remains Goldmann Applanation Tonometry (GAT) [4]. Goldmann IOP measurements errors have been demonstrated as a result of corneal biomechanical variability [5–10]. Clinical correction of GAT for CCT is an incomplete correction of GAT errors and has limited utility [25].

A modified curved Correcting Applanation Tonometry Surface (CATS) prism (CATS Tonometer, Tucson, AZ) has been FDA approved as a replacement prism to the standard flat surfaced prism. The CATS prism technology is the only clinical measurement to challenge the standard-of-care GAT legacy, available in both reusable and sterile single-use variations, depending upon clinical preferences. The CATS prism design differences include a centrally concave and annularly convex applanating surface. **Figure 5** depicts the applanating surface of the CATS prism. The prism has clinically demonstrated decreased sensitivity to CCT and CH when compared to the GAT prism, including comparisons to *in vivo* intracameral pressure [13, 19, 33–36]. The CATS prism applanating shape is a unique mathematical solution to a matrix which incorporates the probability distributions of: Elastic modulus, Corneal Thickness, and Corneal curvature. The solution's shape simultaneously minimizes its sensitivity to all three of the corneal variables [36]. Intraocular pressure differences in CATS and GAT IOP measurements significantly correlated with clinical variations in CH and CCT [33, 34]. Simultaneously, the CATS prism outer annular curvature away from the corneal surface minimizes the effect of the tear-film adhesion error inherent in GAT [35]. Furthermore, the applanation area of the CATS prism was designed and tested so that there is no overall IOP bias between the two prisms over a large standard population retaining historical IOP benchmarks [33, 34]. Future considerations of the CATS prism's improved accuracy utilizing the surface design are under development to be incorporated into the Tonopen design and Pachymeter designs.

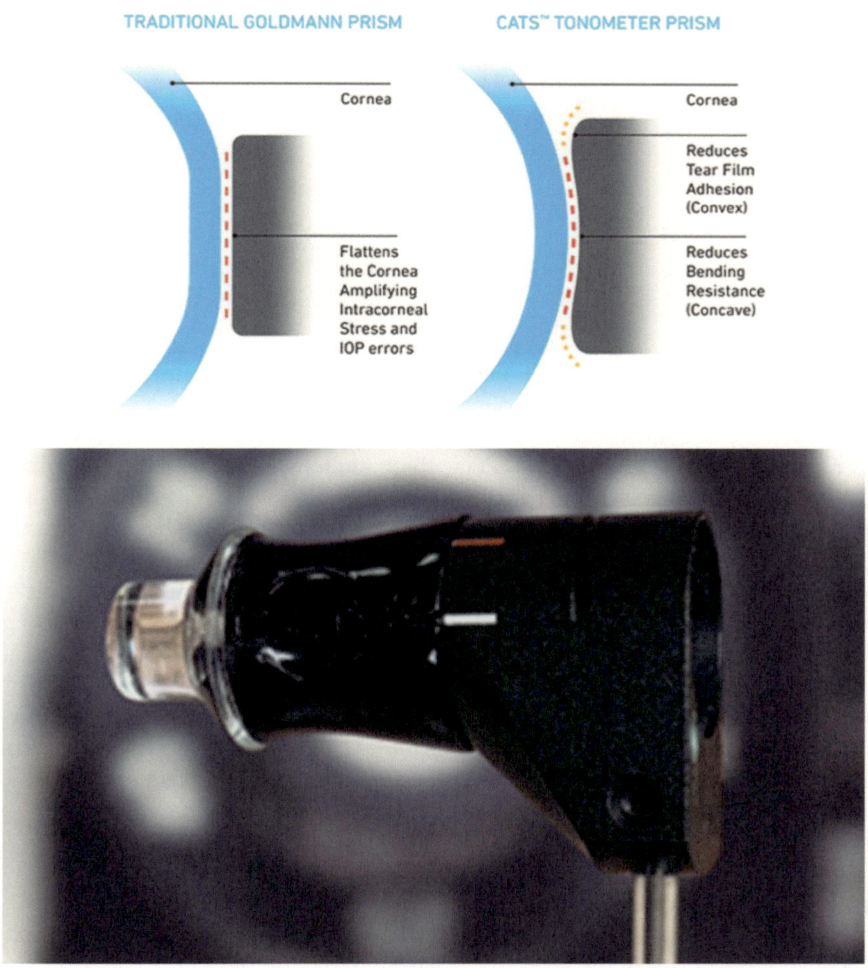

Figure 5.
CATS prism in comparison to the legacy flat Goldmann prism.

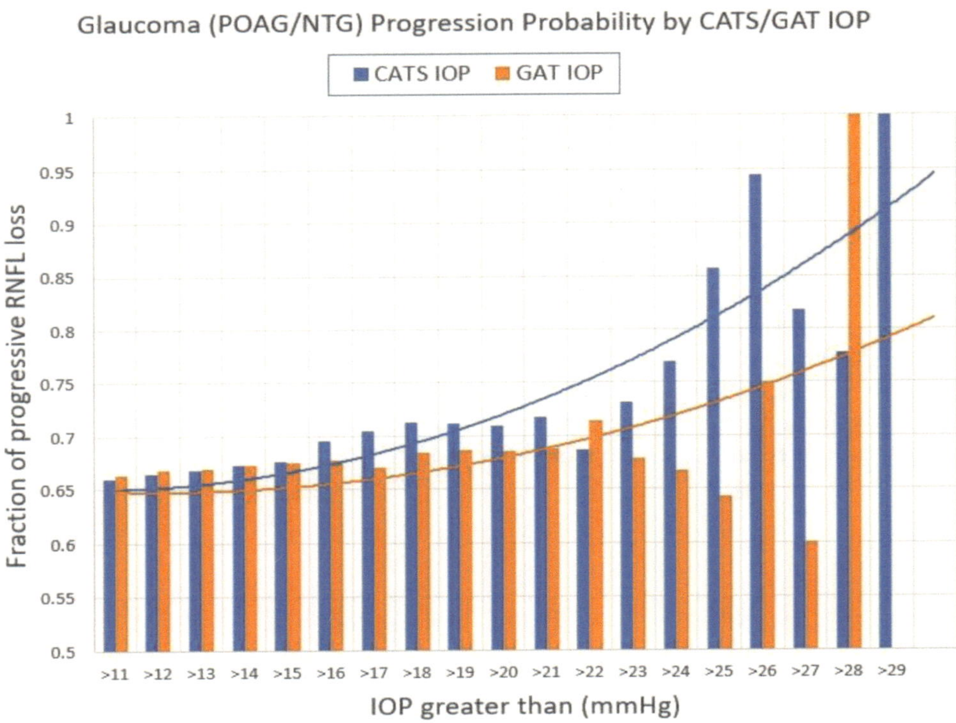

Figure 6.
CATS prism more sensitive than GAT prism to OAG progression, as indicated by continued RNFL loss, above all specified average IOP levels.

Anin-publication Retinal Nerve Fiber Layer (RNFL) progression study was completed examining 1741 eyes on 954 patients with 164 Normal eyes (N), 502 glaucoma suspect (GS), 490 ocular hypertension, 491 primary open angle glaucoma (POAG), and 89 normal tension glaucoma (NTG) in which sequential IOP using a CATS prism and GAT prism was collected along with OCT data over an average of 2.8 years with 3.9 average OCT visits. CATS and GAT IOP measurements are shown to have no significant difference in IOP measurement among normal (N) patients [33]. However, the CATS Tonometer prism picks up an additional 143/490 or 29% more OHT patients translating to 0.875–1.75 million more people in the US being re-classified as OHT. **Figure 6** depicts the fraction of POAG and NTG patients with progressive RNFL loss above the specified IOP levels. The interesting finding of the relationship is two-fold. First, the majority of OAG patients tend to progress despite diligent care. This suggests we generally need earlier and more aggressive treatment for this long-term chronic disease. Second, the CATS prism is significantly more sensitive as a screening tool to predict continued RNFL loss in treated OAG.

8. Ocular response analyzer

The Ocular Response Analyzer (ORA) (Reichert Technologies, Buffalo, NY) senses a reflected infrared signal from the cornea measuring two corneal flattening times during and following the air-impulse. A P1 measurement is made during the air-pulse inward

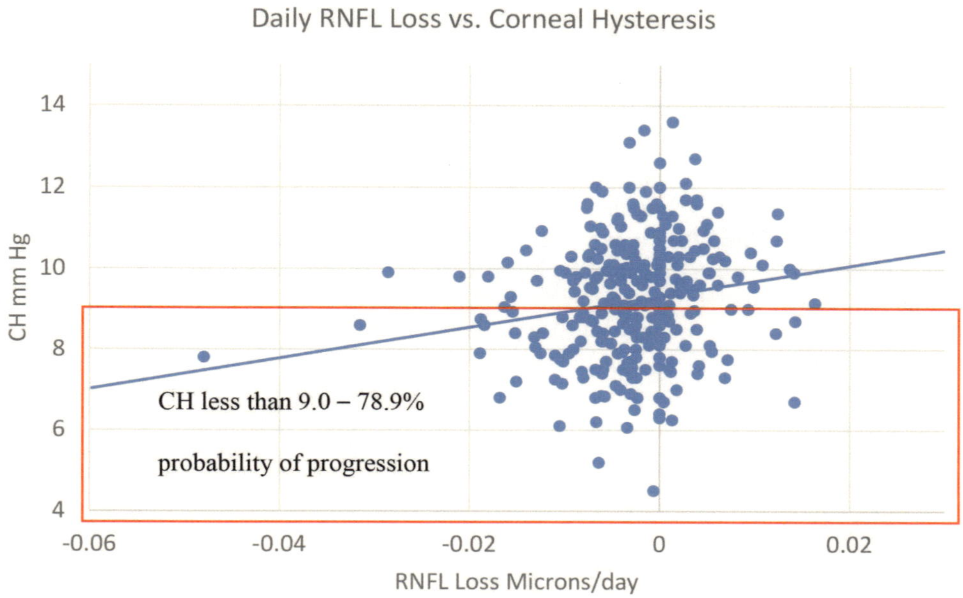

Figure 7.
Lower corneal hysteresis in treated OAG patients associated with increased RNFL loss when CH < 9.0 mmHg.

deformation and a P2 measurement is recorded upon the outward rebound of the cornea returning to its undeformed state. The ORA can measure two corneal mechanical properties: Corneal Hysteresis (CH) and the Corneal Resistance Factor (CRF). Both describe the cornea's viscoelastic properties. Corneal Hysteresis is calculated by the timing difference between P1 and P2. CRF uses an empirical modification of the difference between P1 and P2 [43]. The ORA is designed to measure the dampening constant in an dynamically pulsed system which is hysteresis, but it also utilizes this information to produce an IOP which is significantly independent of the cornea, a corneal corrected IOP (IOPcc). The IOPcc is less affected by corneal thickness and altered biomechanical properties typically seen with LASIK and other corneal surgeries [40, 44].

Corneal hysteresis (CH) represents corneal viscoelastic damping of tissue and is generally not to be interpreted as corneal elasticity. Interpretation of generally high and low CH is clinically important for the management of glaucoma. It has been demonstrated that low CH is significantly associated with an increased risk of glaucomatous progression [45, 46]. Low CCT and low CH are also associated with increased severity of glaucomatous damage in advancing visual field loss [45]. An ongoing longitudinal study of RNFL progression in treated OAG patients found that at CH <9.0 mmHg, there is a 78.9% probability of progression POAG (**Figure** 7).

9. Scheimpflug

More recently, a new technology has been available, which provides an analysis of corneal biomechanics and quantifies the corneal biomechanical profile. The Corvis ST (OCULUS Optikgeräte GmbH, Wetzlar, Germany) is an air-impulse tonometer, which produces a corneal-corrected IOP measurement designed to exclude cornea biomechanical-associated influences, but they also enable the measurement of multiple corneal parameters, for an *in vivo* biomechanical corneal assessment.

The high-speed Scheimpflug Corvis ST technology allows air-impulse deformation corneal imaging of a corneal cross-section. This imaging allows for characterization of the corneal deformation. The Corvis ST is additionally able to measure whole-eye motion along with numerous metrics derived from corneal imaging, including the corneal biomechanical index (CBI) and the tomographic biomechanical index (TBI). The CBI incorporates the corneal pachymetry with the corneal deformation parameters. This CBI has shown a high sensitivity and specificity in detecting keratoconus [47]. The TBI is a composite derived metric generated using Corvis ST parameters and the imaged tomography. Furthermore, the Corvis ST produces a biomechanically correct IOP similar to the ORA (bIOP). Additionally, a stress–strain index (SSI) generates a corneal rigidity parameter using the bIOP. The SSI constructs a deformation stress–strain curve based on imaging and infers a measure of the cornea's intrinsic elastic modulus. A corneal stiffness parameter (SP-A1) is generated by ratio of the loading pressure to the corneal displacement at the time of first applanation. This higher SP-A1 metric has been associated with a stiffer cornea following corneal cross-linking [48].

10. Dynamic contour tonometry

Dynamic contour tonometry (DCT), which is no longer commercially available, may be found as the PASCAL tonometer (Ziemer Ophthalmic Systems Group Co., Port, Switzerland). It is a slit lamp mounted tonometer, which is not significantly influenced by CCT [49]. The PASCAL tonometer also allows simultaneous measurement of the Ocular Pulse Amplitude (OPA), an indirect measure of choroidal perfusion and ocular blood flow.

11. Rebound tonometry

Rebound tonometers are a device which measures the rebound velocity of rounded-tip metallic probe projected toward and bounced off the cornea using a solenoid. IOP is measured using the hand-held device balanced on the patient's forehead. The practitioner actuates the tonometer projecting the probe which must be perpendicular to, and in the center of, the cornea. The return velocity is correlated to GAT IOP measurement. The return velocity, eloquently measured by the solenoid produced current, is microprocessor correlated to GAT IOP. A slow velocity correlates to a low IOP and a high velocity to a high IOP. These measurements are influenced by CH and CCT [50]. The advantages of the rebound tonometer, currently marketed as I-Care, are its portability and lack of need for topical anesthetic, making it suitable for pediatric IOP measurement. Additionally, I-Care has a home use version of the tonometer to better understand variations in IOP. The I-Care was found to have a good correlation applanation tonometry in myopic children [51].

12. Contact Lens transducer

24-hour IOP monitoring measuring the circadian pattern and short-term variations of IOP is valuable to the glaucoma specialist. Spikes and IOP variations have been linked to glaucoma progression measured by progressive visual field loss [52]. In addition to the I-Care Home measurement device, Sensimed (Switzerland) has developed a contact lens sensor (TriggerFISH), which provides continuous IOP monitoring. The device has similar drawback to contact lens wear on an extended basis.

13. Transducer implant

A German company (Implandata Ophthalmic Products, Germany) has developed a permanent intraocular implant for continuous IOP monitoring. This device is currently undergoing human clinical trials and incorporates a wireless transducer measure pressure sensor, which sends a signal to the telemetry unit. In vitro studies demonstrate tolerance and biocompatibility in animal models for up to 25 months [53]. The ARGOS study implanted the Eyemate continuous IOP measurement transducer into the sulcus after cataract surgery in patients with normal-tension glaucoma and primary open-angle glaucoma, and found that all patients had controlled glaucoma without complications [54]. The obvious distinct advantage of this method is that its IOP measurement technique is direct without inference through the cornea or other tissues.

Intraocular pressure remains a critical measure of ocular health and even after over half a century Goldmann remains the standard of care. Newer methods of IOP measurement have clinical advantages and are suitable for many situations. Even the long standing Goldmann may be supplanted for other methods with superior accuracy [19, 54–60].

Disclosure

The Authors have the following disclosures: Sean McCafferty; equity holder in CATS Tonometer. Khin Kilgore; none. Jason Levine; none.

Author details

Sean J. McCafferty[1,2,3*], Khin P. Kilgore[1] and Jason M. Levine[1,3]

1 Arizona Eye Consultants, Tucson, Arizona, USA

2 University of Arizona College of Optical Science, Tucson, Arizona, USA

3 University of Arizona College of Medicine, Tucson, Arizona, USA

*Address all correspondence to: sjmccaff@intuortec.com

References

[1] Quigley H, Broman T. The number of people with glaucoma worldwide in 2010 and 2020. The British Journal of Ophthalmology. 2006;**90**:262-267. DOI: 10.1136/bjo.2005.081224

[2] Friedman D, Roger W, O'Colmain B, Klein, Taylor H, West S, et al. Prevalence of open-angle glaucoma among adults in the United States. Archives of Ophthalmology. 2004;**122**:532-538

[3] Susanna R Jr, De Moraes CG, Cioffi GA, Ritch R. Why do people (still) go blind from glaucoma? Translational Vision Science & Technology. 2015;**4**(2):1

[4] Goldmann H, Schmidt T. Uber Applanationstonometrie. Ophthalmologica. 1957;**134**:221

[5] Liu J, Roberts CJ. Influence of cornea biomechanical properties on intraocular pressure measurement: Quantitative analysis. Journal of Cataract and Refractive Surgery. 2005;**31**:146-155. DOI: 10.1016/j.jcrs.2004.09.031

[6] Kotecha A, Elsheikh A, Roberts C, Haogang Z, Garway-Heath D. Corneal thickness- and age related biomechanical properties of the cornea measured with the ocular response analyzer. Investigative Ophthalmology & Visual Science. 2006;**47**(12):5337-5347

[7] Whitacre M, Stein R. Sources of error with use of Goldmann-type tonometers. Survey of Ophthalmology. 2002;**38**(1):1-30

[8] Kass M, Heuer D, Higginbotham E, Johnson C, Keltner J, Miller J, et al. The ocular hypertension treatment study: A randomized trial determines that topical ocular hypotensive medication delays or prevents the onset of primary open-angle glaucoma. Archives of Ophthalmology. 2002;**120**(6):701-713

[9] Pepose J, Feigenbaum S, Qazi M. Changes in corneal biomechanics and intraocular pressure following LASIK using static, dynamic, and non-contact tonometry. American Journal of Ophthalmology. 2007;**143**:39-47

[10] Elsheikh A, Alhasso D, Gunvant P, Garway-Heath D. Multiparameter correction equation for Goldmann applanation tonometry. Optometry and Vision Science. 2011;**88**(1):E102-E112. DOI: 1040-5488/11/8801-0102/0

[11] Neuburger M, Maier P, Böhringer D, Reinhard T, Jordan JF. The impact of corneal edema on intraocular pressure measurements using goldmann applanation tonometry, Tono-pen XL, iCare, and ORA: An in vitro model. Journal of Glaucoma. 2013;**22**(7):584-590. DOI: 10.1097/IJG.0b013e31824cef11

[12] Orssengo G, Pye D. Determination of the true intraocular pressure and modulus of elasticity of the human cornea in vivo. Bulletin of Mathematical Biology. 1999;**61**(3):551-572

[13] McCafferty SJ, Enikov ET, Schwiegerling J, Ashley SM. Goldmann tonometry tear film error and partial correction with a shaped applanation surface. Clinical Ophthalmology. 2018;**12**:71-78

[14] Tselishchev Y, Val'tsifer V. Influence of the type of contact between particles joined by a liquid bridge on the capillary cohesive forces. Colloid Journal. 2003;**65**(3):385-389 5p

[15] Orr F, Scriven L, Rivas A. Pendular rings between solids: Meniscus properties

and capillary force. Journal of Fluid Mechanics. 1975;**67**(part 4):723-742

[16] Gordon M, Beiser J, Brandt J, et al. The ocular hypertension treatment study: Baseline factors that predict the onset of primary open angle Glaucoma. Archives of Ophthalmology. 2002;**120**:714-720

[17] Kass M, Heuer D, Higginbotham E, et al. The ocular hypertension treatment study: A randomized trial determines that ocular topical hypotensive medication delays or prevents the onset of primary open-angle Glaucoma. Archives of Ophthalmology. 2002;**120**:701-713

[18] Feltgen N, Leifert D, Funk J. Correlation between central corneal thickness, applanation tonometry, and direct intracameral IOP readings. The British Journal of Ophthalmology. 2001;**85**:85-87

[19] McCafferty S, Levine J, Schwiegerling J, et al. Goldmann and error correcting tonometry prisms compared to intracameral pressure. BMC Ophthalmology. 2018;**18**:2

[20] Copt RP, Thomas R, Mermoud A. Corneal thickness in ocular hypertension, primary open-angle glaucoma, and normal tension glaucoma. Archives of Ophthalmology. 1999;**117**:14-16

[21] Ehlers N, Hansen FK. Central corneal thickness in low-tension glaucoma. Acta Ophthalmologica. 1974;**52**:740-746

[22] Brandt JD, Beiser JA, Kass MA, et al. Central corneal thickness in the ocular hypertension treatment study (OHTS). Ophthalmology. 2001;**108**:1779-1788

[23] Miglior S, Pfeiffer N, et al. Predictive factors for open-angle glaucoma among patients with ocular hypertension in the European Glaucoma prevention study. Ophthalmology. 2007;**114**:3-9

[24] Pfeiffer N, Torri V, et al. Central corneal thickness in the European Glaucoma prevention study. Ophthalmology. 2007;**114**:454-459

[25] Brandt JD, Gordon MO, Gao F, et al. Adjusting intraocular pressure for central corneal thickness does not improve prediction models for primary open-angle glaucoma. Ophthalmology. 2012;**119**:437-442

[26] Schwartz NJ, Mackay RS, Sackman JL. A theoretical and experimental study of the mechanical behavior of the cornea with application to the measurement of the intraocular pressure. Bulletin of Mathematical Biology. 1966;**28**:585-643

[27] Jue B, Maurice DM. The mechanical properties of the rabbit and human cornea. Journal of Biomechanics. 1986;**19**:847-853

[28] Schneider E, Grehn F. Intraocular pressure measurement-comparison of dynamic contour tonometry and Goldmann Applanation tonometry. Journal of Glaucoma. 2006;**15**:2-6

[29] Detorakis E, Tsaglioti E, Kymionis G. Non-invasive ocular rigidity measurement: A differential tonometry approach. Acta Medica. 2015;**58**:92-97

[30] Moiseeva I, Stein A, Lyubimov G. Estimating the elastic properties of the eye from differential tonometry by the Schiøtz tonometer: Analysis of the measurement procedure on the basis of a two-component mathematical model. Biophysics. 2016;**61**:1011-1018

[31] Lu SH, Chong IT, Leung SYY, Lam DCC. Characterization of corneal biomechanical properties and determination of natural intraocular pressure using CID-GAT. Translational Vision Science & Technology. 2019;**8**: 1011

[32] Hon Y, Chen G, Lu S, Lam D, Lam A. In vivo measurement of regional corneal tangent modulus eye. Scientific Reports. 2017;7:14974

[33] McCafferty S, Tetrault K, McColgin A, Chue W, Levine J, Muller M. Intraocular pressure measurement accuracy and repeatability of a modified Goldmann prism: Multi-center randomized clinical trial. American Journal of Ophthalmology. 2018;**196**:145-153

[34] McCafferty S, Tetrault K, McColgin A, Chue W, Levine J, Muller M. Modified Goldmann prism intraocular pressure measurement accuracy and correlation to corneal biomechanical metrics: Multicentre randomised clinical trial. British Journal of Ophthalmology. 2019;**0**:1-5

[35] McCafferty S, Enikov E, Schwiegerling J, Ashley S. Goldmann tonometry tear-film error and partial correction with a shaped applanation surface. Clinical Ophthalmology. 2018;**1**:5

[36] McCafferty S, Lim G, Duncan W, Enikov E, Schwiegerling J. Goldmann tonometer prism with an optimized error correcting Applanation surface. Translational Vision Science & Technology. 2016;**5**:1-5

[37] Wang M, Berdahl J, McCafferty S. Cornealcrosslinkingbiomechanicsevaluated by a novel and easily implemented differential tonometry method. Current Eye Research. 2021;**46**:1614-1620

[38] Radcliffe N, Berdahl J, Ibach M, Schweitzer J, Levine J, McCafferty S. Improved efficacy of topical Latanoprost 0.005% demonstrated by corneal biomechanical correcting modified Goldmann prism. Clinical Ophthalmology. 2020;**14**:2245-2253

[39] Chang DH, Stulting RD. Change in intraocular pressure measurements after LASIK: The effect of the refractive correction and the lamellar flap. Ophthalmology. 2005;**112**:1009-1016

[40] Pepose JS, Feigenbaum SK, Qazi MA, et al. Changes in corneal biomechanics and intraocular pressure following LASIK using static, dynamic, and noncontact tonometry. American Journal of Ophthalmology. 2007;**143**:39-47

[41] Song J, Lee Y, Kim J, Lee E, Kim H. Association between corneal refractive surgery and the prevalence of glaucoma: Korea National Health and nutrition examination survey 2010-2012. The British Journal of Ophthalmology. 2022;**106**:172-176

[42] McCafferty S, Levine J, Schwiegerling J, et al. Goldmann applanation tonometry error relative to true intracameral intraocular pressure in vitro and in vivo. BMC Ophthalmology. 2017;**17**:215

[43] Dupps WJ. Hysteresis: New mechanospeak for the ophthalmologist. Journal of Cataract and Refractive Surgery. 2007;**33**(9):1499-1501

[44] Luce DA. Determining in vivo biomechanical properties of the cornea with an ocular 964 response analyzer. Journal of Cataract and Refractive Surgery. 2005;**31**(1):156-162

[45] Medeiros FA, Meira-Freitas D, Lisboa R, Kuang TM, Zangwill LM, Weinreb RN. Corneal hysteresis as a risk factor for glaucoma progression: A prospective longitudinal study. Ophthalmology. 2013;**120**(8):1533-1540

[46] Zhang C, Tatham A, Abe R, et al. Corneal hysteresis and progressive retinal nerve fiber layer loss in glaucoma. American Journal of Ophthalmology. 2016;**166**:29-36

[47] Herber R, Ramm L, Spoerl E, et al. Assessment of corneal biomechanical parameters in healthy and keratoconic eyes using dynamic bidirectional applanation device and dynamic Scheimpflug analyzer. Journal of Cataract and Refractive Surgery. 2019;**45**(6):778-788

[48] Hashemi H, Ambrósio R, Vinciguerra R, et al. Two-year changes in corneal stiffness parameters after accelerated corneal cross-linking. Journal of Biomechanics. 2019;**93**:209-212

[49] Kaufmann C, Bachmann LM, Thiel MA. Comparison of dynamic contour tonometry with 912 Goldmann Applanation tonometry. Investigative Ophthalmology & Visual Science. 2004;**45**(9):3118

[50] Chui W, Lam A, Chen D, et al. The influence of corneal properties on rebound tonometry. Ophthalmology. 2008;**115**(1):80-84

[51] Weng J, Tsai I-L, Kuo L-L, et al. Intraocular pressure monitoring by rebound tonometry in children with myopia. Taiwan Journal of Ophthalmology. 2017;**7**(3):149

[52] Zeimer RC, Wilensky JT, Gieser DK. Presence and rapid decline of early morning intraocular pressure peaks in Glaucoma patients. Ophthalmology. 1990;**97**(5):547-550

[53] Todani A, Behlau I, Fava MA, et al. Intraocular pressure measurement by radio wave telemetry. Investigative Ophthalmology & Visual Science. 2011;**52**(13):9573

[54] Koutsonas A, Walter P, Roessler G, Plange N. Implantation of a novel telemetric intraocular pressure sensor in patients with Glaucoma (ARGOS study): 1-year results. Investigative Ophthalmology & Visual Science. 2015;**56**(2):1063-1069

[55] Ruland K, Olayanju J, Borras T, Grewal DS, Fleischman D. Accuracy of Tonopen versus iCare in human cadaveric eyes with Edematous corneas over a wide range of intraocular pressures. Journal of Glaucoma. 2019;**28**:e82-e85

[56] Termühlen J, Mihailovic N, Alnawaiseh M, Dietlein TS, Rosentreter A. Accuracy of measurements with the iCare HOME rebound tonometer. Journal of Glaucoma. 2016;**25**(6):533-538

[57] Stoor K, Karvonen E, Ohtonen P, Liinamaa MJ, Saarela V. Icare versus Goldmann in a randomised middle-aged population : The influence of central corneal thickness and refractive errors. European Journal of Ophthalmology. 2021;**3**:1231-1239

[58] Prabhakar SK, Mahesh BS, Shanthamallappa M. A comparative study of intraocular pressure measurement by three tonometers in normal subjects. Nepalese Journal of Ophthalmology. 2013;**5**(2):201-206

[59] Bao F, Huang W, Zhu R, et al. Effectiveness of the Goldmann Applanation tonometer, the dynamic contour tonometer, the ocular response analyzer and the Corvis ST in measuring intraocular pressure following FS-LASIK. Current Eye Research. 2020;**45**:144-152

[60] Sedaghat MR, Momeni-Moghaddam H, Yekta A, et al. Biomechanically-corrected intraocular pressure compared to pressure measured with commonly used Tonometers In Normal subjects. Clinical Optometry (Auckl). 2019;**11**:127-133

Chapter 5

Perspective Chapter: Management of Secondary Glaucoma, a Rising Challenge

Julie Pegu, Prerna Garg, Tripti Johri, Shanu Mittal, Surbhi Arora and Suneeta Dubey

Abstract

Secondary glaucoma has increased exponentially in recent times. This is partially due to the increase in complex eye surgeries like corneal transplantation and vitreoretinal surgery and partly due to the increase in life style related diseases like diabetes causing an increase in the prevalence of neovascular glaucoma. The other leading causes of secondary glaucoma are post-trauma, post-cataract surgery, and lens-induced glaucoma. Secondary glaucoma is an important cause of visual morbidity. The management of this complex glaucoma is difficult as they are mostly intractable and do not respond to anti-glaucoma medications. Many patients who are not managed by medical management may require surgical intervention along with vigilant control of their primary pathology. This course would address the stepwise approach to the management of these glaucomas and the tips and tricks to tackle the nuances during management. This chapter would specifically address the management of neovascular glaucoma, Post-PK glaucoma, lens-induced glaucoma, traumatic glaucoma, and uveitic glaucoma.

Keywords: secondary glaucoma, neovascular glaucoma, lens induced glaucoma, uveitic glaucoma, traumatic glaucoma

1. Introduction

Any form of glaucoma with an identifiable cause of increased intraocular pressure, leading to optic nerve damage is referred to as secondary glaucoma. Being acquired conditions, they tend to have a unilateral presentation and the underlying pathology may be that of an open or closed-angle glaucoma. The leading causes of secondary glaucoma were found to be neovascular glaucoma, trauma, post-keratoplasty, uveitic glaucoma, and lens-induced glaucoma.

2. Post PK glaucoma

2.1 Introduction

Penetrating Keratoplasty (PK) involves resecting the host cornea and replacing it with a full-thickness donor graft. In 1969, Irwin and Kaufmann first reported the high incidence of increased IOP following PK [1]. They reported a mean maximum pressure of 40 mmHg in aphakic and 50 mmHg in combined transplants and cataract extraction in the immediate postoperative period. Since then, various authors have reported the incidence of glaucoma in the early postoperative period from 9 to 31 % [2–4] and from 18 to 35 % in the late postoperative period [5, 6]. One of the reasons for this great variation in incidence is the different manner in which glaucoma after PK is defined in various studies [7]. In fact two leading causes of graft failure Post PK are Graft rejection and Secondary Glaucoma. Graft rejection following glaucoma is the second leading cause of graft failure [8]. Glaucoma following keratoplasty can be defined as an increase in the intraocular pressure (IOP) above 21 mmHg with or without associated alteration in visual fields or optic nerve changes that necessitates treatment [9, 10].

Post Penetrating Keratoplasty glaucoma (PPKG) occurs with increased incidence in patients with preoperative glaucoma. Simmons et al noted PPKG in 34% of 229 patients, out of whom 27% had preoperative controlled glaucoma [11]. In another study by Thoft et al, only 10% of patients presenting with PPKG did not have preoperative glaucoma [12].

PPKG is one of the most challenging problems because of its frequent occurrence, difficult diagnosis and monitoring, complexity of its management, irreversible visual loss due to damage to the optic nerve as well as the donor endothelium [5]. Diagnostic difficulty arises due the errors in tonometry recordings of a thick/astigmatic corneal graft [13]. In addition, it is often not possible to assess adequately the optic nerve/visual field before surgery/in the immediate postoperative period because of preoperative media opacification and corneal distortion with high astigmatism [14]. Timely management and diagnosis of post-PK glaucoma with the initiation of appropriate treatment is mandatory to preserve optimal graft clarity and ONH function [15].

2.2 Etiology and risk factors

PK is complicated by a significant incidence of IOP elevation in both the early and late postoperative periods. Early presentation tends to occur within the first few weeks after surgery [16]. Late postoperative period tends to occur >3 months [16]. Pre-existing glaucoma predisposes to increased IOP post-keratoplasty and can become the culprit early/ late following surgery [17].

The most significant risk factors (**Table 1**) noted were pre-existing glaucoma, lens status (i.e. aphakia, pseudophakia), and the disease for which PK is performed [19]. On comparing the incidence of PPKG in phakic, pseudophakic, and aphakic groups, Hemanth et al found that the aphakic group had the highest risk, followed by the pseudophakic and phakic groups; however, there was no statistically significant difference between the last two groups [20]. Kirkness and Ficker published one of the largest studies on the incidence and risk factors associated with post-PK glaucoma, which included 1122 PKs, performed at Moorfields Eye Hospital, London. The

Recipient >60 years
Aph akic and Pseudophakic Bullous Keratopathy [4]
Preexisting glaucoma [3]
Adherent leucoma
Herpes virus infection
Trauma [4]
Repeat PK [18]
ICE syndrome
Perforated corneal ulcer [18]
Combined PK and cataract extraction
Performance of vitrectomy during PK
Anterior segment reconstruction

Table 1.
Risk factors for glaucoma in patients undergoing PK.

Viral keratitis [3]	20–75%
ABK [2]	20–70%
Peters Anamaly [5]	60%
Aniridia [5]	56%
Trauma [6]	9–55%
Pseudophakia [3]	18–53%
Ulcerative diseases	50%
Corneal Regraft [2]	45–50%
Fuchs Dystrophy [5]	0–37%
Kertaoconus [18]	0–12%
CHED & ICE [18]	0–3%

Table 2.
Rates of chronic post PK glaucoma.

incidence of post-PK glaucoma was 14%. Corneal dystrophies and keratoconus had the lowest risk of glaucoma, contrary to bullous keratopathy, anterior segment trauma, iridocorneal endothelial syndrome, and corneal perforations which had an increased risk [21, 22]. In another study, Kirkness and Mashegov demonstrated an increased incidence of post-PK glaucoma after corneal perforations, especially those after bacterial ulcers, was due to the formation of peripheral anterior synechiae (PAS) and secondary angle closure. The longer the period between the perforation and the transplant, the higher the risk of glaucoma [23].

From **Table 2**, it can be seen that the rates of chronic glaucoma after PK differ significantly based on the indication for PK (from a low of 0–12% for keratoconus to a high of 75% after infectious keratitis).

a) Tight suturing
b) Long bites (more compressed tissue)
c) Larger trephine sizes
d) Smaller recipient corneal diameter
e) Increased peripheral corneal thickness

Table 3.
Factors contributing to angle distortion.

a) Less tight sutures
b) Deep sutures
c) Short sutures
d) Suture bites equal on either side of wound
e) Smaller sized grafts
f) Donor corneas larger than that of the recipient
g) Thinner recipient corneas
h) Larger overall corneal diameter

Table 4.
Factors decreasing angle compression.

Early onset	Intermediate onset	Late onset
a) Viscoelastic induced	a) Vitreous in AC	a) POAG
b) Trabecular collapse	b) Hyphema	b) Ghost cell
c) Preexisting OAG	c) Inflammation	c) Epithelial ingrowth
d) Inflammation	d) Steriod induced	d) Steriod induced
e) Hyphema	e) Ghost cell	e) Rejection/inflammation SEQ
	f) Graft rejection	

Table 5.
Mechanism of raised IOP after PK open angle glaucoma.

Early onset	Intermediate onset
a) Preexisting PAS	a) Puppilary block
b) Wound leal with angle closure	b) Malignant glaucoma
c) Operative technique causing compression	c) Progressive synechial closure
d) Puppilary block	
e) Malignant glaucoma	

Table 6.
Mechanism of raised IOP after PK angle closure glaucoma.

2.3 Pathophysiology

The pathophysiology of post-PK glaucoma is multifactorial, the causes being compression of the angle's anatomical elements with the trabecular meshwork's (TM) collapse, incorrect suturing of the graft, postoperative inflammation, and prolonged use of corticosteroids in the postoperative period (**Tables 3–6**).

Olson and Kaufman [6], using a mathematical model, proposed that the elevated IOP following PK in an aphakic patient might be the result of angle distortion secondary to a compressed tissue in the angle. Edema and inflammation after surgery lead to further compromise in the TM function, and the situation is further aggravated by angle distortion.

2.4 Viscoelastic induced

Viscoelastic material is applied in PK procedures in order to ensure maintaining a physical depth between the posterior transplanted cornea and underlying structures including the iris and the lens [24]. The viscoelastic material also decreases the risk of mechanical injury to structures. As much as it is essential to maintain corneal graft survival, the viscoelastic substance is associated with an increased incidence of post-PKP glaucoma [25]. The viscoelastic's high viscosity can cause trabecular meshwork (TM) obstruction, thus hindering aqueous humor outflow from the anterior chamber (AC) [26]. A study conducted by Hozler et al. showed a direct association between increased viscoelastic substance viscosity and increased IOP, but there was no statistical significance [27]. Retained viscoelastic material in the anterior chamber is the most common cause of IOP rise in the immediate post-operative period [28]. Complete removal of viscoelastic should be done at the end of surgery.

2.5 Suturing technique and transplant size

Tight sutures between the recipient and donor tissues would lead to straitening of the two, thus decreasing the corneo-limbal angle and the corneal curvature. This in turn would increase the risk of iridocorneal angle collapse, PAS formation, and out flow obstruction [29–31]. This can be further understood from **Figure 1**. Angle α

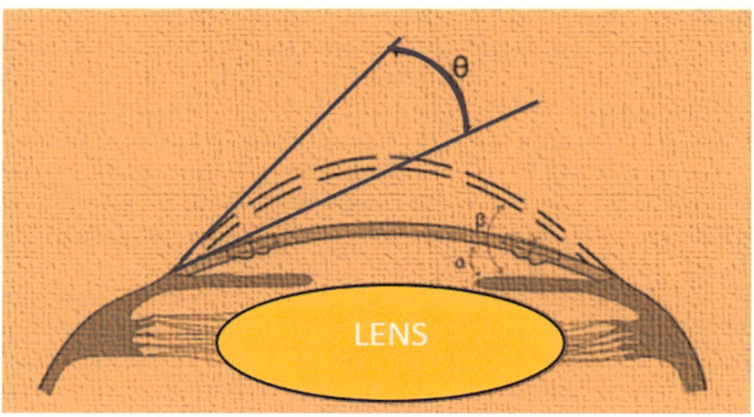

Figure 1.
Effect of suturing technique on development of PPKG.

represents the ideal iridocorneal angle after PK, whereas β is the angle when tight sutures are applied and θ is the difference between the two. More the θ, the more the chance of PPKG. Usually, a combination of same-sized donor button [32], tight sutures, and long bites causes angle crowding that can compromise the TM.

Zimmerman et al demonstrated how through-and-through sutures decreased the aqueous outflow to a lesser extent when compared with mid-stromal sutures (by a factor of 37%) in aphakic patients. In phakic patients, the aqueous outflow did not depend on the depth of sutures, according to their study [33]. They speculated that through-and-through sutures prevented retraction of Descemet's membrane and played a role in keeping the angle taut.

Olson and Kaufmann suggested that the development of PPKG can be avoided by appropriate manipulation of the host and donor sizes [34]. It has been proposed to use a donor button 0.5 mm larger than the host bed. Oversized graft buttons were found to have better control when compared to same-sized buttons in eyes with no pre-existing glaucoma.

Moreover, oversized grafts provide optimal AC depth, which reduces the risk of PAS formation and resultant IOP spike.

2.6 Inflammation and PAS

Late onset post-PK glaucoma is usually due to synechial angle closure with the degree of PAS strongly correlating with the need for surgery. PAS occurs more commonly in eyes undergoing PK for suppurative keratitis and perforated ulcers. In failed, opaque grafts Dada et al concluded that PAS formation was an important cause of secondary angle closure glaucoma post PK [35]. It was also noted that pupilloplasty and iris suturing during keratoplasty decreased the PAS formation [36].

A study by Vajpayee et al. observed that grafts oversized by 1 mm decreased the risk of iridocorneal adhesions [37]. Also, those with pre-existing iridocorneal adhesions were at an increased risk of developing PAS postoperatively in spite of adequate suturing and synechiolysis.

2.7 Corticosteroid usage

Steroids are essential in the postoperative period to prevent endothelial rejection and maintain graft survival. However, steroids themselves are known to cause glaucoma by multiple mechanisms like water retention, inhibition of phagocytic properties, accumulation of cellular debris, and glycosaminoglycans [38–40]. It is known to account for 20–70% of PPKG in different studies [41–44]. The steroid-induced rise in IOP post-PK occurs more commonly in patients with keratoconus and Fuch's Dystrophy (73% and 60.3%, respectively) [25]. It has been suggested to decrease the steroid therapy to the minimum possible to control the IOP spikes [12].

A study done by Mindel et al noted the tendency of different steroids to induce IOP spike over a six-week period. Dexamethasone increased the IOP twice as much as fluorometholone and eight times as much as medrysone [45]. While difluprednate 0.05% was shown to have an IOP rise in 21% of cases [46], fluorometholone and rimexolone caused less IOP elevation but also have decreased anti-inflammatory effects [47]. The efficacy of Cyclosporine A alone to control inflammation and suppress post-PK rejection remains to be determined [48].

2.8 Diagnosis

It is difficult to establish a starting point for the postoperative period because measuring the IOP, optic disc and visual field evaluation are on most occasions difficult to perform preoperatively due to primary corneal disease. After PK, changes in corneal thickness, postoperative astigmatism, and refractive changes often preclude adequate evaluation of the IOP, optic disc, and visual field.

The diagnosis of glaucoma post-PK is primarily based on the IOP measurement in the early postoperative period and on IOP, optic disc changes, and progressive visual field changes in the late postoperative period. In the postoperative period, IOP can be measured especially when the cornea is irregular with a tonopen/ mackaymarg tonometer [49] or a Dynamic contour tonometer (DCT) which works independently of the corneal thickness.

Multiple studies compared DCT with GAT in cases with keratoplasty and proved that DCT was not influenced by thickness, curvature, and corneal astigmatism [50–52]. GAT underestimates the pressure reading post-PK [50, 53]. Kandarakis at al. reported an average IOP measurement by DCT to be 16.6 (SD 2.8) mmHg, while that obtained by GAT to be 15.1 (SD 3.6) mmHg.

On comparing the I-care tonometer with GAT, the values were found to be similar in cases of anterior and posterior lamellar keratoplasty, but in PK patients, I-care underestimated the IOP compared to GAT [54].

The accuracy of GAT is reduced in the presence of corneal edema (underestimation of IOP), corneal scars (overestimation of IOP), blood staining, or any condition which alters corneal thickness or elasticity.

Another device to measure IOP is Ocular Response Analyzer (ORA) which also measures corneal hysteresis, thus taking corneal biomechanical properties into account while measuring IOP. Studies have noted a considerably wide difference in IOP measurements with ORA when compared with GAT [55, 56]. Chou et al. showed a mean of 6.29 mmHg higher reading of IOP with ORA than with GAT. This indicates the need for an adjusted coefficient for GAT IOP reading to become more reliable.

In the presence of tarsorrhaphy, digital palpation [57] can be used or new tonometers which measure the IOP through the lid (Proview Phosphene tonometer) can be used.

PAS formation causing secondary angle closure is an important etiology of raised IOP post-keratoplasty in patients with totally opaque grafts [35]. UBM can be used to view the angle and find the cause of the Post-PK Glaucoma, especially in eyes with a failed graft where the anterior segment details are not visible. The extent of iridocorneal adhesions, the location of IOL, phakic/aphakic status, AC depth, Angle width, and corneal thickness can be determined by UBM. It also helps the glaucoma surgeon in planning the site for a trabeculectomy or a glaucoma drainage device.

2.9 Management

Management of Post-PK Glaucoma is a challenging affair and various steps need to be taken during the surgery to prevent this blinding condition.

2.9.1 Prophylaxis

A. Preoperative factors

Preexisting glaucoma should be well-controlled prior to the surgical intervention. If the IOP is difficult to control with drugs or if the control imposes maximal therapy, the IOP can cause decompensation after keratoplasty. Therefore, in these cases, glaucoma should be controlled surgically and a transplant should be performed afterward [5] because multiple studies revealed a higher incidence of graft failure if the intervention for glaucoma was performed after keratoplasty [18]. Some studies recommend trabeculectomy with mitomycin C (MMC) application or with a GDD concomitantly with PK [18–20].

B. INTRAOPERATIVE FACTORS – During Surgery, the use of the following procedures reduces the risk of Post PK glaucoma

1. 1mm oversize donor corneal button

2. Deep, short, adequately tight bites

3. Goniosynechiolysis

4. Iridoplasty procedures (in cases of atrophic iris)

5. Viscoelastic removal at the end of surgery

6. Careful wound closure to prevent postoperative wound leaks

C. Postoperative factors

1. Judicious use of topical steroids controls PAS and inflammation.

2. Cycloplegics keep the pupil mobile and prevent pupillary block glaucoma.

3. Monitoring of IOP as long-term use of steroids can cause secondary open-angle glaucoma.

2.9.2 Medical management

The use of topical anti-glaucoma medication is still the first line of treatment to control post-PK glaucoma. Beta-blockers, alpha-2 agonists, carbonic anhydrase inhibitors (CAI), topical prostaglandin analogs, miotics, rho-kinase inhibitors as well as systemic CAI can be used to treat post-PK glaucoma.

Adrenergic agents are not used much as they cause chronic conjunctival inflammation. Miotics have little effect in the presence of PAS in cases of angle closure, so they are also not much used. Systemic CAI is very useful as a short-term therapy in the early postoperative period. Long-term therapy is limited by serious side effects such as tinnitus, nausea, gastrointestinal disturbances, paraesthesia, depression, anxiety, weight loss, nephrolithiasis, and blood dyscrasias. Topical CAI should be used with caution as they suppress carbonic anhydrase enzyme in the corneal endothelium and long-term use can lead to graft rejection.

Preservatives such as benzalkonium chloride are epitheliotoxic and one should avoid and use preservative-free unims for long-term therapy.

When using topical anti-glaucoma medication, one has to be aware of the local side effects of the drugs as these side effects can be detrimental to the state of the graft.

In the cases of steroid-induced glaucoma, the dose of steroids should be tapered to the minimum possible dose. High-potency steroids should be replaced with low-potency steroids such as fluorometholone and loteprednol. Cyclosporine 0.5–2% can be substituted for steroids and this can help in IOP control.

2.9.3 Laser therapy

Selective/ Argon laser trabeculoplasty (SLT/ALT) has been used quite infrequently in this subset of patients. There are few reports indicating a significant reduction with laser trabeculoplasty in areas of the angle without PAS [58, 59]. Van Meter et al. reported an average IOP reduction of 9.1 mm Hg in 10 patients with ALT persisting till a follow-up of two years [58].

2.9.4 Surgical management

Surgical options include trabeculectomy with mitomycin C, glaucoma drainage devices, and cyclophotocoagulation. Ayyala et al reported no significant difference in IOP control and graft failure when comparing the above three procedures [60]. Sekhar et al. reported a preference for trabeculectomy in phakic eyes because of higher success in a patient with a previously undisturbed angle. Endothelial cell loss is also reported to be negligible compared to Ahmed valves [61]. Overall, the success rates for IOP control range from 87% (14 of 16 eyes) with 1-year follow-up to 50% (12 of 24 eyes) after 2 years of follow-up based on various small studies [62, 63]. Graft clarity has been reported to be 60% after 2 years in a series of 24 patients and 62% after 22 months in a series of 26 patients [63, 64]. Glaucoma drainage implants (GDIs) are possibly the most successful modality for control of IOP after the fewest treatment procedures [65]. IOP control has been reported to be 62–96% after 2 years of follow-up [66, 67]. The rate of graft failure has been reported to be 35–74% after 2 years of follow-up [68, 69]. The tube of these devices can be placed in the anterior chamber (AC), posterior chamber (ciliary sulcus), or in the anterior vitreous via the pars plana route. Placing the tube in the AC has been associated with an increased risk of corneal endothelial damage and decompensation, with the reported frequency between 7% and 27%. Pars plana insertion would require additional vitreoretinal surgery and thus pose an increased risk of retinal damage. Rumelt and Rehany reported a safer alternative technique of tube insertion into the ciliary sulcus in patients with glaucoma secondary to corneal transplantation [70].

For eyes with intractable glaucoma and poor visual potential, cyclodestructive modalities have been advocated.

3. Lens induced glaucoma

Lens induced glaucoma (LIG) is a common form of secondary glaucoma in which the crystalline lens is involved in the mechanism of raised IOP. It was first reported by two clinicians independently; Gifford and von Reuss [71]. Later various workers described such types of cases under different names like LIG, lens-induced uveitis and glaucoma, phacotoxic glaucoma, phacogenic glaucoma, phacolytic glaucoma etc. At present, LIG is a clinical condition characterized by

- a violent secondary glaucoma (resembling acute angle closure glaucoma) in one eye with a senile mature cataract, hyper mature senile cataract (rarely immature senile cataract)

- normal intraocular pressure and open angle in other eye,
- and prompt relief of symptoms and restoration of vision after cataract extraction in the affected eye

The late reporting for treatment of cataracts thus leads to serious complications like LIG and it remains one of the most important causes of irreversible loss of vision, especially so in the rural population.

3.1 Epidemiology

The epidemiology varies across developed and developing countries. In developing countries with more limited resources, acquired LIG from advanced senile cataracts is the more prevalent subtype. The incidence of LIG is up to 2.4% at the time of the presentation of senile cataracts with a female preponderance [72].

3.2 Classification

LIG can be classified into the following subtypes based on their pathogenesis:

1. Lens protein-related: Leakage of lens protein across an intact or a breached lens capsule.

   This form includes

   - Phacolytic glaucoma (PLG)
   - Lens-particle induced glaucoma (LPIG)
   - Phacoanaphylactic glaucoma (PAG)

2. Secondary angle closure: Anatomical obstruction of aqueous flow from the posterior to the anterior chamber

   - Phacomorphic glaucoma (PMG)

3.3 Phacolytic glaucoma

Phacolytic glaucoma was first described by Flocks and colleagues [73]. The condition occurs chiefly in the setting of a senile hypermature, or Morgagnian, cataract with leakage of lenticular material through microscopic openings in an apparently intact lens capsule. The raised IOP was originally thought to be caused by obstruction of the trabecular meshwork by macrophages distended by engulfed lens material and Morgagnian fluid that had escaped from an intact crystalline lens. Later much of the evidence showed the role of high-molecular-weight soluble lens protein, leaked from an intact capsule, in causing direct obstruction of aqueous outflow channels and thus elevation of the IOP. In very rare scenarios, the cataract may be immature, with the liquefaction of the posterior cortex.

3.3.1 Clinical features

Patients present with sudden onset of severe pain and redness of the eye with a history of a gradual decrease in vision over a few months to years. They may complain of a further acute reduction of vision, usually due to the corneal edema due to the high IOP.

On examination, the presenting signs are high IOP, microcystic corneal edema, and open angles on gonioscopy with few scattered endothelial precipitates. The cellular reaction is usually present in the anterior chamber ranging from mild cells and flare to intense reaction with pseudohypopyon. The cells are usually larger than those seen in other uveitis, as the cells are swollen macrophages with the engulfed lenticular matter.

Diagnosis: Phacolytic glaucoma is usually a clinical diagnosis, but microscopic examination of aspirated anterior chamber fluid can aid in suspected cases. Biochemical studies can help to identify high-molecular-weight lens proteins that have leaked out of the cataract. Engorged macrophages may be seen as well [74].

3.3.2 Treatment

Phacolytic glaucoma is a surgical semi-emergency. After decreasing the inflammation and IOP with topical steroids and topical and oral anti-glaucoma medications, the patient should be posted for cataract surgery removal ideally within a week. Cycloplegic agents aid in decreasing inflammation and pain. Usually, miotics and prostaglandin analogs are avoided in anti-glaucoma therapy for these conditions, due to their pro-inflammatory roles.

Cataract extraction can be done by ECCE, SICS, or phacoemulsification depending upon the surgeon's expertise. Even in patients presenting with No Perception of light, cataract surgery can be performed to decrease inflammation, IOP, and pain.

3.4. Phacomorphic glaucoma

Phacomorphic glaucoma is a type of secondary glaucoma caused by lens swelling in eyes with mature or intumescent cataracts who otherwise are not predisposed to angle closure [75]. When the lens swells, acute angle closure with pupillary block occurs in the acute phase; in the late phase, it can occur even without pupillary block as a result of forward movement of the peripheral iris. Phacomorphic glaucoma is encountered more commonly in developing countries, where cataracts tend to get neglected by the patient because of the general belief that cataract surgery is neither indicated nor feasible unless the cataract becomes matured or 'ripe'.

Clinical features: The presentation of phacomorphic glaucoma is similar to acute angle-closure glaucoma. Patients may experience severe pain and headache secondary to elevated IOP, blurred vision, perception of halos around lights, nausea, vomiting, bradycardia, and sometimes diaphoresis [76]. Clinical features may include corneal edema, conjunctival injection, and a mid-dilated pupil. The intumescent lens may be observed pushing the iris forward and reducing the anterior chamber depth. The cellular reaction may be present in the anterior chamber, usually mild in nature, with angles typically closed on gonioscopy. The diagnosis is made on the basis of typical clinical features.

Management is similar to that of phacolytic glaucoma, involving initial control of IOP and inflammation followed by cataract surgery. The initial lowering of IOP is commonly done with medical treatment with combinations of topical anti-glaucoma medications (AGM), oral acetazolamide, and intravenous mannitol but it has been documented that in 37.5% of cases medical treatment had failed to lower IOP [77]. This may be because of the poor corneal drug penetration and relative ischemia caused by raised IOP leading to the failure of topical therapy. IOP lowering is however desired to prevent the risks of operating on an eye with corneal edema and high IOP.

Cataract surgery in these patients poses several challenges: the high IOP, sometimes quite refractory to medical management increases the risk of posterior capsular rupture and expulsive hemorrhage. The pre-existing corneal haze and shallow AC further increase the risk. The increased intra-lenticular pressure makes anterior capsulotomy difficult, with a high chance of extension or an Argentinian Flag Sign. Formation of the Anterior chamber with a high viscosity OVD and aspirating fluid from the lenticule through a small opening in the anterior capsule decreases the intralenticular pressure and allows a more controlled capsulorrhexis. Different techniques of performing capsulorrhexis have been described in literature like two-step capsulorrhexis, sewing needle microcapsulotomy, phaco-capsulotomy etc.

Role of laser peripheral iridotomy (LPI) Preoperative laser peripheral iridotomy (LPI) may offer multiple benefits in such patients. LPI helps in lowering IOP by releasing the pupillary block and may facilitate surgery by increasing the peripheral AC depth. Moreover, by equalizing the pressures in anterior and posterior chambers the effect of relative ischemia is negated allowing the topical medications to work. But doing an LPI in such patients may be challenging. Corneal edema due to raised IOP may hamper visibility. As the lens is positioned in close proximity to the iris there is a risk of lens capsule rupture with subsequent leakage of lenticular material into the AC.

Although these patients present early to the hospitals because of the acute symptoms, the visual prognosis remains unpredictable due to the irreversible optic nerve damage that may have incurred in a matter of few days. Also, a delay in the treatment causes a permanent synechial closure of the anterior chamber angle as a result of which IOP spikes can be seen even after cataract extraction.

3.5 Lens particle glaucoma

Lens-particle-induced glaucoma was previously mislabelled as 'phacotoxic uveitis'. In lens-particle glaucoma, IOP elevation is caused by obstruction of aqueous outflow by lens particles, which can occur either after cataract surgery (with retained cortical matter/ epinuclear matter), trauma to lens, or YAG posterior capsulotomy.

It is a type of secondary open-angle glaucoma similar to phacolytic glaucoma, the difference being that the lens capsule is grossly disrupted instead of micro ruptures present in phacolytic glaucoma.

Clinical features: Clinical findings of lens-particle glaucoma are similar to those of phacolytic glaucoma with conjunctival injection, corneal edema, elevated IOP, and anterior chamber reaction. However, lens particles cause more inflammation, usually leading to anterior and posterior synechiae and pupillary membranes.

Diagnosis: The diagnosis of lens-particle glaucoma can be made based on a history of recent intraocular surgery or trauma, along with the presence of gross lens material in the anterior chamber.

Treatment: The course of treatment depends upon the severity of the disease upon presentation. If only minimal cortical material is present, cycloplegics, corticosteroids, and IOP lowering agents (aqueous suppressants) usually suffice. However, if there is significant lens matter with high levels of inflammation and poorly controlled IOP, urgent removal of the residual lens cortex is necessary. Prompt treatment is required to avoid serious consequences.

Inflammation persisting for a longer duration can lead to the development of pupillary membranes, pupillary block, and subsequent PAS formation and intractable glaucoma.

Cystoid macular edema and even tractional retinal detachments may also occur.

3.6. Phacoantigenic glaucoma

Also known as Phacoanaphylactic glaucoma, it is the rarest type of lens-induced glaucoma which is often difficult to diagnose. It is an Arthus-type immune complex reaction, mediated by IgG and the complement system against lens proteins. These lens proteins are normally sequestered within the lens capsule and are thus immune-privileged. Either during a complicated cataract surgery involving loss of vitreous or following trauma, these lens proteins get admixed with vitreous and result in retention of these lens proteins followed by their slow release [74]. This usually presents at least after a period of 2 weeks, as this is the time period required for sensitization of the lens protein [78].

3.6.1 Clinical features

Presenting signs include lid edema, conjunctival congestion, corneal stromal/microcystic edema with an intense fibrinous anterior chamber reaction with posterior synechiae with characteristic mutton-fat keratic precipitates. Anterior vitritis also usually occurs. A confirmed diagnosis is established by visualizing the polymorphonuclear leukocytes in the aqueous or vitreous specimen, along with the presence of circulating lens proteins within the aqueous humor. The diagnosis is difficult to establish without aqueous/vitreous tap analysis as the lens proteins seen in the anterior chamber are quite less as compared to the severity of glaucoma.

Treatment: It is similar to other forms of lens-induced glaucoma, involving anti-inflammatory and anti-glaucoma medications and usually requiring surgical removal of the remaining lens material.

3.7 Prognosis of lens induced glaucoma

A good visual prognosis can be expected if the patient presents early and is managed promptly. After controlling the inflammation and IOP, patients should be taken early for surgical management. The presence of PAS post-operatively is associated with a poor prognosis and requires regular IOP monitoring. Usually, the primary surgery involves only cataract extraction or lens matter wash, as trabeculectomy combined at this stage has poor success due to the presence of inflammation at the time of surgery. If IOP remains uncontrolled in the postoperative period on multiple anti-glaucoma medications, then a glaucoma surgery is done.

4. Traumatic glaucoma

4.1 Introduction

Glaucoma is a common complication following trauma. It can occur either after open or closed globe injury.

The 6-month risk of developing glaucoma was estimated to be 2.67% after penetrating injury [79] and 3.4% after blunt injury according to the U.S. Registry [80]. In children <15 years, it is estimated that about 3.3–5.7 million suffer from ocular trauma annually and 160,000–280,000 children/year sustain ocular trauma serious enough to require hospitalization [81].

Risk factors predicting the development of traumatic glaucoma include- elderly, baseline visual acuity < 6/60, elevated baseline IOP, hyphema, angle recession > 180 degrees, iris injury, injury/ displacement of lens [80, 82, 83].

Glaucoma after penetrating injuries is more common in presence of adherent leucoma or lens injury/ displacement [79].

4.2 Closed globe injury

4.2.1 Pathophysiology

Blunt trauma causes momentary anatomic deformation of the globe on impact, leading to sudden posterior displacement of the cornea and anterior sclera and a compensatory expansion at the equator. This can lead to separation at seven rings of tissue anterior to the equator (Rings of Campbell)-

1. Sphincter Pupillae – Radial sphincter tears (**Figure 2**)

2. Trabecular meshwork- Tears/ splits/disruption

3. Iris root – Iridodialysis

4. Split between longitudinal and oblique ciliary muscle – Angle recession

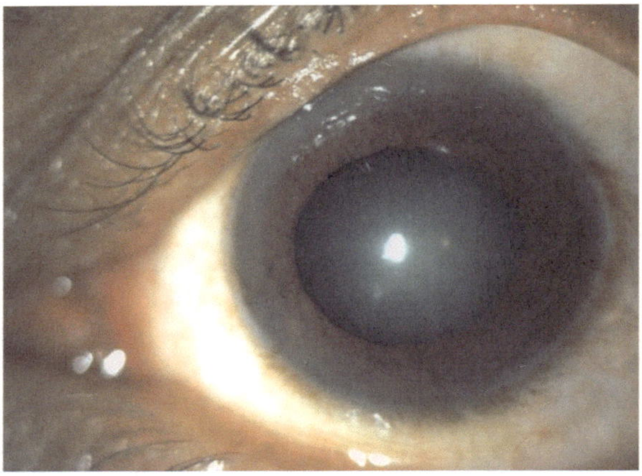

Figure 2.
Multiple sphincter tears causing traumatic mydriasis.

Early onset	Delayed onset
Trabeculitis	Angle recession
Uveitis	Peripheral anterior synechiae
TM disruption	Ghost cell glaucoma
Hyphema	Phacolytic and lens particle glaucoma
Lens-induced glaucoma- Phacomorphic / lens displacement	Delayed closure of a cyclodialysis cleft
Massive choroidal hemorrhage	Rhegmatogenous retinal detachment

Table 7.
Causes of IOP elevation post-ocular trauma.

5. Attachment of ciliary body to scleral spur- Cyclodialysis cleft

6. Zonules – Lens displacement

7. Attachment of retina to ora Serrata – Retinal dialysis and detachment

Causes of IOP elevation post-trauma have been enumerated in **Table 7**.

4.3 Causes of early onset traumatic glaucoma

4.3.1 Trabeculitis and uveitis

Anterior uveitis accounts for 20% of cases of traumatic glaucoma [84]. Subcellular iris and TM trauma trigger an innate immune response, leading to increased vascular permeability and release of inflammatory mediators. Obstruction of the TM by these circulating precipitates or by the primary trabecular swelling can cause an increase in IOP. However, this is self-limiting in nature with the mainstay of treatment being topical steroids and cycloplegic agents.

4.3.2 Trabecular disruption

Acute blunt trauma to the globe can produce partial/full thickness tears in the TM, which lead to hemorrhage in the Schlemm's Canal and scarring over time. They can lead to acute as well as chronic intraocular pressure (IOP) elevation. These changes have been documented in a study when a gonioscopy was performed within 2 days post-injury [85].

4.3.3 Hyphema

The presence of hyphema indicates significant ocular injury. Bleeding most commonly occurs from fine vessels in the angle. The mechanisms by which hyphema can cause glaucoma include- contusion/inflammation of the trabecular meshwork, physical disruption of the meshwork, plugging with red blood cells, or by a large clot in the anterior chamber producing pupillary block.

The extent of bleeding correlates with the incidence of elevated IOP, risk of secondary bleeding, and visual outcomes (**Table 8**) [86–88]. Secondary bleeding is caused by clot lysis and retraction and typically occurs between day 2 and day 7 following the

Grade of hyphema	Risk of elevated IOP [8]	Chance of recovering vision 20/50 or better [9]	Risk of secondary bleeding [10]
I – 1/3rd of anterior chamber	13.5%	75–90%	25%
II – 1/3–1/2	13.5%	65–70%	
III - >1/2	27%	25–50%	60–70%
IV- Full anterior chamber	50%	25–50%	60–70%

Table 8.
Prognosis depending on the grade of hyphema.

initial injury, during which time close monitoring is advised. Rebleeds are typically worse than the initial bleed and are associated with a worse visual prognosis.

Management is usually conservative in the form of topical and oral steroids, cycloplegic agents, and antiglaucoma medications (other than PGA and miotics). Oral aminocaproic acid and tranexanemic acid have been advocated by few, as they decrease the risk of re-bleeding, however, they are associated with systemic side effects and are known to decrease the rate of clearance of hyphema [89].

The most commonly cited surgical indications for all patients with hyphema are based largely on two studies done by Read and Goldberg from 1970–1972 [90, 91]. Their surgical indications are:

1. corneal blood staining at any time;

2. total hyphemas with IOP ≥ 50 mmHg for five days to prevent optic atrophy;

3. total hyphemas that do not clear by 50% after six days with an IOP ≥ 25 mmHg (to prevent corneal blood staining);

4. unresolved hyphemas after eight days to prevent PAS; and

5. IOP ≥ 60 mmHg for 48 hours despite intravenous mannitol.

History of sickle cell disease/ trait should be elicited in all patients, particularly those of African American lineage, as these patients experience higher IOP elevation with even minimal hyphema and increase risk of re-bleeds. Goldberg et al recommended surgery (AC wash) in these patients after only 24 hours with a mean IOP ≥ 25 mmHg or several spikes ≥ 30 mmHg [92].

In cases of refractory glaucoma, trabeculectomy has been used to achieve IOP normalization [93, 94].

4.3.4 Massive choroidal hemorrhage

This is a rare cause of acute IOP elevation post-trauma, presenting as a shallow anterior chamber, both centrally and peripherally with a reduced red reflex and choroidal elevation seen on indirect ophthalmoscopy or B scan ultrasonography.

Initial treatment includes topical and oral antiglaucoma medications, cycloplegics, and steroids. Miotics should be avoided as they can cause further anterior chamber shallowing

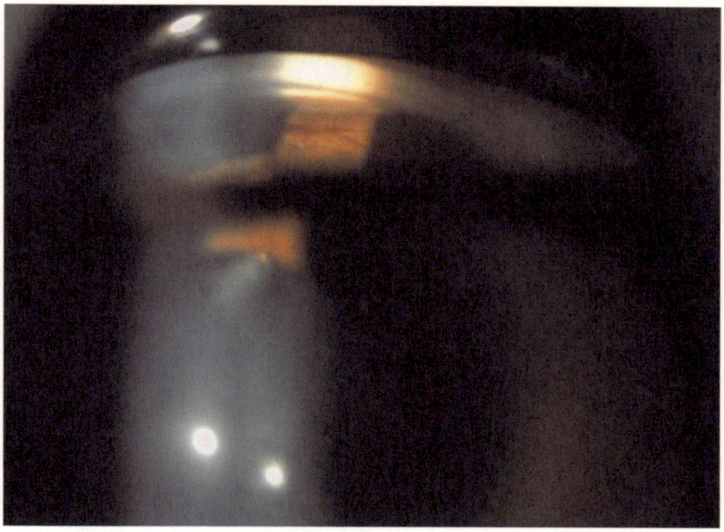

Figure 3.
Angle recession (green arrow) with clotted blood on iris (red arrow).

due to ciliary spasms. Persistent angle closure with pressure elevation, lenticulo-corneal touch, and kissing choroidal with retinal apposition warrants surgical drainage.

4.4 Causes of delayed onset traumatic glaucoma

4.4.1 Angle recession

It is defined as the separation between the longitudinal and circular fibers of the ciliary muscle, causing a posterior displacement of the iris root, giving an appearance of widened ciliary body band on gonioscopy. It is indicative of damage to the trabecular meshwork following trauma and is not per se responsible for the increase in intraocular pressure. Its reported incidence ranges from 70 to 100% [95, 96] following traumatic hyphema, however, glaucoma occurs in 7–9% of patients [97]. Glaucoma has been reported to occur either within the first year or after 10 years of trauma [95] with it being more common when angle recession of >180 degrees is present. Spaeth et al reported that 50% of patients with unilateral angle recession glaucoma had frank or probable glaucoma in their fellow eye [97], indicating an inherent predisposition for developing glaucoma in these patients. Treatment is usually medical, with laser trabeculoplasty having some role when IOP is not too high [98]. Refractory glaucoma is treated surgically with either filtering surgery (provided that the conjunctiva is not scarred) or drainage devices. The success of trabeculectomy was found to be lower (43% vs 75%) in these patients when compared to patients with primary open-angle glaucoma [99]. However, routine use of antimetabolites like mitomycin C or 5-FU either intraoperatively or postoperatively has been associated with higher success [100, 101]. A recent study has evaluated the role of AGV implant in angle recession glaucoma with a success of 90% at the mean follow-up duration of 29.47 ± 3.39 months (**Figure 3**) [102].

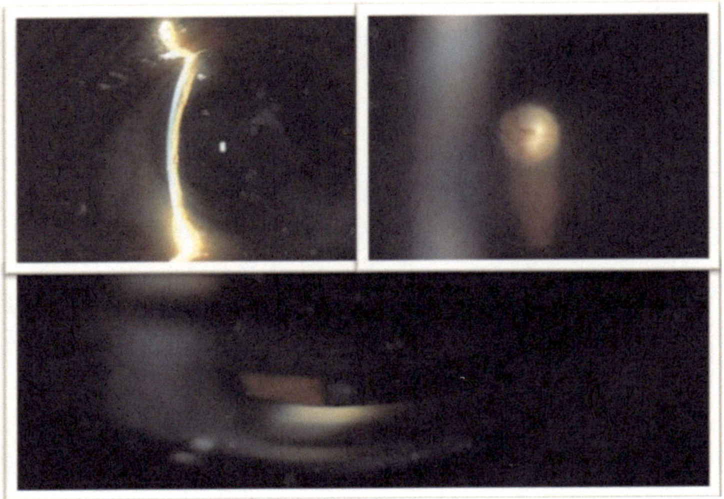

Figure 4.
Secondary angle closure glaucoma following closed globe injury.

4.4.2 Peripheral anterior synechiae

Following blunt trauma, the organization of blood and inflammatory debris can lead to either PAS formation or endothelization of the angle. Persistent hyphema for >8 days was found to be associated with PAS formation [91]. Presence of massive choroidal hemorrhage causing AC shallowing can also lead to permanent angle closure. Treatment in these cases often requires surgical therapy, when the IOP is not controlled medically (**Figure 4**).

4.4.3 Ghost cell glaucoma

Degeneration of red blood cells in an anaerobic chamber like the vitreous leads to the formation of khaki-colored cells, known as ghost cells, as they become depigmented due to the loss of intracellular hemoglobin. Disruption of the anterior hyaloid face after trauma, vitrectomy, cataract surgery, or even spontaneously allows these cells to circulate in the anterior chamber and obstruct the trabecular meshwork due to their rigid nature. This typically occurs 1–3 months after trauma. It is usually self-resolving and managed medically, however, it may require repeated anterior chamber lavage and glaucoma surgery.

4.4.4 Lens-induced glaucoma: can occur in an acute or chronic setting

a. Lens dislocation- Severe trauma can cause zonular disruption and thus anterior or posterior displacement of the lens. Both conditions can cause a pupillary block, either by the lens itself or by vitreous blocking the pupillary margin. Treatment is laser iridotomy/ surgical iridectomy to relieve the pupillary block followed by lensectomy.

b. Lens swelling- Phacomorphic glaucoma: The impact from blunt trauma can cause an immature cataract to become intumescent, causing either pupillary block or a forward push of the iris-lens diaphragm leading to angle closure glaucoma. Treatment is the same as in the above condition.

c. Phacolytic and lens particle glaucoma: Microruptures in the fragile anterior capsule of a hyper mature cataract induced by trauma, cause leakage of high molecular weight proteins into the anterior chamber and clog the trabecular meshwork causing secondary open-angle glaucoma. Similarly, a complete rupture of the anterior capsule will cause leakage of lens fragments which in turn will obstruct the trabecular meshwork. Treatment in both these conditions is by surgical removal of the lens after decreasing the inflammation and lowering the intraocular pressure medically.

4.4.5 Delayed closure of a cyclodialysis cleft

Closed globe injury may be associated with acute hypotony in some instances. These include severe cyclitis causing ciliary body shutdown or development of a cyclodialysis cleft. Separation of the ciliary muscle from the scleral spur creates this cleft, which acts as an alternative outflow pathway for aqueous humor, causing a decrease in IOP. Over time, this cleft undergoes fibrosis, which may cause an elevation in IOP. Goldmann hypothesized that a decrease in the flow through the conventional trabecular meshwork pathway results in its decreased permeability, and thus it fails to function after the closure of the cleft. Treatment is aimed at controlling the IOP either medically or surgically. Miotics and phenylephrine may be effective in reopening the cleft in the early stages (**Figure 5**).

4.4.6 Rhegmatogenous retinal detachment

The retinal tear usually causes a decrease in IOP due to an increase in the uveoscleral outflow through the tear. In 5–10% of cases, ocular hypertension can

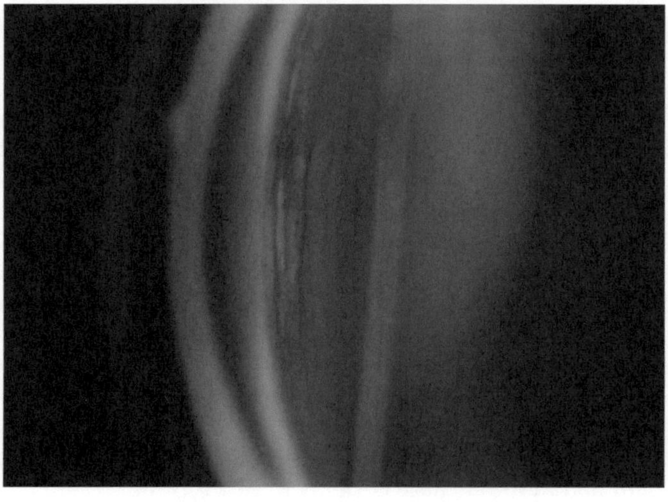

Figure 5.
Cyclodialysis cleft with co-existent angle recession.

occur, possible causes being pre-existing open-angle glaucoma, presence of inflammation and rarely Matsuo-Shwartz Syndrome [103] (obstruction of trabecular meshwork with photoreceptor outer segment cells).

4.5 Open globe injury

Risk factors for developing glaucoma after open globe injury include advancing age, hyphema, lens injury, perforating injury, zone 2 injury, vitreous hemorrhage, lens dislocation, presence of the intraocular foreign body, and cataract surgery following primary repair. The incidence was found to range from 2.6% to 17% in various studies [104–107].

4.5.1 Causes of glaucoma following open globe injury

Osman et al classified glaucoma after open globe injury into three stages namely early (<1 month), intermediate (1–6 months), late stage (>6 months). They found the cause of glaucoma in the early stage to be un-removed lens particles, inflammation, and hyphema. In the intermediate stage, glaucoma was due to synechial angle closure, ghost cell glaucoma, and unremoved lens particles. In the late stage, the causes noted were angle recession and synechial angle closure [107]. Other causes include epithelial down growth, fibrous ingrowth, and retained intraocular foreign body. A few of these conditions will be discussed subsequently.

A. Epithelial downgrowth

A rare cause of delayed glaucoma following open globe injury, it can present either as epithelial cysts or pearls, or membranes. Risk factors include inadequate wound closure, wound fistula, presence of iris incarceration or vitreous incarceration in a full-thickness wound, and iatrogenic implantation of epithelial cells into the anterior chamber while repairing ocular lacerations. While cysts and pearls, usually do not cause glaucoma, the membrane can obstruct the drainage from the angle, first by growing over it and later by undergoing contraction and causing synechial closure. It appears as a grey translucent membrane with scalloped edges and presents as a retro corneal membrane with corneal edema and glaucoma. Treatment is challenging and aimed at controlling intraocular pressure. Glaucoma drainage devices are preferred due to the high rate of failure with trabeculectomy. In recalcitrant cases, cyclophotocoagulation is often required.

B. Fibrous ingrowth

Presents either as a focal, thick, vascularized membrane inside the anterior chamber or as an extensive membrane covering the corneal endothelium, trabecular meshwork, and iris surface. Glaucoma is usually refractory to medical and surgical treatment and requires cyclodestructive procedures.

C. Retained intraocular foreign body

A retained foreign body can cause ocular hypertension and glaucoma by various mechanisms. Angle-closure glaucoma can occur due to synechiae formation following shallowing or flattening of the anterior chamber after penetrating injury, due to epithelial /fibrous ingrowth or due to pupillary block from an anteriorly dislocated or intumescent lens. Rupture of the anterior lens capsule with the foreign body can cause lens particle glaucoma. A delayed type of glaucoma is siderotic glaucoma, due to fibrosclerosis of trabecular meshwork from the intraocular toxicity of the iron-containing foreign body [108]. These patients have a typical presentation with iris heterochromia, mydriasis, rust-like discoloration of anterior chamber structures, nyctalopia, and reduced electroretinogram responses. The mainstay of management is the removal of the foreign body. Few cases with similar manifestations have been reported without any evidence of an intraocular foreign body. This has been attributed to the iron derived from the degradation of red blood cells in patients with a history of hyphema or vitreous hemorrhage. The hemoglobin from the lysed red blood cells is phagocytosed and degraded into hemosiderin which accumulates in ocular tissues causing degeneration and sclerosis. This has been termed as hemosiderotic glaucoma [109].

5. Uveitic glaucoma

5.1 Introduction

Uveitic glaucoma also known as inflammatory glaucoma is an acquired clinical entity that causes secondary glaucoma. Intraocular inflammation and intraocular pressure share a complex relationship as they can alter both aqueous production as well as its drainage. Inflammation leads to alteration in aqueous composition resulting in increased resistance to outflow, blockage of trabecular outflow facility by cells and debris, structural changes of trabecular meshwork due to corticosteroid use and pupillary block [110]. It is estimated that 38–730 people per 100,000 are affected with uveitis worldwide. Approximately 20% of patients develop ocular hypertension and many of these progress to glaucomatous optic nerve damage [111].

5.2 Pathogenesis

An equilibrium between aqueous production and drainage maintains a normal IOP, which is distorted in patients with uveitis [112]. Inflammation in the eye leads to the breakdown of the blood-aqueous barrier, thereby releasing inflammatory cells, proteins, debris, or fibrin in the eye causing mechanical obstruction of trabecular meshwork and alteration of aqueous composition thus, increasing resistance to outflow. Glaucoma can present in an open-angle stage or a closed-angle stage [113, 114].

5.3 Physiological changes in aqueous composition in uveitis

Intraocular inflammation leads to increased vascular permeability which results in the release of inflammatory cells, proteins, prostaglandins, and cytokines into the aqueous [112, 115]. The inflammatory cells narrow the trabecular pores resulting in dysfunction and swelling of trabecular lamellae and endothelial cells, hence disrupting aqueous outflow [116]. Prostaglandins contribute to elevated IOP by increasing the aqueous viscosity and are known to cause aqueous hypersecretion via PGE_1 and PGE_2 [117]. Cytokines stimulate neovascularisation and have a direct influence on aqueous humor dynamics [112]. The elevated protein content can result in aqueous sludging, causing compromise of aqueous outflow [118].

5.4 Anatomical changes seen at outflow facility

The cellular and biochemical changes result in morphological alteration at the level of the trabecular meshwork. On gonioscopic evaluation, uveitic glaucoma can be classified as a closed or open-angle stage. Open-angle stage is more frequently encountered [119, 120]. Increased vascular permeability and disrupted blood-aqueous barrier lead to infiltration of TM with inflammatory cells and proteins, which results in mechanical blockage and swelling of trabecular lamellae and endothelial cells. This eventually causes scarring and damage to the TM [121].

Intraocular inflammation leads to adhesions of pupillary margins with the anterior lens capsule forming posterior synechiae. It leads to pupillary block if they extend 360 degrees, obstructing the passage of aqueous humor into the anterior chamber and hence forming iris bombe and causing angle closure glaucoma. Another mechanism of the pupillary block is caused by occlusio pupillae, where the inflammatory cells and protein form a fibrin membrane covering the pupillary margin and adhering to the anterior lens capsule, hence causing occlusion of the transfer of aqueous humor into the anterior chamber. Iris bombe formation eventually leads to the formation of PAS, thereby, closing the angle structures. Neovascularisation induced by cytokines may be witnessed at the angle in chronic uveitis, which pulls the iris and causes angle closure. Inflammation and swelling of the ciliary body lead to its forward rotation and hence causing non-pupillary block angle closure [122, 123].

5.5 Ocular conditions associated with inflammatory glaucoma

Uveitic glaucoma can be due to idiopathic ocular conditions, infective causes or systemic causes. With the advent of antimicrobial therapy, there is a drastic reduction in uveitic glaucoma due to infective pathology. The mechanism and progression of glaucoma depend on the etiology of uveitis and has been reported as more common in Fuchs heterochromic uveitis, Posner-Schlossman syndrome, herpetic uveitis, and Juvenile idiopathic arthritis (JIA) [124–128].

Ocular conditions:

- Fuch's Heterochromic Iridocyclitis
- Posner-Schlossman Syndrome
- Sympathetic ophthalmitis

Infective conditions:

- Viral (Herpes simplex, zoster, CMV)
- Syphilis
- Hansen disease

Systemic conditions:

- Juvenile Idiopathic Rheumatoid Arthritis
- Tuberculosis
- Sarcoidosis
- Behcet's

5.6 Signs and symptoms

The patient may present with symptoms of blurred vision, ocular pain, redness, brow ache, redness, and other ocular disturbances like photophobia and colored halos due to corneal edema in patients with markedly elevated IOP. The corneal examination may show band-shaped keratopathy, healed herpetic scars, and keratic precipitates on the endothelium. The anterior segment may reveal iris nodule, neovascularization, heterochromia, iris atrophy, posterior synechiae, and peripheral anterior synechiae. The lens may reveal pigment on the anterior lens capsule and development/ progression of cataracts. Gonioscopy may show the presence of PAS and the degree of angle closure. May show features of fine vascularization in the trabecular meshwork, occasional trabecular precipitates, hypopyon, hyphaema, or fibrin deposition. Optic nerve evaluation and visual field assessment for glaucomatous damage must be done and recorded. Other possible posterior segment findings may include cystoid macular edema, retinitis, perivascular sheathing, choroidal infiltrates, or retinal detachment.

5.7 Management of uveitic glaucoma

The treatment approach in a case of uveitic glaucoma depends on various factors, but most importantly on a careful diagnosis of underlying etiology, strict control of inflammation and IOP, and constant monitoring for early glaucomatous damage and progression to initiate appropriate management. A rheumatologist's opinion to control systemic disease is a must. The main aim of the therapy is providing symptomatic relief, preventing glaucomatous damage, reducing the recurrence of uveitis, preventing the formation of synechiae or neovascularization, and reducing the need for surgical intervention.

5.8 Medical management

The control of uveitis is necessary to minimize any further complications that occur due to uveitis. An immediate and aggressive anti-inflammatory therapy prevents IOP rise and adverse events of uveitis [129].

5.8.1 Corticosteroids

Corticosteroids are the first line of treatment for addressing non-infectious ocular inflammation. The mechanism of action is by inhibiting the release of arachidonic acid and subsequent production of prostaglandins, thus reducing inflammation. It can be administered through various routes like topically, peri ocularly, intravitreally, and systemically depending on the severity of inflammation. Anterior segment inflammation is addressed by the use of localized drug delivery, which reduces systemic side effects [130–132]. Posterior segment inflammation can be addressed by periocular, intravitreal, or systemic application of steroids [133].

Immunosuppressive drugs: These drugs are generally reserved for refractory cases or when systemic side effects of chronic uses of corticosteroids are suspected. Most immunosuppressive agents take a minimum of 6 weeks to achieve maximum efficacy, so should be used in conjunction with corticosteroids in the beginning. It includes the use of drugs such as methotrexate, azathioprine, cyclosporine, tacrolimus, and other immunosuppressive agents [134–138].

Immunomodulatory agents: These biological agents are monoclonal antibodies, which are used as third-line drugs in recent times [139]. Favorable results have been seen with the usage of biological modulators, especially Adalimumab in the treatment of treating JIA-associated and pediatric refractory panuveitis [140].

Anti-inflammatory treatment must be given in association with topical cycloplegic drugs in acute uveitic episodes. Topical cycloplegics (atropine 1%, homatropine 1%, tropicamide 1%, cyclopentolate 1%) are used to relieve ciliary spasms, break acutely formed posterior synechiae, or prevent them from forming if started early in the disease process [141]. Treatment of specific etiologies such as herpes simplex or varicella-zoster requires prescription of antiviral therapy along with antiglaucoma medications [142].

5.8.2 Antiglaucoma treatment

Traditionally, beta blockers and CAI have been used as a first-line therapy to control IOP spikes in uveitic glaucoma patients. Beta-blockers are considered the drug of choice to lower the IOP elevation in patients of uveitic glaucoma by reducing aqueous humor production [143, 144]. CAIs are frequently used as 1st line management along with beta-blockers in uveitic glaucoma [142] or in cases where beta blockers are contraindicated. CAIs lead to the alteration of the ion transport mechanism in the ciliary epithelium thereby, reducing the production of aqueous humor [144]. Brimonidine is an Alpha-2 adrenergic agonist which leads to the reduction of IOP via a dual mechanism. They reduce aqueous production at ciliary epithelium and also enhance uveoscleral outflow [145, 146] and their mydriatic effect is useful in preventing posterior synechiae formation in uveitic eyes [110]. The role of PGA in the management of uveitic glaucoma is controversial because of the high risk of inducing anterior uveitis, blood-aqueous barrier disruption, cystoid macular edema, and reactivation of Herpes simplex keratitis [110]. Ripasudil, a Rho-associated protein kinase inhibitor shown to lower IOP by altering trabecular meshwork, has been approved in Japan in 2014. It has been effective in lowering IOP in approximately 50% of eyes of UG [147]. Hyperosmotic agents like glycerol and mannitol are used in acute elevation of IOP.

Laser therapy: Laser peripheral iridotomy (LPI) must be performed for eyes that have a narrow anterior chamber angle susceptible to a primary acute angle closure attack [148]. An ideal peripheral iridotomy of 300– 350 microns is required to prevent acute angle-closure glaucoma [149].

5.8.3 Surgical management

Clinically about 30% of uveitic eyes do not respond to maximal medical therapy and require surgical intervention [150]. Inflammation-induced accelerated scarring is a challenging problem as it is associated with a higher risk of surgical failure. Adequate control of inflammation, both pre-operative and post-operative, and IOP control are desirable prior to surgical intervention for better results [151]. A quiescent phase of a minimum 3 months is considered ideal, which can be attained by the use of corticosteroid therapy. The risk of post-operative hypotony is more in uveitic glaucoma cases as chronic and relapsing intraocular inflammation leads to ciliary body impairment. Both trabeculectomy (with and without adjunctive antifibroblast medications) and aqueous drainage implants are used to control IOP [152]. Glaucoma drainage implants are preferred in patients with extensive conjunctival scarring, or after failed trabeculectomy [153–155]. The other significant risk factors for surgical failure are male sex, age younger than 45 years, and non-granulomatous uveitis [156].

Trabeculectomy is considered gold standard surgery for UG with uncontrolled IOP with maximal medical therapy and in cases of angle closure with extensive PAS formation. A bleb-dependent fistula is formed that helps aqueous drainage from the anterior chamber into subconjunctival space. Adequate control of IOP (< 21 mm Hg) has been seen in various studies in patients with uveitis who underwent trabeculectomy [157–159]. Studies have reported failure of the procedure in patients with significant post-op inflammation [157].

The results of unaugmented trabeculectomy are variable and are particularly poor in young patients with UG [160], as a result of an accelerated wound-healing response. Trabeculectomy augmented with MMC or 5-FU has shown good surgical success rates in patients with a high risk of failure, due to its effect of minimizing scarring of the filtering bleb [161].

Glaucoma Drainage Devices: Glaucoma drainage implants have been used increasingly in the treatment of uveitic glaucoma. They are especially useful in cases with unhealthy conjunctiva as primary surgery or after failed trabeculectomy surgery. Drainage devices may be valved (AGV), or non-valved (Baerveldt glaucoma implant, BGI, and Molteno implant). A study has reported AGV to have success rates of up to 94% at 4 years follow-up in chronic UG [162]. The AGV is considered effective in reducing IOP, decreasing the number of glaucoma medications, and preserving vision [162].

Cyclophotocoagulation: Laser cytophotocoagulation is used to destroy the ciliary body where aqueous humor is produced. Unfortunately, it leads to the aggravation of intraocular inflammation, and is reserved as the last step for eyes with uncontrolled IOP and poor visual potential [158].

5.9 Conclusion

Strict control of Inflammation and finding the root cause that triggers inflammation is one of the first steps in controlling the adversaries caused by Uveitis. With the advent of more aggressive and comprehensive medical control of uveitis, the prognosis for UG patients has drastically changed compared to a few years ago. Management is directed at the diagnosis of the underlying condition and appropriate management of the local or systemic disease for adequate control of inflammation and deferring repeated attacks. Better medical and surgical options are available for patients suffering from UG. Apart from traditional trabeculectomy, various implantable drainage devices are available, which have proven to be effective and successful. Long-term large prospective studies are warranted for a better understanding of long-term efficacy. Non-penetrating Goniotomy procedures appear to be a lucrative option in pediatric patients and even adults. Other glaucoma surgical options like minimally invasive glaucoma surgery (MIGS) may also be effective in these patients, but those approaches are still under evaluation. A booming role of stem cell therapy has shown effectiveness in the management of various diseases, but its role is yet to be discovered in patients with uveitic glaucoma.

6. Neovascular glaucoma

6.1 Introduction

Neovascular glaucoma (NVG) is a sight-threatening condition, especially in developing countries. NVG occurs secondary to several diseases that affect the eye, the most common being proliferative diabetic retinopathy (PDR) [163], ischemic retinal vein occlusion [164], and less frequently CRAO and ocular ischemic syndrome (OIS). It is a significant cause of visual morbidity due to its aggressive nature and resistance to the currently available medical therapy, especially in the latter stages of the disease. Only 3% of cases of NVG are caused by inflammation without retinal ischemia [165].

The central mechanism is a hypoxic posterior segment, leading to increased vascular endothelial growth factor (VEGF) formation. VEGF, an endothelial cell mitogen is synthesized by several types of retinal cells, but under ischemic conditions, Muller cells are the primary source.

The cytokine-rich environment promotes the formation of fibrovascular tissue that gradually covers the trabecular meshwork causing impairment of AH outflow and a resultant increase in IOP [166]. In the initial stages, the angles remain open, but the myofibroblasts' proliferation eventually creates a synechial angle-closure [167] and further IOP elevation. Many other substances that might be involved in angiogenesis are under investigation. These include insulin-like growth factors I and II [168], insulin-like growth factors binding proteins 2 and 3 [169], basic fibroblast growth factors [170], platelet-derived growth factors [169], and interleukin 6 [169].

1. Clinical manifestations

Although there is a certain degree of overlap, it is convenient to divide the stages of NVG into the following:

1. Stage of Rubeosis iridis

2. Stage of Secondary open-angle glaucoma

3. Stage of Secondary synechial angle-closure glaucoma

2. Early stage (Rubeosis Iridis)

The first visible sign of incipient NVG is tiny tufts of new vessels at the pupillary margin which may at times appear just as tiny red dots. One should maintain a high index of suspicion and carefully examine under high magnification at the slit lamp. These small vessels can be easily overlooked, especially in darkly pigmented irises if casually viewed. In case a contact gonioscopy is used at the initial examination, the light pressure on the lens is sufficient to collapse these neovascular tufts and render them clinically invisible. Similarly, these vessels will be missed if a dilated examination is done. The new vessels will continue to grow radially over the surface of the iris in an irregular meandering manner toward the angle, sometimes joining dilated blood vessels at the collarette. At this stage, the IOP is usually normal and the new vessels may regress with the treatment of the primary pathology or may progress to involve the angle. At times, neovascularization of the angle (NVA) can occur with or without neovascularization of the iris (NVI), so a careful gonioscopy is a must in all eyes at high-risk for NVG, even in the absence of pupillary and iris involvement. NVI tends to begin where the greatest aqueous-tissue contact occurs, so, it is important to examine the other passageways for aqueous to enter the AC bypassing the pupil, for example, a peripheral iridotomy.

All patients diagnosed with severe NPDR should also be examined for early NVI as the presence of NVI may direct the clinician to look for CNP areas in the retina with an FFA.

3. Stage of secondary open-angle glaucoma

If the process of rubeosis continues, the new vessels continue to grow across the iris surface and join the circumferential ciliary body artery. On reaching the angle, the new vessels cross the ciliary body band and scleral spur onto the TM. Until a significant portion of the TM is covered by NVA, the IOP may be completely normal. A fibrovascular membrane, which is invisible on gonioscopy, commonly accompanies NVA and may block enough of the TM and raise the IOP thus causing a secondary form of open-angle glaucoma. Pathological NVA is differentiated from normal NVA by the former crossing the scleral spur (diagnostic) and the latter as a visible circumferential blood vessel over the peripheral iris seen during gonioscopy.

4. Stage of secondary synechial angle-closure glaucoma

If the second stage continues the fibrovascular membrane contract producing peripheral anterior synechiae (PAS). As these PAS coalesce, synechial angle closure occurs and the IOP may remain continuously elevated.

6.2 Clinical features

The prototypic picture of NVG is quite characteristic. In the stage of rubeosis iridis, a careful examination would reveal the new vessels at the pupillary area with normal IOP. The second stage of open-angle of NVG would have NVI/ NVA with or without elevated IOP. As the third stage of angle closure ensues, the IOP is usually elevated. The vision may be severely reduced due to an edematous cornea and the primary disorder underlying the NVG. There is congestion of the globe with marked pain. The IOP can be very high (>40 mm Hg or higher), but in some cases, such as carotid artery obstructive disease, it may be normal or even subnormal. However, if the patient is young and the endothelium is healthy, the cornea may remain clear with a high IOP. In case of very elevated IOP with corneal edema, the NVI/NVA may be missed thus causing a diagnostic dilemma. So, a repeat slit-lamp examination is very important to note the NVI/NVA when the cornea clears on treatment. There can be associated aqueous flare due to leakage of proteins from the new iris vessels and seen only when the cornea clears. There can be a distortion of the pupil and ectropion uvea due to the radial contraction of fibrovascular tissue during the late changes. Gonioscopy may show synechial angle closure at different levels with NVA. At the burnt-out stage, the picture of a smooth zippered-up line of iridocorneal adhesion is pathognomonic, at which stage NVA may be absent but other signs like ectropion uvea and the fundus pathology should help in making the diagnosis.

6.3 Role of fluorescein angiography

Iris fluorescein angiography (FA) demonstrates leakage from damaged iris vessels long before new vessels can be detected on slit-lamp examination. This is due to the production of VEGF, which is also a potent Vaso permeability factor and is likely to be 50,000 times more potent than histamine [170]. The fluorescein leakage occurs throughout the iris which persists and increases with time, unlike in the benign forms of capillary incompetence (e.g. pseudoexfoliation). In one study, NVI could be detected in 37% of eyes before the development of clinically visible new vessels [171].

Grading of Iris Neovascularization [172] – as proposed by Teich and Walsh

Grade 0- No iris neovascularisation

Grade 1- Less than 2 quadrants of NV at iris pupillary zone

Grade 2- More than 2 quadrants of NV at iris pupillary zone

Grade 3- Grade 2 + less than 3 quadrants of NV at iris ciliary zone and/or ectropion uveae

Grade 4- More than 3 quadrants of NV at ciliary zone and/or ectropion uveae

NVA grading [173] is as follows:

Grade 1 - Fine neovascular twigs cross scleral spur and ramify on the trabecular meshwork, involving ≤2 quadrants;

Grade 2 - Neovascular twigs cross scleral spur and ramify on the trabecular meshwork, involving ≥2 quadrants;

Grade 3 - In addition to the trabecular meshwork, PAS involving 1 to 3 quadrants;

Grade 4 - PAS involving ≥3 quadrants.

6.4 Management

The management of NVG involves decreasing the primary ischemic drive by either pan-retinal photocoagulation (PRP) and/or anti-angiogenic injection and control of IOP by ocular hypotensive therapy [167]. In the early open-angle glaucoma stage, AGMs or PRP may be effective. However, an overwhelmingly great number of patients do not respond to medical treatment in the closed-angle stage. The exact reason is not known but presumably, the high IOP inhibits the drug to penetrate the cornea in the presence of corneal epithelial edema and the ischemic status further prevents the absorption of the drug from the AH to the ciliary circulation. Surgical options include trabeculectomy, and GDD in eyes with vision potential while cyclodestructive procedures are reserved when the former is not feasible or in absolute eyes. Both trabeculectomy and GDD act by creating alternative channels for AH drainage and thus reducing the IOP whereas cyclodestructive techniques are based on partial destruction of the ciliary body which decreases AH production, and therefore lowers the IOP.

6.4.1 Medical management

Management of NVG mainly targets treatment of the underlying disease process responsible for rubeosis and treatment of the increased IOP.

6.4.2 Treatment of the primary pathology

A. Pan retinal photocoagulation (PRP)

A.1. Early-stage therapy

During the stage of early NVI (Rubeosis iridis), the mainstay in therapy is pan-retinal photocoagulation (PRP). The most widely accepted mechanism by which PRP works is by destroying the retinal outer layer and thereby decreasing oxygen demand since the outer photoreceptor-retinal pigment epithelium complex accounts for the majority of total retinal oxygen consumption. This allows choroidal oxygen to diffuse into the inner retina, decreasing not only inner retinal hypoxia but also reducing the stimulus for the release of angiogenic factors. There is sufficient documentation that PRP decreases ocular VEGF levels and subsequent regression of the NVI in CRVO [174] and PDR [175].

It has been noted that treatment with approximately 1,200–1,600 spots is required to cause regression of NVI. Ohnishi and colleagues [176] documented regression of rubeosis in 68% of patients and normalization of IOP in 42% of patients treated with PRP. There is also a higher success rate for glaucoma filtering procedures when PRP is performed [176]. However, the results of PRP in CRAO are not as effective as in CRVO and PDR [177].

A.2. Late-stage therapy

In this stage usually, synechial angle closure has set in, and the management of glaucoma becomes increasingly difficult. In the presence of clear media, PRP should be performed as soon as possible to eliminate the stimulus for new vessel formation; otherwise, filtration surgery is more likely to fail. Regression of NVI can occur within days to weeks of completed PRP. Filtration surgery should be done at least 1 week and preferably 3 to 4 weeks after completion of PRP.

A.3. Endophotocoagulation

Intraoperative PRP is useful in situations where routine PRP cannot be done due to hazy media. It is done in conjunction with intraocular surgery like cataract extraction or vitrectomy and can be just as effective as standard photocoagulation and hence extensively used, especially during vitrectomy [178].

B. Role of anti-VEGF agents

B.1. Intravitreal bevacizumab

In situations where PRP cannot be done due to associated ocular conditions such as poor pupillary dilatation, corneal edema, cataract, or vitreous hemorrhage, intravitreal Bevacizumab (IVB) has been shown to cause marked and rapid regression of anterior segment neovascularization in NVG. Marked regression of iris neovascularization has been noted in various case reports within a median of 8 days (range 1 to 10 days) [179]. Although the long-term effectivity is not known, even a transient effect could be of benefit in the preoperative preparation of filtering surgery for NVG." Bevacizumab is applied in the dose of 1.25 mg/0.05 ml intravitreally and 0.25 mg/0.02 ml intracamerally [180].

6.4.3 Treatment of elevated IOP

A. Medical therapy

In the secondary open-angle glaucoma stage, all the standard antiglaucoma medications will be effective to some degree in lowering the IOP. However, in all stages of NVG, one must avoid the usage of pro-inflammatory drugs like Prostaglandin analogs and Pilocarpine eye drops. With extensive synechial angle closure, medications that decrease aqueous production, such as topical β-blockers and carbonic anhydrase inhibitors, are beneficial but do not lower the IOP to a normal range in the face of a highly inflamed state of the eye. Frequently, oral acetazolamide may be required to control IOP. Intravenous mannitol at a dosage of 1mg/kg/body weight may temporarily reduce IOP but should be used judiciously in hypertensive patients. Oral glycerol may not be as effective as mannitol but can help to reduce IOP till a definitive filtration surgery can be planned. It is, however, contraindicated in diabetics. The two other medications that are of the greatest benefit clinically are topical atropine 1% three times per day to decrease ocular congestion, and topical steroids four times per day to decrease ocular inflammation [181].

B. Conventional surgery

B.1. Trabeculectomy

Filtration surgery in NVG should be reserved for eyes that have the potential for useful vision and when the extent of the PAS is >180°. It should be preferably performed when the eye is quiet; otherwise, intraoperative and postoperative hemorrhages are likely to occur. Also, the presence of active neovascularization may lead to late bleb failure through conjunctival scarring at the filtration site.

Higashide T [182] et al studied 61 eyes of 54 patients with NVG treated by trabeculectomy following intraocular bevacizumab injection. The surgical success rate at a mean follow-up of 45+ 22.2 months was 86.9 + 4.3%, 74.0 + 6.1%, and 51.3 + 8.6% at 1,3, and 5 years. Effects of adjunctive use of intraocular anti-VEGF agents on glaucoma filtration surgeries for NVG have been evaluated in several studies [183, 184]. Less post-operative hemorrhagic complications and better surgical outcomes were anticipated because of the remarkable rapid and steady suppression of rubeosis after intraocular injection of bevacizumab. Indeed, postoperative hyphema was significantly less frequent when bevacizumab was used before trabeculectomy [185] or tube shunt surgery [186].

Risk factors for surgical failure of trabeculectomy in eyes with NVG were found to be younger age, previous pars plana vitrectomy (PPV), extensive peripheral anterior synechia, pseudophakia, and postoperative hyphema [187, 188].

B.2. Glaucoma drainage implants

When conventional surgery fails or is not possible because of excessive conjunctival scarring, insertion of a drainage device may be indicated. GDIs can be valved like the Ahmed Glaucoma valve and non-valved like the Baerveldt / Molteno and Aurolab aqueous drainage implant. Sevim et al. [189] assessed the efficacy of preoperative IVB injection before AGV implantation in NVG and found a better surgical success rate in the study group (79%) than in the control group (64%), with reduced early postoperative complications such as fibrinous reaction in the AC as well as hyphema. Shen et al. [188] found similar surgical outcomes in neovascular glaucoma patients who underwent trabeculectomy with MMC versus AGV implantation, with 20 patients in each group and an average follow-up of 31 months for the AGV group and 25 months for the trabeculectomy group. Success was 70% and 65% at 1 year and 60% and 55% at 2 years after AGV and trabeculectomy, respectively. Hyphema was the most common complication in both groups.

B.3. Ciliodestructive procedures

In end-stage NVG, when there is total synechial angle closure and no useful vision remaining, there is no indication for surgical intervention, and control of pain becomes the primary therapeutic aim. Ciliodestructive procedures were widely used before the advent of antifibrotic agents and anti-VEGF agents in the management of NVG. Although they may be highly effective in lowering IOP, the visual results are disappointing, especially with cyclocryotherapy (CCT). Sympathetic ophthalmia, RD, anterior segment ischemia, and phthisis have all been reported with cyclocryotherapy [190]. Direct laser cyclophotocoagulation seems to have better control and titration of the ciliary processes destroyed and a lower complication rate, but the percentage of patients with NVG who lose total vision remains high, with a long-term vision loss of 46.6% as reported by Shields and Shields [191]. Transscleral Cyclophotocoagulation (TSCPC) is another method. There is less elevation of IOP in the immediate postoperative period, along with less inflammation and pain than after CCT. With the contact system, there is a report of 140 eyes treated, 45 of which had NVG. An IOP of less than 19 mm Hg was achieved in 40% of the eyes with NVG. It was also noted that 50% of the serious complications were in eyes with NVG, including one eye with phthisis and one with traction RD [192].

In the meta-analysis of the surgical management of NVG by Shchomak et al [193]

there was no statistically significant difference in IOP-lowering capacity between the GDDs vs cyclophotocoagulation group. However, failure rates and proportion of patients with loss of LP were favorable to the GDDs group.

6.4.4 Conclusion

Neovascular glaucoma remains a therapeutic challenge. Despite many advances in the treatment of NVG, the visual prognosis remains poor. Early detection of neovascularization and prophylactic treatment with PRP directed at the ischemic retina are key elements in preventing a visually devastating outcome of this disease. Once IOP becomes elevated, successful management of the disease may be extremely difficult. Although the ideal surgical management of the neovascular glaucoma procedure has yet to be determined, trabeculectomy with antimetabolite therapy, aqueous shunt implants, and diode laser cyclophotocoagulation is the best surgical options. Current research on ocular angiogenesis and the advent of new pharmacological agents with activity against vascular endothelial growth factors have increased our treatment options for combating this serious disease. Bevacizumab may be a valuable addition to the treatment of NVG by hastening the resolution of anterior segment neovascularization and thereby improving the results of glaucoma surgeries.

Abbreviation list

PK	penetrating keratoplasty
IOP	intraocular pressure
PPKG	post penetrating keratoplasty glaucoma
PAS	peripheral anterior synechiae
TM	trabecular meshwork's
AC	anterior chamber
DCT	dynamic contour tonometer
GAT	Goldmann applanation tonometry
ORA	ocular response analyzer
UBM	ultrasound biomicroscopy
IOL	intraocular lens
CAI	carbonic anhydrase inhibitors
MMC	mitomycin C
5-FU	5-fluorouracil
GDD	glaucoma drainage device
SLT	selective laser trabeculoplasty
ALT	argon laser trabeculoplasty
GDIs	glaucoma drainage implants
LIG	lens induced glaucoma
PAG	phacoanaphylactic glaucoma
PLG	phacolytic glaucoma
LPIG	lens-particle induced glaucoma
PMG	phacomorphic glaucoma
PGA	prostaglandin analogues
AGM	anti-glaucoma medications
LPI	laser peripheral iridotomy
IgG	immunoglobulin G
AGV	Ahmed glaucoma valve
BGI	Baerveldt glaucoma implant
PGE_1	prostraglandin E_1
PGE_2	prostraglandin E_2
JIA	juvenile idiopathic arthritis

CMV	Cytomegalo virus
UG	uveitic glacucoma
MIGS	minimally invasive glaucoma surgery
NVG	neovascular glaucoma
PDR	proliferative diabetic retinopathy
CRAO	central retinal artery occlusion
CRVO	central retinal vein occlusion
OIS	ocular ischemic syndrome
VEGF	vascular endothelial growth factor
NVA	neovascularization of the angle
NVI	neovascularization of the iris
FA	fluorescein angiography
PRP	pan-retinal photocoagulation
IVB	intravitreal bevacizumab
PPV	pars plana vitrectomy
CCT	cyclocryotherapy
RD	retinal detachment
TSCPC	transscleral cyclophotocoagulation

Author details

Julie Pegu*, Prerna Garg, Tripti Johri, Shanu Mittal, Surbhi Arora and Suneeta Dubey
Dr. Shroff's Charity Eye Hospital, New Delhi, India

*Address all correspondence to: juliepegu2003@yahoo.co.in

References

[1] Irvine AR, Kaufman HE. Intraocular pressure following penetrating keratoplasty. American Journal of Ophthalmology. 1969;**68**:835-891

[2] Goldberg DB, Schanzlin DJ, Brown SI. Incidence of increased intraocular pressure after keratoplasty. American Journal of Ophthalmology. 1981;**92**: 372-377

[3] Karesh JW, Nirankari VS. Factors associated with glaucoma after penetrating keratoplasty. American Journal of Ophthalmology. 1983;**96**:160-164

[4] Chien AM, Schmidt CM, Cohen EJ, Rajpal RK, Sperber LT, Rapuano CJ, et al. Glaucoma in the immediate postoperative period after penetrating keratoplasty. American Journal of Ophthalmology. 1993;**115**:711-714

[5] Foulks GN. Glaucoma associated with penetrating keratoplasty. Ophthalmology. 1987;**94**:871-874

[6] Olson RJ, Kaufman HE. A mathematical description of causative factors and prevention of elevated intraocular pressure after keratoplasty. Investigative Ophthalmology & Visual Science. 1977;**16**:1085-1092

[7] Lim MC, Brandt JD, O'Duny DG. Glaucoma after Penetrating Keratoplasty. Mosby: Elsevier Inc; 2011. pp. 1441-1454

[8] Arroyave CP, Scott IU, Fantes FE, et al. Corneal graft survival and intraocular pressure control after penetrating keratoplasty and glaucoma drainage device implantation. Ophthalmology. 2001;**108**:1978-1985

[9] Raj H, Bhanushree G, Hulinaykar RM, Vijayanath V. Preoperative risk factors and incidence of glaucoma after penetrating keratoplasty. International Journal of Opthalmology. 2014;**1**(2):55

[10] Dada T, Aggarwal A, Minudath KB, et al. Post-penetrating keratoplasty glaucoma. Indian Journal of Ophthalmology. 2008;**56**(4):269

[11] Simmons RB, Stern RA, Teekhasaenee C, Kenyon KR. Elevated intraocular pressure following penetrating keratoplasty. Transactions of the American Ophthalmological Society. 1989;**87**:79-91

[12] Thoft RA, Gordon JM, Dohlman CH. Glaucoma following keratoplasty. Transactions - American Academy Ophthalmology and Otolaryngology. 1974;**78**:352-364

[13] Kaufmann C, Bachmann LM, Thiel MA. Comparison of dynamic contour tonometry with Goldmann applanation tonometry. Investigative Ophthalmology & Visual Science. 2004;**45**:3118-3121

[14] Ayyala RS. Penetrating keratoplasty and glaucoma. Survey of Ophthalmology. 2000;**45**:91-105

[15] Wilson SE, Kaufman HE. Graft failure after (1990)penetrating keratoplasty. Survey of Ophthalmology;**34**:325-356

[16] Rumelt S. Glaucoma in Cases of Penetrating Keratoplasty, Lamellar Procedures and Keratoprosthesis. In: Rumelt S, editor. Glaucoma - Basic and Clinical Concepts. IntechOpen; 2011. DOI: 10.5772/23895

[17] Greenlee EC, Kwon YH. Graft failure: III. Glaucoma escalation after penetrating keratoplasty. International Ophthalmology. 2008;**28**(3):191-207

[18] Kirkness CM, Moshegov C. Postkeratoplasty glaucoma. Eye. 1988;**2** (Suppl):S19-S26

[19] Gupta P, Sharma A, Ichhpujani P. Post penetrating keratoplasty glaucoma. Nepalese Journal of Ophthalmology. 2014;**6**(11):80-90

[20] Hemanth Raj MN, Bhanushree G, Hlinaykor RM, Vijayanath V. Preoperative risk factors and incidence of glaucoma after penetrating keratoplasty. International Journal of Clinical Trials. 2014;**1**(2):55-61

[21] Kirkness CM, Ficker LA. Risk factor for the development of postkeratoplasty glaucoma. Cornea. 1992;**11**(5):427-432

[22] Kirkness CM, Moshegov C. Postkeratoplasty glaucoma. Eye. 1998;**2**: 19-26

[23] Keroday O, Kugu S, Erdogan G, Kandenir B, Odzil SE. Incidence of and risk factors for increased intraocular pressure after penetrating keratoplasty. Cornea. 2010;**29**:278-282

[24] Sugar A, Sugar J. Techniques in penetrating keratoplasty. Cornea. 2000; **19**(5):603-610

[25] Al-Mahmood AM et al. Glaucoma and corneal transplant procedures. Journal of Ophthalmology. 2012;**2012**:1-9

[26] Stamper R et al. Effect of intraocular aspiration of sodium hyaluronate on postoperative intraocular pressure. Ophthalmic Surgery, Lasers and Imaging Retina. 1990;**21**(7):486-491

[27] Holzer MP et al. Effect of healon5 and 4 other viscoelastic substances on intraocular pressure and endothelium after cataract surgery. Journal of Cataract & Refractive Surgery. 2001;**27** (2):213-218

[28] Burke S, Sugar J, Farber MD. Comparison of the effects of two viscoelastic agents, Healon and Viscoat, on postoperative intraocular pressure after penetrating keratoplasty. Ophthalmic Surgery. 1990;**21**:821-826

[29] Zimmerman T. Transplant size and elevated intraocular pressure. Archives of Ophthalmology. 1978;**96**(12):2231

[30] Bourne WM, Davidson A, O'Falon WM. The effects of oversize donor buttons on postoperative intraocular pressure and corneal curvature in aphakic penetrating keratoplasty. Ophthalmology. 1982;**89**:242-246

[31] Perl T, Charlton KH, Binder PS. Disparate diameter grafting, astigmatism, intraocular pressure, and visual acuity. Ophthalmology. 1981;**88**: 774-781

[32] Olson RJ. Aphakic keratoplasty. Determining donor tissue size to avoid elevated intraocular pressure. Archives of Ophthalmology. 1978;**96**:2274-2276

[33] Zimmerman TJ, Krupin T, Grodzki W. The effect of suture depth on outflow facility in penetrating keratoplasty. Archieves in Ophthalmology;**91**:505-506

[34] Olson RJ, Kaufman HE. Prognostic factors of intraocular pressure after aphakic keratoplasty. American Journal of Ophthalmology. 1975;**86**:510-515

[35] Dada T, Aggarwal A, Vanathi M, et al. Ultrasound biomicroscopy in opaque grafts with post-penetrating keratoplasty glaucoma. Cornea. 2008;**27**:402-405

[36] Cohen EJ, Kenyon R, Dohlman CH. Iridoplasty for the prevention of postkeratoplasty angle closure and glaucoma. Ophthalmic Surgery. 1982;**13**: 994-996

[37] Vajpayee R. Oversized corneal grafts for corneal opacities with iridocorneal adhesions. Ophthalmology. 2001;**108** (11):2026-2028

[38] Kersey JP, Broadway DC. Corticosteroid-induced glaucoma: A review of the literature. Eye. 2005;**20**(4): 407-416

[39] Francois J. Corticosteroid glaucoma. Annals of Ophthalmology. 1977;**9**:1075-1080

[40] Armaly MF. Effect of corticosteroids on intraocular pressure and fluid dynamics: I. The effect of dexamethasone in the normal eye. Archives of Ophthalmology. 1963;**70**:482-491

[41] Baltaziak M et al. Glaucoma after corneal replacement. Survey of Ophthalmology. 2018;**63**(2):135-148

[42] Nguyen TD, Chen P, Huang WD, Chen H, Johnson D, Polansky JR. Gene structure and properties of TIGR, an olfactomedin-related glycoprotein cloned from glucocorticoid-induced trabecular meshwork cells. The Journal of Biological Chemistry. 1998;**273**:6341-6350

[43] Alward WLM, Fingert JH, Coote MA, Johnson T, Lerner SF, Junqua D, et al. Clinical features associated with mutations in the chromosome 1 open-angle glaucoma gene (GLC1A). The New England Journal of Medicine. 1998;**338**: 1022-1027

[44] Erdurmus M, Cohen EJ, Yildiz EH, et al. Steroid induced intraocular pressure elevation or glaucoma after penetrating keratoplasty in patients with keratoconus or Fuchs dystrophy. Cornea. 2009;**28**:759-764

[45] Mindel JS et al. Comparative ocular pressure elevation by medrysone, fluorometholone, and dexamethasone phosphate. Archives of Ophthalmology. 1980;**98**(9):1577-1578

[46] Sorkin N et al. Outcomes of difluprednate treatment for corneal graft rejection. Canadian Journal of Ophthalmology. 2020;**55**(1):82-86

[47] Stewart RH, Kimbrough RL. Intraocular pressure response to topically administered fluorometholone. Archives of Ophthalmology. 1979;**97**: 2139-2140

[48] Perry HD, Donnenfeld ED, Kanellopoulos AJ, Grossman GA. Topical cyclosporine A in the management of postkeratoplasty glaucoma. Cornea. 1997;**16**:284-288

[49] McMillan F, Forster RK. Comparison of MacKay-Marg, Goldmann, and Perkins tonometers in abnormal corneas. Archives of Ophthalmology. 1975;**93**: 420-424

[50] Geruti P, Morbib R, Marraffe M, Marchini G. Comparison of dynamic contour tonometry and Goldmann applanation tonometry in deep lamellar and penetrating keratoplasties. American Journal of Ophthalmology. 2008;**145**(2):215-221

[51] Zemba M, Stamate A-C. Glaucoma after penetrating keratoplasty. Romanian Journal of Ophthalmology. 2017;**61**(3):159-165

[52] Ismail A.. Comparison of dynamic contour tonometry with goldmann applanation tonometry for measurement of IOP in patients following penetrating keratoplasty; 2012

[53] Ismail AR, Lamont M, Perera S, et al. Comparison of IOP measurement using GAT and DCT in patients with penetrating keratoplasties. The British

Journal of Ophthalmology. 2007;**91**:980-981

[54] Salvetat ML, Zeppori M, Miani F, Tosoni C, Parisi L, Brusini P. Comparison of I Care tonometer and Goldmann applanation tonometry in normal corneas and in eyes with automated lamelar and penetrating keratoplasty. Eye. 2011;**25**:642-650

[55] Bezerra BDPS et al. Intraocular pressure measurement after corneal transplantation. Survey of Ophthalmology. 2019;**64**(5):639-646

[56] Huang J et al. Comparison of intraocular pressure measurement using 4 different instruments following penetrating keratoplasty. American Journal of Ophthalmology. 2012;**153**(3):580

[57] Rubinfeld RS, Cohen EJ, Laibson PR, et al. The accuracy of finger tension for estimating intraocular pressure after penetrating keratoplasty. Ophthalmic Surgery and Lasers. 1998;**29**:213-215

[58] Van Meter WS, Allen RC. Waring 3rd GO, Stulting RD. Laser trabeculoplasty for glaucoma in aphakic and pseudophakic eyes after penetrating keratoplasty. Archives of Ophthalmology. 1988;**106**:185-188

[59] Nakakura S, Imamura H, Nakamura T. Selective laser trabeculoplasty for glaucoma after penetrating keratoplasty. Optometry and Vision Science. 2009;**86**:e404-e406

[60] Ayyala RS, Pieroth L, Vinals AF, et al. Comparison of mitomycin C trabeculectomy, glaucoma drainage device implantation, and laser neodymium:YAG cyclophotocoagulation in the management of intractable glaucoma after penetrating keratoplasty. Ophthalmology. 1998;**105**:1550-1556

[61] Sekhar GC, Vyas P, Nagarajan R, et al. Post-penetrating keratoplasty glaucoma. Indian Journal of Ophthalmology. 1993;**41**:181-184

[62] Sharma A, Kumar S, Ram J, Gupta A. Trabeculectomy with mitomycin-C for postkeratoplasty glaucoma: A preliminary study. Ophthalmic Surgery and Lasers. 1997;**28**(11):891-895

[63] WuDunn D, Alfonso E, Palmberg PF. Combined penetrating keratoplasty and trabeculectomy with mitomycin C. Ophthalmology. 1999;**106**(2):396-400

[64] Ishioka M, Shimazaki J, Yamagami J, Fujishima H, Shimmura S, Tsubota K. Trabeculectomy with mitomycin C for post-keratoplasty glaucoma. The British Journal of Ophthalmology. 2000;**84**(7):714-717

[65] Elhofi A, Helaly HA. Graft survival after penetrating keratoplasty in cases of trabeculectomy versus ahmed valve implant. Journal of Ophthalmology. 2018;**2018**:1-6. DOI: 10.1155/2018/9034964

[66] Sidoti PA, Mosny AY, Ritterband DC, Seedor JA. Pars plana tube insertion of glaucoma drainage implants and penetrating keratoplasty in patients with coexisting glaucoma and corneal disease. Ophthalmology. 2001;**108**(6):1050-1058

[67] Sherwood MB, Smith MF, Driebe WT Jr, Stern GA, Beneke JA, Zam ZS. Drainage tube implants in the treatment of glaucoma following penetrating keratoplasty. Ophthalmic Surgery. 1993;**24**(3):185-189

[68] Rapuano CJ, Schmidt CM, Cohen EJ, Rajpal RK, Raber IM, Katz LJ, et al. Results of alloplastic tube shunt procedures before, during, or after penetrating keratoplasty. Cornea. 1995;**14**(1):26-32

[69] Alvarenga LS, Mannis MJ, Brandt JD, Lee WB, Schwab IR, Lim MC. The long-term results of keratoplasty in eyes with a glaucoma drainage device. American Journal of Ophthalmology. 2004;**138**(2):200-205

[70] Rumelt S. Implantation of glaucoma drainage implant tube into the ciliary sulcus in patients with corneal transplants. Archives of Ophthalmology. 1998;**116**(5):685. DOI: 10.1001/archopht.116.5.685

[71] Kothari R, Tathe S, Gogri P, Bhandari A. Lens-induced glaucoma: The need to spread awareness about early management of cataract among rural population. ISRN Ophthalmology. 2013;**2013**:581727

[72] Shah SS, Meyer JJ. Lens Induced Glaucoma. Treasure Island (FL): StatPearls Publishing; 2022

[73] Laurenti K, Salim S. Lens-Induced glaucoma: Diagnosis and management. Eye Net Magazine, 2016

[74] Conner IP et al. Lens-induced glaucoma. In: Kahook M et al., editors. Chandler and Grant's Glaucoma. 5th ed. Thorofare, N.J: Slack; 2013. pp. 441-447

[75] Kumar S, Pegu J, et al. Retrospective audit of phacomorphic gluacoma in last 12 years in a Tertiary Eye Care Cenre, New Delhi, India. JCDR. 2021;**15**(4):18-21

[76] Papaconstantinou D et al. Lens-induced glaucoma in the elderly. Clinical Interventions in Aging. 2009;**4**:331-336

[77] Rajkumari V, Kaminibabu KS, Bhabanisana RD, Victor R. Manual small incision cataract surgery in phacomorphic glaucoma: Surgical technique and outcome in North-eastern India. Journal of Current Glaucoma Practise. 2013;**7**(2):43-48

[78] Perlman EM, Albert DM. Clinically unsuspected phacoanaphylaxis after ocular trauma. Archives of Ophthalmology. 1977;**95**(2):244-246

[79] Girkin CA, McGwin G Jr, Morris R, Kuhn F. Glaucoma following penetrating ocular trauma: A cohort study of the United States Eye Injury Registry. American Journal of Ophthalmology. 2005;**139**(1):100-105. DOI: 10.1016/j.ajo.2004.08.052

[80] Girkin CA, McGwin G Jr, Long C, Morris R, Kuhn F. Glaucoma after ocular contusion: A cohort study of the United States Eye Injury Registry. Journal of Glaucoma. 2005;**14**(6):470-473. DOI: 10.1097/01.ijg.0000185437.92803.d7

[81] Abbott J, Shah P. The epidemiology and etiology of pediatric ocular trauma. Survive in Ophthalmology. 2013;**58**:476-485

[82] Sihota R, Sood NN, Agarwal HC. Traumatic glaucoma. Acta Ophthalmologica Scandinavica. 1995;**73**(3):252-254

[83] Sihota R, Kumar S, Gupta V, et al. Early predictors of traumatic glaucoma after closed globe injury: Trabecular pigmentation, widened angle recess, and higher baseline intraocular pressure. Archives of Ophthalmology. 2008;**126**(7):921-926. DOI: 10.1001/archopht.126.7.921

[84] Gutteridge IF, Hall AJ. Acute anterior uveitis in primary care. Clinicaal and Experimental Optometry. 2007;**90**(2):70-82

[85] Herschler J. Trabecular damage due to blunt anterior segment injury and its relationship to traumatic glaucoma.

Transactions of Ophthalmology. 1977;**83**(2):239-248

[86] Coles WH. Traumatic hyphema: An analysis of 235 cases. Southern Medical Journal. 1968;**61**(8):813-816

[87] Berrios RR, Dreyer EB. Traumatic hyphema. International Ophthalmology Clinics. 1995;**35**(1):93-103

[88] Brandt MT, Haug RH. Traumatic hyphema: A comprehensive review. Journal of Oral and Maxillofacial Surgery. 2001;**59**(12):1462-1470

[89] Gharaibeh A, Savage HI, Scherer RW, Goldberg MF, Lindsley K. Medical interventions for traumatic hyphema. Cochrane Database System Review. 2019;**1**(1):CD005431

[90] Read J, Goldberg MF. Comparison of medical treatment for traumatic hyphema. Transactions on American Academy Ophthalmology Otolaryngology. 1974;**78**:799-815

[91] Read J. Traumatic hyphema: Surgical vs medical management. Annals of Ophthalmology. 1975;**7**(5):659

[92] Baig MS, Ahmed J, Ali MA. Role of trabeculectomy in the management of hypertensive traumatic total hyphaema. Journal of the College of Physicians and Surgeons–Pakistan. 2009;**19**(8):496-499

[93] Kaplowitz K, Nobe M, Abazari A, Honkanen R. Trabeculectomy for traumatic hyphema in sickle cell trait. Seminars in Ophthalmology. 2015;**30**(4):297-304. DOI: 10.3109/08820538.2013.847108

[94] Blanton FM. Anterior chamber angle recession and secondary glaucoma. A study of 847 the aftereffects of traumatic hyphema. Archives of Ophthalmology. 1964;**72**:39-43

[95] Canavan YM, Archer DB. Anterior segment consequences of blunt ocular injury. British Journal of Ophthalmology. 1982;**66**:549-555

[96] Kaufman JH, Tolpin DW. Glaucoma after traumatic angle recession: A ten-year prospective study. American Journal of Ophthalmology. 1974;**78**(4):648-654

[97] Tesluk GC, Spaeth GL. The occurrence of primary open-angle glaucoma in the fellow eye of patients with unilateral angle-cleavage glaucoma. Ophthalmology. 1985;**92**(7):904-911. DOI: 10.1016/s0161-6420(85)33936-2

[98] AlObaida I, Aljasim LA. Selective laser trabeculoplasty in patients with angle recession glaucoma: A small case series. American Journal of Ophthalmology. 2020;**19**:100835

[99] Mermoud A, Salmon JF, Straker C, Murray AD. Post-traumatic angle recession glaucoma: A risk factor for bleb failure after trabeculectomy. The British Journal of Ophthalmology. 1993;**77**(10):631-634. DOI: 10.1136/bjo.77.10.631

[100] Senthil S, Dangeti D, Battula M, Rao HL, Garudadri C. Trabeculectomy with Mitomycin-C in post-traumatic angle recession glaucoma in phakic eyes with no prior intraocular intervention. Seminars in Ophthalmology. 2022;**37**(2):171-176. DOI: 10.1080/08820538.2021.1945116

[101] Manners T, Salmon JF, Barron A, Willies C, Murray AD. Trabeculectomy with mitomycin C in the treatment of post-traumatic angle recession glaucoma. The British Journal of Ophthalmology. 2001;**85**(2):159-163. DOI: 10.1136/bjo.85.2.159

[102] Kaushik J, Parihar JKS, Singh A, et al. Evaluation of primary Ahmed

Glaucoma valve implantation in post-traumatic angle recession glaucoma in Indian eyes. International Journal of Ophthalmology. 2021;**10**:1007

[103] Matsuo T. Photoreceptor outer segments in aqueous humor: Key to understanding a new syndrome. Survey of Ophthalmology. 1994;**39**:211-233

[104] Bojikian KD, Stein AL, Slabaugh MA, Chen PP. Incidence and risk factors for traumatic intraocular pressure elevation and traumatic glaucoma after open-globe injury. Eye (London). 2015; **29**(12):1579-1584. DOI: 10.1038/eye.2015.173. Epub: 2015 Sep 18. PMID: 26381097; PMCID: PMC5129804

[105] Osman EA, Al-Fawaz N, Al-Otaibi AG. Glaucoma after open globe injury at a tertiary care university hospital in Central Saudi Arabia. Cumulative incidence and risk factors. Saudi Medical Journal. 2013;**34**:374-378

[106] Turalba AV, Shah AS, Andreoli MT. Predictors and outcomes of ocular hypertension after open-globe injury. Journal of Glaucoma. 2014;**23**:5-10

[107] Osman EA, Mousa A, Al-Mansouri SM, Al-Mezaine HS. Glaucoma after open-globe injury at a tertiary care university hospital: Cumulative causes and management. Journal of Glaucoma. 2016; **25**(3):e170-e174. DOI: 10.1097/IJG.0000000000000162. PMID: 25265009

[108] Ballantyne JF. Siderosis bulbi. The British Journal of Ophthalmology. 1954; **38**(12):727-733

[109] Vannas S. Hemosiderosis in eyes with secondary glaucoma after delayed intraocular hemorrhages. Acta Ophthalmology. 1960;**38**:254-267

[110] Muñoz-Negrete FJ, Moreno-Montañés J, Hernández-Martínez P, et al. Current approach in the diagnosis and management of uveitic glaucoma. Biomedical Research International. 2015; **2015**:742792

[111] Sng CC, Ang M, Barton K. Uveitis and glaucoma: New insights in the pathogenesis and treatment. Progress in Brain Research. 2015;**221**:243-269

[112] Moorthy R, Mermoud A, Baerveldt G, et al. Glaucoma associated with uveitis. Survive in Ophthalmology. 1997; **41**:361-394

[113] Toris CB, Pederson JE. Aqueous humor dynamics in experimental iridocyclitis. Investment in Ophthalmological Visual Science. 1987; **28**(3):477-481

[114] Kok H, Barton K. Uveitic glaucoma. Ophthalmological Clinical North America. 2002;**15**(3):375-387

[115] Freddo TF, Patterson MM, Scott DR. Influence of mercurial sulfhydryl agents On aqueous outflow pathway in enucleated human eyes. Investigative Ophthalmology & Visual Science. 1984; **25**:278-285

[116] Roth M, Simmons RJ. Glaucoma associated with precipitates on the trabecular meshwork. Ophthalmology. 1979;**86**:1613-1619

[117] Chiang TS, Thomas RP. Ocular hypertension following infusion of prostaglandin E_1. Archives of Ophthalmology. 1972;**88**:418-420

[118] Epstein DL, Hashimoto JM, Grant WM. Serum obstruction of aqueous outflow in enucleated eyes. American Journal of Ophthalmology. 1978;**86**:101-105

[119] Panek WC, Holland GN, Lee DA, Christensen RE. Glaucoma in patients

with uveitis. British Journal of Ophthalmology. 1990;**74**:223-227

[120] Krupin T, Feite ME. Glaucoma associated with uveitis. In: Ritch R, Shields MB, Krupin T, editors. The Glaucomas. CV Mosby: St Louis; 1989. pp. 1205-1223

[121] Oguz E, Alasehirli B, Pehlivan Y, et al. Association between Rho-kinase (ROCK2) gene polymorphisms and Behçet's disease. Translational Research. 2012;**160**:428-434

[122] Brooks AMV, Grant G, Young T, et al. Cyclitic glaucoma. Australian New Zealand Journal of Ophthalmology. 1989; **17**:1.57-1.1164

[123] Pavlin CJ, Easterbrook M, Harasiewicz K, Foster FS. An ultrdsound biomicroscopic analysis of angle-closure gbducomd secondary to ciliochoroidal effusion in IgA nephropathy. American Journal of Ophthalmology. 1993;**116**:341-345

[124] Renfro L, Snow JS. Ocular effects of topical and systemic steroids. Dermatologic Clinics. 1992;**10**:505-510

[125] Kimura SJ, Hogan MJ, Thygeson P. Fuch's syndrome of heterochromic cyclitis. A.M.A. Archives of Ophthalmology. 1955;**54**:179-186

[126] Hirose S, Ohno S, Matsuda H. HLA Bw 54 and glaucomocyclitic crisis. Archives of Ophthalmology. 1985;**103**: 1837-1839

[127] Matsuda K, Izawa Y, Mishima S. Prostaglandins and glaucomatocyclitic crisis. Japan Journal of Ophthalmology. 1975;**19**:368-375

[128] Foster CS et al. Secondary glaucoma in patients with juvenile rheumatoid arthritis-associated iridocyclitis. Acta Ophthalmologica Scandinavica. 2000;**78** (5):576-579

[129] Becker B. Intraocular pressure response to topical steroids. Invest Ophthalmology. 1965;**4**:198-205

[130] Yaylali V, Ozbay D, Tatlipinar S. Efficacy and safety of rimexolone 1% versus prednisolone acetate 1% in the control of postoperative inflammation following phacoemulsification cataract surgery. International Ophthalmology. 2004;**25**:65-68

[131] Rothova A. Corticosteroids in uveitis. Ophthalmology Clinics of North America. 2002;**15**:389-394

[132] Friedman DS, Holbrook JT, Ansari H, Alexander J, Burke A, et al. Risk of elevated intraocular pressure and glaucoma in patients with uveitis: Results of the multicenter uveitis steroid treatment trial. Ophthalmology. 2013; **120**(8):1571-1579

[133] Sen HN, Vitale S, Gangaputra SS, Nussenblatt RB, Liesegang TL, et al. Periocular corticosteroid injections in uveitis: Effects and complications. Ophthalmology. 2014 Nov;**121**(11):2275-2286

[134] Jones NP. The Manchester Uveitis Clinic: The first 3000 patients, 2: Uveitis Manifestations, Complications, Medical and Surgical Management. Ocular Immunology and Inflammation. 2015;**23** (2):127-134

[135] Larkin G, Lightman S. Mycophenolate mofetil. A useful immunosuppressive in inflammatory eye disease. Ophthalmology. 1999;**106**:370-374

[136] Hesselink DA, Baarsma GS, Kuijpers RW. Experience with cyclosporine in endogenous uveitis

posterior. Transplantation Proceedings. 2004;**36**:372-377

[137] Durrani K, Papaliodis GN, Foster CS. Pulse IV cyclophosphamide in ocular inflammatory disease: Efficacy and short-term safety. Ophthalmology. 2004;**111**:960-965

[138] Goldstein DA, Fontanilla FA, Kaul S. Long-term follow-up of patients treated with short-term high-dose chlorambucil for sight-threatening ocular inflammation. Ophthalmology. 2002;**109**:370-377

[139] Diederen RM, Hulsman CA, Zegers RH, Verbraak FD. Outcomes and complications of Baerveldt glaucoma drainage implants for the treatment of uveitisrelated glaucoma. Acta Ophthalmologica. 2018;**96**(6):e752-e753

[140] Ku WN, Lin CJ, Tsai YY. The rescue effect of adalimumab in the treatment of refractory pediatric panuveitis complicated with steroid-induced glaucoma. Taiwan Journal of Ophthalmology. 2018;**8**(3):164-167

[141] Kulkarni A, Barton K. Uveitic glaucoma. In: Shaarawy TM, Sherwood MB, Hitchings RA, Crowston JC, editors. Glaucoma Volume I. 2nd ed. St. Louis, MO: Saunders Ltd.; 2015

[142] Siddique SS, Suelves AM, Baheti U, et al. Glaucoma and uveitis. Survive in Ophthalmology. 2013;**58**:1-10

[143] Ohno S, Ichiishi A, Matsuda H. Hypotensive effect of carteolol on intraocular pressure elevation and secondary glaucoma associated with endogenous uveitis. Ophthalmologica. 1989;**199**:41-45

[144] Dailey RA, Brubaker RF, Bourne WM. The effects of timolol maleate and acetazolamide on the rate of aqueous formation in normal human subjects. American Journal of Ophthalmology. 1982;**93**:232-237

[145] Sponsel WE, Paris G, Trigo Y, et al. Latanoprost and brimonidine: therapeutic and physiologic assessment before and after oral nonsteroidal antiinflammatory therapy. American Journal of Ophthalmology. 2002;**133**: 11-18

[146] Toris CB, Camras CB, Yablonski ME. Acute versus chronic effects of brimonidine on aqueous humor dynamics in ocular hypertensive patients. American Journal of Ophthalmology. 1999;**128**:8-14

[147] Kusuhara S, Katsuyama A, Matsumiya W, Nakamura M. Efficacy and safety of ripasudil, a Rho-associated kinase inhibitor, in eyes with uveitic glaucoma. Graefe's Archive for Clinical and Experimental Ophthalmology. 2018 Apr;**256**(4):809-814

[148] Ramdas WD, Pals J, Rothova A, Wolfs RCW. Efficacy of glaucoma drainage devices in uveitic glaucoma and a meta-analysis of the literature. Graefe's Archive for Clinical and Experimental Ophthalmology. 2019;**257**(1):143-151. DOI: 10.1007/s00417-018-4156-9. Epub: 2018 Oct 11. PMID: 30310971; PMCID: PMC6323086

[149] Agraval U, Qi N, Stewart P, Luo X, Williams G, Rotchford A, et al. Optimum size of iridotomy in uveitis. Clinical & Experimental Ophthalmology. 2015;**43**(7):692-696

[150] Kalin-Hajdu E, Hammamji K, Gagne S, Harasymowycz P. Outcome of viscodilation and tensioning of Schlemm's canal for uveitic glaucoma. Canadian Journal of Ophthalmology. 2014;**49**(5):414-419

[151] Sung VC, Barton K. Management of inflammatory glaucomas. Current Opinion in Ophthalmology. 2004; **15**:136-140

[152] Netland PA, Denton NC. Uveitic glaucoma. Contemporary Ophthalmology. 2006;**5**:1-26

[153] Da MA et al. Management of uveitic glaucoma with Ahmed glaucoma valve implantation. Ophthalmology. 1999;**106**: 2168-2172

[154] Ceballos EM, Parrish RK, Schiffman JC. Outcome of Baerveldt glaucoma drainage implants for the treatment of uveitic glaucoma. Ophthalmology. 2002; **109**:2256-2260

[155] Kuchtey RW, Lowder CY, Smith SD. Glaucoma in patients with ocular inflammatory disease. Ophthalmology Clinics of North America. 2005;**18**: 421-430

[156] Shimizu A, Maruyama K, Yokoyama Y, Tsuda S, Ryu M, Nakazawa T. Characteristics of uveitic glaucoma and evaluation of its surgical treatment. Clinical Ophthalmology. 2014;**8**:2383-2389

[157] Hill RA, Nguyen QH, Baerveldt G, et al. Trabeculectomy and molteno implantation for glaucomas associated with uveitis. Ophthalmology. 1993;**100**: 903-908

[158] Hoskins DH, Hetherington J, Shaffer RN. Surgical management of the inflammatory glaucomas. Perspect Ophthalmol. 1977;**1**: 173-181

[159] Stavrou P, Misson GP, Rowson NJ, et al. Trabeculectomy in uveitis: Are antimetabolites necessary at the first procedure? Ocular Immunology and Inflammation. 1995;**3**:209-216

[160] Stavrou P, Murray PI. Long-term follow-up of trabeculectomy without antimetabolites in patients with uveitis. American Journal of Ophthalmology. 1999;**128**:434-439

[161] Wright MM, McGehee RF, Pederson JE. Intraoperative mitomycin-C for glaucoma associated with ocular inflammation. Ophthalmic Surgery and Lasers. 1997;**28**:370-376

[162] Bao N, Jiang ZX, Coh P, Tao LM. Long-term outcomes of uveitic glaucoma treated with Ahmed valve implant in a series of Chinese patients. International Journal of Ophthalmology. 2018;**11**(4): 629-634

[163] Brown GC, Magargal LE, Schachat A, et al. Neovascular glaucoma: Etiologic considerations. Ophthalmology. 1984;**91**: 315

[164] The Central Retinal Vein Occlusion Group. A randomized clinical trial of early panretinal photocoagulation for ischemic central vein occlusion- The central vein occlusion study group report. Ophthalmology. 1995;**102**:1434-1444

[165] Cairns JE. Rationale for therapy in neovascular glaucoma. Transaction on Ophthalmological Society U K. 1981;**101**: 184-185

[166] Christakis PG, Tsai JC, Kalenak JW, et al. The Ahmed Versus Baerveldt Study. Ophthalmology. 2013;**120**:2232-2240

[167] Ma KT, Yang JY, Kim JH, et al. Surgical results of ahmed valve implantation with intraoperative bevacizumab injection in patients with Neovascular glaucoma. Journal of Glaucoma. 2012;**21**:331-336

[168] Meyer-Schwickerath R, Pfeiffer A, Blum WF, et al. Vitreous levels of the

insulin-like growth factors I and II, and the insulin-like growth factor binding proteins 2 and 3, increase in neovascular eye diseases.Studies in nondiabetic and diabetic subjects. Journal of Clinical Investment. 1993;**92**:2620-2625

[169] Chen KH, Wu CC, Roy S, et al. Increased interleukin-6 in aqueous humor of neovascular glaucoma. Investment in Ophthalmological Visual Science;**40**:2627-2632

[170] Senger D, Connolly D, Van de Walter L, et al. Purification and NH2-terminal amino acid sequence of guinea pig tumor-secreted vascular permeability factor. Cancer Research. 1990;**50**:1774

[171] Sanborn GE, Symes DJ, Margargal LE. Fundus-iris fluorescein angiography: Evaluation of its use in the diagnosis of rubeosis iridis. Annals of Ophthalmology. 1986;**18**:52

[172] Teich SA, Walsh JB. A grading system for iris neovascularization. American Academy of Ophthalmology. 1981:1102-1106

[173] Weiss DI, Gold D. Neofibrovascularization of iris and anterior chamber angle: A clinical classification. Annals of Ophthalmology. 1978;**10**(4):488-491

[174] Callahan MA, Hilton GF. Photocoagulation and rubeosis iridis. American Journal of Ophthalmology. 1974;**78**:873

[175] Jaffe GJ, Burton TC. Progression of nonproliferative diabetic retinopathy following cataract extraction. Archives of Ophthalmology. 1988;**106**:745

[176] Bellows AR. Cyclocryotherapy for glaucoma. International Ophthalmology Clinics. 1981;**21**:99

[177] Brown GC. Isolated central retinal artery obstruction in association with ocular neovascularization. American Journal of Ophthalmology. 1983;**96**:110

[178] Duker JS, Sivalingam A, Brown GC. A prospective study of acute central retinal artery obstruction: The incidence of secondary ocular neovascularization. Archives of Ophthalmology. 1991;**109**: 339

[179] Brucker AJ, Hoffman ME, Neuyas HJ, et al. New instrumentation for fluid-air exchange. Retina. 1983;**3**:135

[180] McGuire D, Crowston J, Weinreb R, Goldbaum M. Managing neovascular glaucoma with bevacizumab. Glaucoma Today. 2006;**4**(4):23-24

[181] Moataz E, Gheith ME, Siam GA, de Barros DS, Garg SJ, Moster MR. Role of intravitreal bevacizumab in neovascular glaucoma. Journal of Ocular Pharmacology and Therapeutics. 2007; **23**(5):487-491. DOI: 10.1089/jop.2007.0036. PMID: 17900231

[182] Higashide T, Ohkubo S, Sugiyama K. Long-term outcomes and prognostic factors of trabeculectomy following intraocular bevacizumab injection for neovascular glaucoma. PLoS One. 2015 Aug 14;**10**(8):e0135766

[183] Wakabayashi T, Oshima Y, Sakaguchi H, Ikuno Y, Miki A, Gomi F, et al. Intravitreal bevacizumab to treat iris neovascularization and neovascular glaucoma secondary to ischemic retinal diseases in 41 consecutive cases. Ophthalmology. 2008;**115**(9):1571-1580

[184] Saito Y, Higashide T, Takeda H, Ohkubo S, Sugiyama K. Beneficial effects of preoperative intravitreal bevacizumab on trabeculectomy outcomes in neovascular glaucoma. Acta Ophthalmology. 2010;**88**(1):96-102

[185] Takihara Y, Inatani M, Kawaji T, Fukushima M, Iwao M, et al. Combined intravitreal bevacizumab and trabeculectomy with Mitomycin C Versus Trabeculectomy With Mitomycin C alone for neovascular glaucoma. Journal of Glaucoma. 2011;**20**(3):196-201

[186] Mahdy RA, Nada WM, Fawzy KM, Alnashar HY, Almosalamy SM. Efficacy of intravitreal bevacizumab with panretinal photocoagulation followed by Ahmed valve implantation in neovascular glaucoma. Journal of Glaucoma. 2013;**22**(9):768-772

[187] Nakatake S, Yoshida S, Nakao S, Arita R, Yasuda M, Kita T, et al. Hyphema is a risk factor for failure of trabeculectomy in neovascular glaucoma: A retrospective analysis. BMC Ophthalmology. 2014;**14**:55. DOI: 10.1186/1471-2415-14-55. PMID: 24766841; PMCID: PMC4026882

[188] Shen CC, Salim S, Du H, Netland PA. Trabeculectomy versus Ahmed Glaucoma Valve implantation in neovascular glaucoma. Clinical Ophthalmology. 2011;**5**:281-286

[189] Sevim MS, Buttanri IB, Kugu S, Serin D, Sevim S. Effect of intravitreal bevacizumab injection before Ahmed glaucoma valve implantation in neovascular glaucoma. Ophthalmologica. 2013;**229**(2):94-100

[190] Krupin T, Johnson MF, Becker B. Anterior segment ischemia after cyclocryotherapy. American Journal of Ophthalmology. 1977;**84**:426-428

[191] Shields MB, Shields SE. Non-contact transscleral Nd:YAG cyclophotocoagulation: A long-term follow-up of 500 patients. Transactions of the American Ophthalmological Society. 1994;**92**:271-283

[192] Schuman JS, Puliafito CA, Allingham RR, et al. Contact transscleral continuous wave neodymium: YAG laser cyclophotocoagulation. Ophthalmology. 1990;**97**:571

[193] Shchomak Z, Cordeiro Sousa D, Leal I, Abegão Pinto L. Surgical treatment of neovascular glaucoma: A systematic review and meta-analysis. Graefe's Archive for Clinical and Experimental Ophthalmology. 2019;**257**(6):1079-1089

Section 4

Glaucoma: New Frontiers

Chapter 6

Molecular Genomics of Glaucoma: An Update

Govindasamy Kumaramanickavel, Siddhita Jadhav, Sugirdhana Parthiban Ramsait and Pinakin Gunvant Davey

Abstract

Glaucoma is in the top five age-related eye disorders with increasing prevalence globally. Past research has led to the understanding of glaucoma as a neurodegenerative disease. Glaucoma phenomics could be syndromic or non-syndromic. Globally primary open angle, primary angle closure and primary pseudoexfoliation glaucomas are widely present. The genetics and genomics of glaucoma are heterogeneous, both clinically and genetically. Glaucoma has heritability associations, particularly with central corneal thickness, retinal nerve fibre layer and peripapillary atrophy. Ocular embryogenesis genes when mutated could cause either local (*in situ*), pan-ocular or systemic syndromic glaucoma phenomics. In glaucoma, except for a few single gene causes, most of the associations have been shown with innumerable gene single-nucleotide polymorphisms and epigenetic factors. The biological mechanisms in glaucoma are mechanical strain, inflammation, oxidative stress, vascular dysregulation, and immune imbalance, which independently or collectively contribute to the neurodegeneration and visual morbidity. Biomarkers in glaucoma have experimental study biases and therefore today we cannot apply them effectively in clinical practice and henceforth that demands further research to understand the fundamental basis of the disease. However, the knowledge gained in research will translate into early detection and biomolecular interventional strategies, having traction toward personalised medicine.

Keywords: age-related eye diseases, biomarkers, biomechanisms, epigenetics, glaucoma, genomewide associations, genetics, gene therapy, neurodegeneration, neuroprotection, personalised medicine

1. Introduction

Genetics is usually the study of a gene and the corresponding physiological trait or disease phenotype, which is inherited through generations; whereas genomics is the study of all the genes, genes expressed in the person's genome which are responsible for a physiological or pathophysiological phenotype (phenomics) in the health or disease. The phenotype of glaucoma is heterogeneous, varying from a spectrum of normal tension, high tension to retinal ganglion cell death and visual morbidity. Similarly, the molecular genomics of glaucoma is complex, which is unlike corneal, lens or retinal genomics, where the seat of the disease is localised to the site of the respective tissues. However, in contrast glaucoma is pan ocular – extending from the anterior segment to posterior segment of the eye and the optic nerve, and thus, several anatomical regional tissues of the eye and genes, gene expressions are the stakeholders in the molecular mechanism of glaucoma. In addition, the disease outcome is measurable in the tears, aqueous humour, ciliary body, trabecular meshwork, vitreous body, lamina cribrosa (superficial nerve fibre layer, retinal ganglion cells, prelaminar region, laminar region, retrolaminar region), retina, optic nerve, serum and blood, which collectively blurs a single cause and effect of the glaucoma machinery [1, 2]. At the same time, these candidates remain to be the barriers and opportunities in glaucoma screening measures, early clinical detection, effective clinical management, valuable prognostication and futuristic molecular interventions.

The genetics of glaucoma is less of Mendelian and more of complex nature, perhaps more diverse compared to any other age-related eye diseases (ARED), like for example, age-related macular degeneration (AMD). In glaucoma genomics, there are very few genes which behave as a Mendelian single gene disease, while several genes and single nucleotide polymorphisms (SNPs), gene expression modulations, correspond to the pathophysiological traits as a neurodegenerative disease. There are a couple of hundred genes, several hundred SNPs, and many microRNAs which all are associated with ARED glaucoma phenomics. Many of the genomewide association studies are robust, where large collaborative sample sizes, validation studies, across different populations have been designed, executed and published. The molecular mechanisms of glaucoma are a spectrum of clinical outcomes played by several biological actors, beginning from inflammation, oxidative stress, extracellular matrix dysregulation, immune system imbalance, neuroprotection, neurodegeneration, apoptosis, metabolites accumulation, to abnormal lipid factors. However, most of the molecular genomic factor studies are not robust and are unfortunately poorly validated. Besides, glaucoma manifests in the elderly as a result of mix and match with other AREDs visual morbidities like cataract, corrected or uncorrected refractive errors, AMD, and diabetic retinopathy and therefore usually may not be isolated. For example, a person with glaucoma may have cataracts and/or AMD as well, again this could be another bias factor in the molecular genomics laboratory studies. Nevertheless, in this review, we shall have an in-depth overview of the molecular genetics and genomic factors associated with the pathophysiological mechanisms of glaucoma. However, the review also provides a larger insight into the visual impairment, prevalence, and comorbidities, besides the genetics and genomics of glaucoma. However, it is beyond the scope of the review to provide a gist of all the biological, experimental, epidemiological, genetic and genomic studies in glaucoma and hence, kindly refer to the references provided at the end, for further information.

2. Glaucoma in general

2.1 Visual impairment, age-related disorders and the central role of glaucoma

In the elderly, glaucoma cannot be viewed as an isolated pathology and it is frequently associated with other age-related visual and systemic comorbidities like ocular (cataracts, age-related macular degeneration, type 2 diabetes mellitus and its complications, visual impairments, diabetic retinopathy) and non-ocular (airways diseases, coronary artery disease, hypertension, heart failure, dementia, depression, et cetera). Besides, the treatment of glaucoma will have an effect on some of the morbidities mentioned [3]. As the population of the aged increase, common causes of visual morbidity increase significantly. In 2015, the three top causes of blindness were preventable - cataract, uncorrected refractive error (URE) and glaucoma, whereas for visual impairment it is URE, cataract and AMD. Effective and largescale eyecare service is required to combat these problems [4]. In 2017, Ackland et al., published that 253 million people are visually impaired with 217 million moderately or severely visually impaired (MSVI) and 36 million blind and they estimate that by 2050 these numbers would climb sharply to 588 million MSVI and 115 million blind globally [5]. About 89% of the VI live in low or middle-income countries and 55% of them are women. About 1.1 billion people have uncorrected functional presbyopia. Though the prevalence of VI has reduced from 4.58% to 3.38%, more thrust has to be given to reduce it further [5]. Eckert et al., estimated the cost of blindness as US$ 7.8 billion in the US and the cost of MSVI as US$ 16.5 billion, however, Gordois et al., estimated the cost of VI as a staggering US$ 3 trillion and the direct costs as US$ 2.3 trillion and also mentions that these figures could increase by 20% by the year 2020 [6]. Another non-profit organisation of Prevent Blindness in America estimates that the economic burden of adult vision problems (AMD, cataract, diabetic retinopathy, glaucoma, refractive errors, VI and blindness) in the US in 2007 as US$ 54.1 billion annually, which includes direct medical, direct-other and loss of productivity costs, however, they revised the figure to US$ 139 billion in a 2013 report [7].

In 2015, it was estimated that the moderate to severe VI affected 216.6 million globally, with the URE being the leading cause, and blindness prevalent amongst 36 million with cataract outnumbering the other causes [4]. The proportion of those with preventable or treatable blindness and VI is reducing in trend over the decades, fortunately, as mentioned earlier, due to the control of infectious and nutritional causes. And amongst those with visual morbidity, aged individuals comprise the maximum, having the distribution variable between the developed and developing countries [8, 9]. ARED, such as AMD, cataract, diabetic retinopathy (DR), glaucoma and refractive errors are the key components of global visual morbidity and cataract forms more than half of all those affected in the group. Amongst those, 70–74 years of age 37% have cataract, 10% AMD, 3% glaucoma and 2% DR [10]. Out of the 285 million with VI and blindness, those above 50 years of age constitute 65% of the VI and 82% of blindness. In addition, due to poor socio-economic status and biological element like longevity, 75% of those affected with ARED are women and this factor is consistent irrespective of the fact that whether women live in developed or developing countries [11, 12].

In Germany, ARED commonly found were cataract, dry eye, AMD and glaucoma, furthermore, they found that the aged individuals had different combinations of these conditions [13]. Asia has one of the highest representations of the blind, with India having the highest prevalence of 11.9% and Malaysia with the lowest of 0.3% [14]. Due to the robust epidemiological studies, ARED in Asia includes, along similar lines to that of the West, cataract, refractive errors, glaucoma, DR and AMD. AMD is prevalent in both the developed and developing countries as being the cause of blindness and VI, the prevalence of the disease is higher in the West, but the emerging trends and patterns from China, India, Japan, Mongolia, Singapore to Taiwan are echoing the West, due to the growing aged populations [14]. ARED in Iran had a similar pattern to most Asian countries with 35.8% having either cataract, AMD, glaucoma or DR and moreover one in two of those over 75 years of age have these conditions [15]. In the US, a third of the subjects were either 80 years or over who had cataract, AMD, primary open-angle glaucoma (POAG), DR or VI and two-thirds had late AMD. In addition, POAG, VI and DR were prevalent at a higher age amongst

Hispanics and Blacks, whereas cataract and late AMD prevalence were higher amongst the Whites [16]. The prevalence of ARED in Canada increased alarmingly after the age of 75 years [17]. In high-income Eastern and Central European countries, blindness and mild to severe VI reduced between 1990 and 2015 from 0.26% to 0.15% and from 1.74% to 1.27%, respectively and similar trends were observed in Australasia, North America and Western Europe. One in 28, above 40 years have low vision in the USA [18]. Conflicting reports are available in the US demonstrating that vision screening methods could improve the visual status of a community, in older adults [19]. In Britain, Prasad et al., observed that diabetes was not the primary factor for the prevalence of blindness and MSVI, whereas non-diabetes factors were particularly responsible [20, 21]. In Latin America for the elderly, 50 years of age or above, the prevalence of blindness varied from 1.1% in Argentina to 4.4% in Guatemala, with cataract being the foremost reason, however, DR and glaucoma are rising and infectious diseases are declining [22]. In the population of Indian origin in Singapore, 40 years or above, the prevalence of VI and blindness were 3.4% and 0.4% respectively, far lower than in India, for which cataract, DR, AMD and glaucoma were the leading causes and the first was the primary cause [23, 24]. ARED in Singapore Indians 40 years or above irrespective of education level, literacy or immigration types were deteriorating and active screening measures should be implemented rather than voluntary enrolment is emphasised [25].

With the ageing population, rising in proportion across the world despite the fall in birth rates, the corresponding increase in morbidity and mortality amongst the group is worrying. Universal health coverage and eye health objectives are persevering to reduce global visual morbidity for which robust databases are key to achieving the goals [26–28]. Biological understanding of ARED, not only clinical screening, is equally important for the prevention and management of the diseases. Oxidative stress and inflammation are the key causative mechanisms for ARED. Autophagy mechanisms also play both protective and detrimental outcomes in ARED and therefore nurturing preventive and therapeutic strategies [29]. Malnutrition and anaemia have been associated with poor vision besides other systemic disorders in the elderly, in a study from southern India [30]. In a southern Indian glaucoma study, primarily around three-quarters were due to cataract and the remaining were because of glaucoma, cystoid macular oedema, optic atrophy and corneal scars and these were significantly associated with ageing ($p < 0.0001$) [31].

2.2 Prevalence of glaucoma

Globally, the five leading causes of visual impairment are, URE, cataract, AMD, glaucoma and DR. However, glaucoma is the second leading cause of loss of vision in the world. About 60.5 million people are estimated to be affected globally by glaucoma in 2010, which is equivalent to the population of Italy, and about 8.4 million of them will be suffering from bilateral irreversible blindness and there are closely varying estimates according to other studies [32]. These figures could rise to 111.8 million in 2040 and the global prevalence of glaucoma presently is around 3–4% [33, 34]. POAG is highest amongst African and Hispanic races and is found amongst all races, whereas primary angle closure glaucoma (PACG) is the highest in Asia [35, 36]. Primary congenital glaucoma (PCG) is a less common type, however primary exfoliative glaucoma (PXFG) is a comparatively more frequent disorder resulting in most common glaucoma related blindness, rather than the other types. In a focused metanalysis of five glaucoma prevalence studies in India by Geroge et al., it was estimated that in 2010 about 11.2 million would be affected with the disease and out of which 6.48 million would have POAG and 2.54 million, PACG and these figures should have increased in the decade that has passed since the publication [37]. The economic burden of glaucoma in the United States calculated by Rein et al., in 2006 was around US$ 2.9 billion, in this context we should take note that the majority of glaucoma cases are undiagnosed [38]. Studying five major prevalence studies in India, the age-standardised prevalence ranges of those 40 or 50 years or above with POAG was—1.29% to 4.24% and for PACG—0.5% to 1.11% and the reason for the wide range of variations are largely due to disparities in clinical and epidemiological study methodologies. Childhood glaucoma is constituted by primary congenital glaucoma and juvenile open angle glaucoma, which affects 1 in 10,000 to 100,000 children worldwide and the former is more prevalent in high consanguineous marriage geographical regions [33]. Pigmentary glaucoma or pigment dispersion syndrome is caused by PMEL gene variants only less than 50% of those with the variants get affected. PMEL is involved in melanin pigment synthesis, storage and transport and these pigments get deposited in the trabecular meshwork and increase the IOP.

3. Genetics and genomics of glaucoma

'Glaykoseis', a blindness in the elderly, as mentioned by Hippocrates—the Father of Modern Medicine, dates back to 400 years before Christ emerged and Amida, a Byzantine physician, named it as 'Amaurosis' [39]. Before 1850, POAG was termed as amaurosis, black cataract or gutta serena. The eyes were observed to be hard and angle-closure glaucoma caused green or grey pupils and hence the name glaucoma (blue, green or grey and viriditate occuli) and in 1850 after the ophthalmoscope invention, the scenario changed, when the term 'Glaucoma' was christened to the disease, which has not changed until today [39]. Ganglionic optic neuropathy is the pathological defect of glaucoma which leads to a painless visual loss. The molecular genetics and medical biology of glaucoma have intrigued scientists for a while, however, whatever knowledge that we have gained today is not yet as clear as compared to the inherited retinal degenerative diseases (IRDD).

3.1 Heritability of glaucoma

In the earlier days, twin studies were the proof to establish if a disease is caused by heritable or environmental factors. The twin studies in 1987 established that the heritability of POAG at 0.135 [40]. In addition, two recent robust studies with genomewide array data though parked the heritability of POAG between a wide range of 24–42% [41, 42]. The risk factors for developing glaucoma are age, ethnic origins (African Americans, Hispanics), gender (women), genetics, hypertension and increased intraocular pressure prescription drugs [43]. The prevalence of POAG was highest amongst the African race descent, then Asians, but the lowest was amongst the Europeans, showing racial and genetic preponderance. However, the genetics of the disease is complex with only 10% having Mendelian inheritance.

Central corneal thickness, intra-ocular pressure (IOP), optic disc area and vertical cup/disc ratio (VCDR) have high heritability associations across populations. Asefa et al., looked at the anterior chamber size, central corneal thickness (CCT), corneal hysteresis, cup-to-disc ratio, cup-shape, cup-size, disc-size, intraocular pressure, peripapillary atrophy (PA) and retinal never fibre layer thickness (RFNLT) in a metanalysis [44]. And the highest heritability was observed in CCT (h^2 = 0.81), RFNLT (h^2 = 0.73) and PA (h^2 = 0.73) [44].

3.2 Mendelian genetics of glaucoma

There are very few single gene defect causations in non-syndromic glaucoma, so far, four PCG loci have been located—GLC3A, B, C and D. The GLC3A region in 2p21 has the CYP1B1 gene and about 150 or so autosomal recessive mutations have been associated with PCG. The majority of patients with PCG/CYP1B1 mutations are found in Saudi Arabia and Slovakia gypsy population and these mutations have variable expressivity and incomplete penetrance with a wide range of clinical phenotypes [45]. PCG is present across the world and being an autosomal recessive disease, is more frequent in consanguineous populations, has a widely varying incidence of 1 in 1250 to 1 in 22,000 in different parts of the world and is one of the paediatric causes of blindness in India [46–48]. A consanguineous south Indian family with PCG was investigated by using homozygosity analysis. The microsatellite markers D2S177 and D2S1346 were tightly linked to CYP1B1 and the Q110X mutation in exon 2 of the gene was co-segregating in all the affected [49]. A newborn in the family was found to be a heterozygous carrier to the relief of the family during genetic counselling [45]. CYP1B1 plays a critical role in the development of the trabecular meshwork (TM) and acts in the removal of reactive oxygen species, regulating oxidative stress and production of periostin which influences the mechanical strength and structural integrity of the TM [45]. GLC3B and C have not resulted in any gene till date, but GLC3D location at 14q24 has resulted in null mutations in LTBP2 and PCG phenotype correlation. LTBP2 (latent transforming growth factor beta binding protein 2) is a matrix protein that performs cell adhesion and tissue repair processes.

Optineurin (OPTN) gene mutation is one of the causes of POAG in various populations, though it is rate. In OPTN, M98K variation is associated with POAG across populations and in our study, was less frequent cause of the disease as it was found that in 4% of HTG and 6% of NTG patients compared to the controls [50]. OPTN plays critical role in Golgi complex maintenance, membrane trafficking, exocytosis, interacts with myosin VI and Rab8.

A sensational MYOC gene location for glaucoma was identified by Stone et al. in 1997 and is one of the most investigated in glaucoma genetics [51]. The sensational was though short-lived in the history of genetics of glaucoma and it lost its steam as the frequency of the mutations started to fall to very small proportions amongst the global glaucoma populations. When we screened 100 POAG/JOAG patients for the MYOC gene, we found a G144A, Gln48His substitution, which was novel at that time, in 2% of the patients, the change was also found in another four affected members of a JOAG family. MYOC was found to not play a significant role amongst glaucoma patients in India [52]. Juvenile open angle glaucoma (JOAG) was described in a large pedigree in the US seventy years ago and today the Phe369Leu MYOC mutation was identified in the family [53].

3.3 Molecular genetics of syndromic glaucoma

Syndromic glaucoma, which are also Mendelian in nature, may not be uncommon in the paediatric age group, hence glaucoma may be associated with additional ocular and systemic phenotypes like aniridia, anterior segmental dysgenesis, collagen or vascular disorders, immunogenetic diseases, metabolic disorders and nanophthalmos. The embryogenesis of the eye is complex with both the ectoderm and neuroectoderm involved together in the formation. Mutation in genes, infections acquired during or after pregnancy, ageing and systemic disorders affect the development of the eye [45]. Axenfeld-Rieger syndrome, a disorder is prevalent in 1:200,000 individuals, which affects the anterior segment like defective cornea, iris and the extraocular features include facial, dental and skeletal abnormalities. Peters' anomaly, an autosomal dominant disorder, is another common condition affecting the anterior segment development where cornea, iris and lens resist to separate, leading to central corneal opacity and non-ocular features like cleft lip/palate, short stature, physical and mental retardation. Aniridia is another developmental condition accompanied by photophobia and poor visual acuity. The genetics of syndromic glaucoma is Mendelain.

WAGR syndrome with **W**ilms tumour, **a**niridia, **g**enitourinary anomalies and intellectual disability earlier mentioned as mental **r**etardation. In WAGR syndrome there will be chromosomal deletion at the 11p13 region which harbours many genes including mutated WT1 and/or PAX6 genes and the affected have glaucoma as well. Hence, aniridia patients should undergo an abdominal ultrasound to rule out WAGR syndrome and renal tumour. There is a rare condition of Gillespie syndrome, where patients have aniridia, ptosis and corectopia with mutation in the ITPR1 gene [54].

Collagen vascular diseases like Stickler syndrome and osteogenesis imperfecta patients have glaucoma due to trabecular meshwork impedance. Stickler syndrome patients have myopia, cataract and retinal giant tear, the iris ciliary process is long and covers the trabecular meshwork blocking the aqueous flow. The gene variants in COL2A1 and COL11A1 cause autosomal dominant Stickler syndrome, whereas variations in COL9A1 cause autosomal recessive type. Osteogenesis imperfecta has COL1A1 and COL1A2 gene variants manifesting in an autosomal dominant manner. Osteogenesis imperfecta is a collagen bone disorder with a variable five phenotypes, all mostly have low mineral density leading to bone fragility (hence the name brittle-bone disease), blue sclera, abnormal cornea, glaucoma, poorly formed dentine, the ligaments are hyper lax, cardiovascular disease and hearing loss [55]. Immune-related disorders like Aicardi-Goutieres syndrome (AGS) and Singleton-Merten syndrome (SGMRT), are severe and fatal conditions with a plethora of genes involved in RNA processing like ADAR, RNASEH2A, RNASEH2B, RNASEH2C, SAMHD1, TREX1 and the gene IFIH1 responsible for innate immunity. In a severe type, patients could have cerebral atrophy, congenital glaucoma, hepatosplenomegaly, intracranial calcification, leukodystrophy, microcephaly, thrombocytopenia and death are not uncommon. Singleto-Merten syndrome is caused by variants in the DDX58 and IFIH1 genes and has glaucoma as a clinical feature.

Nanophthalmos, with small fully formed eyes, could be inherited as both autosomal dominant and recessive types. There are several genes involved in this condition (CRB1, BEST1, FAM111A, MFRP, MYRF, PRSS56 and TIMEM98), which has additional systemic features like congenital diaphragmatic hernia, cardio-pulmonary abnormalities, glaucoma and urogenital anomalies, causing some rare genetic disorders like Kenny-Caffey syndrome [56]. MYRP, CRB1 and BEST1 are genes associated with retinal degenerative genetic disorders. TEK/ANGPT1 genes' variants independently resulted in haploinsufficiency-based primary congenital glaucoma. The genes have a critical role in the structure and function of Schlemm's canal and trabecular meshwork [57].

PITX2 (Paired Like Homeodomain 2) in chromosome 4q25 and FOXC1 Forkhead Box C1 are transcription factors jointly involved in the anterior segment development. Mutations or copy number variations in these genes result in anterior segment anomalies, due to haploinsufficiency, like Axenfeld Reiger syndrome or Peters' anomaly [58]. Axenfeld first described the anomaly in 1920 and later was added more by Reiger in 1934 [56]. A majority of the children with mutations in PITX2 and FOXC1 develop glaucoma [56]. Non-ocular systemic features include variable phenotypes like facial/dental anomalies, pituitary involvement, umbilical anomalies, syndromes like SHORT, short FRAME, cardiac defects, sensorineural deafness and myotonic dystrophy [56]. The development of the eye is highly complicated and well-studied in Drosophila and humans [59]. PAX6 gene in humans or ey gene in drosophila is the chief conductor of the biological symphony of eye development. PAX6 (Transcription factor Paired Box 6) gene in chromosome 11p13 mutation is associated with mostly aniridia but rarely Peters' anomaly and other ocular defects have also been reported [58]. Peters' anomaly could be caused by a variety of genes like PAX6, PITX2, FOXC1, CYP1B1 and B3GALTL as they all collectively during embryogenesis orchestrate the anterior segment development [56].

FOXC1 (forkhead box) gene mutation and haploinsufficiency cause anterior segment anomalies [59]. The MAF basic region leucine zipper (bZIP) transcription factors perform anterior segment and lens development and mutations in the gene in humans cause cataract and ocular developmental defects. CPAMD8 (C3 and PZP-like alpha-2-macroglobulin domain-containing protein 8) mutation causes anterior segment dysgenesis (ectropion uveae, cataract, corectopia, iridodonesis with ectopia lentis) in an autosomal recessive manner [56]. CPAMD8 is involved in the dynamics of aqueous humour.

B3GALTL (Beta-3-Glucosyltransferase) gene in 13q12.3 which glycosylates proteins and when mutated causes Peter Plus syndrome manifesting with ocular and systemic features like abnormal ears, brachydactyly, cleft lip/palate, dextrocardia, dysmorphic face, hydrocephalus and Potter syndrome [56]. SOX2 (SRY-like box2) involved in eye development is mapped to 3q26.3-27 and mutations in the gene cause sclerocornea and anophthalmia [60]. CHRDL1 (Chordin like 1) mutation causes megalocornea and Neuhauser syndrome and the gene is X-linked and located in the Xq23 region [61]. Keratoconus, myopia and glaucoma are associated with glaucoma and hence mutations in the autosomal dominant gene associated with the former is the VSX1 (Visual System Homeobox 1), a transcription factor located in 20p11.21 [62]. Genes like COL4A1, CYP1B1, FGFR2, BMP4, BMP7, FOXE3, MYOC LAMBB2 and LTBP2 are involved in anterior segment anomalies [63].

SIX3 gene mutation causes holoprosencephaly or microphthalmia and iris coloboma [59]. SIX3 interacts with Groucho-related proteins 4 and 5 and functions as an eye development repressor. Besides, PAX6 and SIX3 regulate each other during eye development. Along with FOXE3, MAF, MITF, LHX2, PITX3, PROX1, and SIX3, PAX6 forms the cornea and lens, whereas along with CHX10, EYA1 and PAX2 forms the retina and optic nerve. In addition, genes like BMP4, BMP7, RX and SHH also regulate PAX6 in eye development and mutations in them affects eye development which may result in glaucoma.

In metabolic disorders, the X-linked recessive and autosomal recessive mucopolysaccharidoses [Hurler syndrome (alpha-L-iduronidase), Hunter syndrome (iduronate2-sulfatase), Sanfilippo syndrome (heparin sulphate), Morquino syndrome (N-acetyl galactosamine-6-sulfatase), Maroteauz-Lamy syndrome (N-acetyl galactosamine-4-sulfatase), Natowicz syndrome (hyaluronidase)] gene mutations could result in defective enzyme causing cataract and glaucoma and the latter by blocking the trabecular meshwork with the glycosaminoglycans [56].

4. Complex genetics and genomics of glaucoma

Syndromic glaucoma is well understood genetically and genomically, with the fundamental knowledge of the cause and effect. However, POAG is a multifactorial disease, where embryological development, genetics, epigenetics, genetic polymorphisms, variable gene expressivity, inflammation and environmental modifiers play a collective complex role and in addition, the penetrance and expressivity may vary between affected individuals [64]. All mentioned earlier, is applicable to most of the lifestyle related complex genetic disorders. This means that the person with a genetic risk may or may not manifest the disease and hence, it is completely unlike the Mendelian genetics. Hence, the disease aetiology, onset, duration, drug response and inheritance are dependent on genetics and environmental modifiers. In addition, some non-genetic modifiers complicate the glaucoma disease status, like smoking, and comorbidities (diabetes, untreated high blood pressure) and near-sightedness [64].

Genetic Epidemiology Research in Adult Health and Ageing (GERA) is part of the UK Biobank (UKB) that has phenotype and genotypes of 500,000 participants aged 40–69 years, which has multi-ethnic glaucoma cases of 7329 and 169,561 controls [65]. Choquet et al., in a GERA study, having 4986 POAG cases and 58, 426 controls comprising of African-Americans, non-Hispanic whites, Hispanic/Latinos, and East-Asian races and ethnicities, identified 24 loci for POAG, out of which 14 were novel and 9 replicated near the genes FMNL2, PDE7B, TMTC2, IKZF2, CADM2, DGKG, ANKH, EXOC2, and LMX1B, across races, but was found higher in African-Americans. Some of the genes had functional influence like FMNL2 and LMX1B – Lmx1b mutations increase the IOP and POAG in mice. A metanalysis of GERA and UKB further identified 24 additional loci expanding the spectrum of the genetics of POAG, however, most of the variants have minimal genetic risk [66]. Burdon et al., have associated the following genes with ocular physiological traits, which are key in maintaining the IOP in POAG - ZNF469, FOXO1, COL5A1, AKAP13, AVGR8, COL8A2, IBTK, LRRK1/CHSY1, C7orf42, ATOH7, TGFBR3, CARD10, CDC7/TGFBR3, SALL1, CDKN2A/B, SIX1/SIX6, FERM8/SCYL1, DCLK1 and CHEK2 [67]. Furthermore, POAG associated candidate genes have been identified, CAV1/CAV2, TMCO1, CDKN2B-AS1, TXNRD2, ATXN2, FOXC1 and GAS7 [68, 69]. Some of the genes are consistent across various studies besides ATOH7, CAV1/CAV2, CDC7-TGFBR3, CDKN2B-AS1, GAS7, SIX1/SIX6 and TMCO1; these are not only associated with POAG but also with the quantitative traits (endophenotypes) [68]. However, some genes having mutations do affect a small proportion of those with POAG, such as cyclin-dependent kinase inhibitor 2B, myocilin (MYOC), neurotrophin 4, optineurin (OPTN), tank binding kinase 1 (TBK1) and WDR 36. Other types of glaucoma like PXFG are associated with LOXL1 and CNTNAP2 and PCG with CYP1B1 and LTBP2 [69, 70]. MYOC, OPTN and TBK1 are used in genetic diagnosis, counselling and clinical management, in addition to this list even CYP1B1 could be added [69]. Verma et al., in a complex gene–gene interaction modelling using NEIGHBOUR, eMERGE datasets and tissue expressing databases identified a new set of genes like GNG7, ROBO1, SUMF1, RYR3, SLC24A3, CCDC3, CARS2, RPS6KA, SETDB1 not only associating with POAG, but also showed that they were expressing in the eye and particularly in the trabecular meshwork [71, 72]. Transforming growth factor-β

(TGFβ) has the basic property of regulating and remodelling the extracellular matrix and hence is one of the candidate genes for glaucoma. TGFB1 –509C > T polymorphism is associated with POAG and therefore we looked at 104 patients with the disease but found no association of the SNP with VCDR, IOP and POAG [73]. VCDR is associated in glaucoma with ABCA1, ASAP1, ATOH7 and ELN gene polymorphisms [68]. GLIS1 (GLIS Family Zinc Finger 1 Kruppel-like transcription factor) variant rs941125 has shown to be associated with glaucoma in humans [74].

Though PXFG and POAG are the leading causes of blindness in glaucoma, PACG is one of the leading causes of blindness particularly in Asia and the blindness due to the latter (PACG) is 10 times more than that of POAG [75]. *PLEKHA7, COL11A1, PCMTD1 and ST18 genes related SNPs located in chromosomes* 11p15, 1p21 and 8q11.23 *were first associated with PACG* [76–78]. In major five Asian countries, a collaborative study was conducted in which 854 cases and 9608 controls (Singapore, Hong Kong, India, Malaysia and Vietnam) with replication studies on 1917 cases and 8943 controls (China, Singapore, India, Saudi Arabia and the UK, including that of the first author [GKM] team) GWAS was conducted to identify genetic factors' associated with the PACG. In the GWAS, three SNPs were significantly associated with PACG in our collaborative cohort - rs11024102 in PLEKHA7 [Pleckstrin Homology Domain Containing A7] (per-allele odds ratio (OR) = 1.22; P = 5.33 × 10(−12)), rs3753841 in COL11A1 [Collagen Type XI Alpha 1 Chain] (per-allele OR = 1.20; P = 9.22 × 10 (−10)) and rs1015213 located between PCMTD1 [Protein-L-Isoaspartate (D-Aspartate) O-Methyltransferase Domain Containing 1] and ST18 [ST18 C2H2C-Type Zinc Finger Transcription Factor] on chromosome 8q (per-allele OR = 1.50; P = 3.29 × 10(−9)) [76]. PLEKHA7 (Pleckstrin Homology Domain Containing, Family A Member 7) protein is require for zonule adherens biogenesis and maintenance, *COL1A1 implicated in myopia and MMP9 have been also associated with ACG predisposing traits* [79, 80]. COL11A1 (Collagen Type XI Alpha 1 Chain) protein may play a role in fibrillogenesis regulating the lateral growth of collagen II fibrils. PCMTD1 (Protein-L-Isoaspartate (D-Aspartate) O-Methyltransferase Domain Containing 1) protein is of the methyltransferase superfamily and ST18 (ST18 C2H2C-Type Zinc Finger Transcription Factor) protein inhibits basal transcription activity through target promoters. *There are a myriad of players implicated in PACG as predisposing traits, (extensively reviewed by Ahram et al., Aboobakar and Wiggs) like MTHFR, MFRP, CHX10, HGF, RS; PO1, C3orf26, LAMA2, GJD2, ZNRF3, CD55, MIP, ALPPL2, ZC3H11B, PRSS56, ABCC5, MYOC, CYP1B1, eNOS, PCMTD1, ST18, HSP70, SPARC, CALCRL, EPDR1, CHAT, FERMT2, DPM2, FAM102A and NEB* [77, 81]. A variety of anatomical, physiological, genetic and environmental factors individually or collectively result in PACG and hence, these associations reveal the larger etiopathogenesis network. There are many SNPs associated with PACG predisposing traits, however, the only gene so far identified which causes ACG is NNO1, which leads to nanophthalmos and hyperopia as well [77].

Primary pseudoexfoliation syndrome (PXFS) has fibrogranular extracellular debris in the anterior segment (besides systemic manifestations) which is made up of complex glycoprotein–proteoglycan that causes glaucoma in many but not all, with a preponderance in Scandinavian and Greek populations. In our cohort, we looked at *LOXL1* [Lysyl Oxidase-Like Protein 1] gene exon 1 polymorphisms - allele G of rs1048661 (R141L) and allele G of rs3825942 (G135D), which are significantly associated with XFS in various populations [82]. About 52 XFS including those with glaucoma were screened for the variations and found that allele G of rs3825942 was significantly associated (p = 0.0001) and genotype GG (p = 0.000305) with XFS in our population, which was the first Asian study [83]. Pseudo-exfoliation glaucoma is caused by polymorphisms in the lysyl oxidase like 1 (LOXL1) gene in chromosome 15 with significant associations through GWAS in many populations across the world [81]. Pseudo-exfoliation syndrome, due to the deposition of extracellular fibrillar material (basement membrane, clusterin, elastic fibre contents, elastin, fibrillin-1, laminin, fibronectin, latent TGF-B proteins) crosslinking with LOXL1, hence systemically, it may be associated with cardiovascular diseases, cerebrovascular disorders, dementia like Alzheimer's, pelvic organ prolapse and sensory neural deafness [84]. Non-coding variants in exons 1 and 2 of LOXL1 had conflicting reports [78]. CACN1A1 (Calcium Voltage-Gated Channel Subunit Alpha1 A) gene SNP variant was found to be significantly associated with ACG in the Japanese population which was validated in 17 other countries [78]. CACN1A1 helps calcium ion channel function and hence any dysregulation leads to the accumulation of XFS material on the trabecular meshwork. However, neurological disorders, familial hemiplegic migraine, epilepsy, cerebellar atrophy and episodic ataxia are associated with mutations in this gene. Another large 24 countries study significantly associated with POMP (proteasome maturation protein), TMEM136 (transmembrane protein 136), AGPAT1 (1-acylglyceroal-3phosphate O-acyltransfrase), RMBS3 (RNA binding motif single stranded interacting protein 3), SEMA6A (semaphorin 6A) and they were dysregulated [78]. In another Chinese study, The SNPs associated with the genes DENND1A (rs2479106), INSR (rs2059807), THADA (rs12478601), and TOX3 (rs4784165) [85].

5. Genomic mechanisms of glaucoma

The mechanisms of glaucoma is not understood clearly, however, increased IOP is significantly associated with structural (histopathological) and functional (physiological and molecular) distortions leading to neurodegeneration and glaucomatous modifications [86]. The mechanical physical strain and in addition collective stress effects (oxidative, reduced vascular flow, neurotrophic factors deprivation, metabolic, circulatory, immune, mitochondrial dysfunction, excitotoxicity, neuroinflammation, genetic susceptibility, vascular dysregulation) imposed on the lamina cribrosa, retinal ganglion cells and nearby optic nerve cells prevents the free flow of the axonal transport [86, 87]. Zukerman et al., in a review gave the list of genes associated with increased IOP, namely (in the same order)—*ABCA1* (ATP-Binding Cassette, Sub-Family A (ABC1), Member 1), *ABO* (alpha 1–3-N-acetylgalactosaminyltransferase and alpha 1–3-galactosyltransferase), *ADAMTS8* (ADAM Metallopeptidase With Thrombospondin Type 1 Motif 8), *ADAMTS17* (ADAM Metallopeptidase With Thrombospondin Type 1 Motif 17), *ADAMTS18-NUDT7*,(ADAM Metallopeptidase With Thrombospondin Type 1 Motif 18- Nudix Hydrolase 7), *AFAP1(*Actin Filament Associated Protein), *ANGPT1(*Angiopoietin 1), *ANTXR1(*ANTXR Cell Adhesion Molecule 1), *ARHGEF12* (Rho Guanine Nucleotide Exchange Factor 12), *ARID5B* (AT-Rich Interaction Domain 5B), *ATXN2* (Ataxin 2), *CAV1-CAV2(*Caveolin 1- Caveolin 2), *CDKN2B-AS1*(CDKN2B Antisense RNA 1), *CELF1* (CUGBP Elav-Like Family Member 1), *CYP26A1-MYOF* (Cytochrome P450 Family 26 Subfamily A Member 1- Myoferlin), *FAM125B*, (Family With Sequence Similarity 125, Member B) *FNDC3B(*Fibronectin Type III Domain Containing 3B), *FOXC1* (Forkhead Box C1), *FOXP1* (Forkhead Box P1), *GAS7* (Growth Arrest Specific 7), *GLCCI1-ICA1*

(Glucocorticoid Induced 1- Islet Cell Autoantigen 1), *GLIS3* (GLIS Family Zinc Finger 3), *GMDS* (GDP-Mannose 4,6-Dehydratase), *HIVEP3* (HIVEP Zinc Finger 3), *INCA1* (Inhibitor Of CDK, Cyclin A1 Interacting Protein 1), *LMX1B* (LIM Homeobox Transcription Factor 1 Beta), *LOC171391*, *MADD* (MAP Kinase Activating Death Domain), *MIR548F3* (MicroRNA 548f-3), *MYBPC3* (Myosin Binding Protein C3), *NDUFS3* (NADH:Ubiquinone Oxidoreductase Core Subunit S3), *NR1H3* (Nuclear Receptor Subfamily 1 Group H Member 3), *PDDC1* (Parkinson disease 7 domain containing 1), *PKHD1* (PKHD1 Ciliary IPT Domain Containing Fibrocystin/Polyductin), *PTPRJ* (Protein Tyrosine Phosphatase Receptor Type J), *RAPSN* (Receptor Associated Protein of the Synapse), *RPLP2-PNPLA2* (Ribosomal Protein Lateral Stalk Subunit P2- Patatin Like Phospholipase Domain Containing 2), *SIX1/SIX6* (SIX Homeobox 1/SIX Homeobox 6), *SEPT9* (Septin 9), *SEPT11* (Septin11), *TFEC-TES* (Transcription Factor EC- Testin LIM Domain Protein), *TMCO1* (Transmembrane And Coiled-Coil Domains 1) and *TXNRD2* (Thioredoxin Reductase 2) [2]. Majority of the genes' mechanism to cause glaucoma is not understood, however, LMX1B (LIM homeodomain) alters anterior segment development and aqueous humour dynamics; MADD (MAP kinase activating death domain) performs through TNF-a-mediated microglial activation; NR1H3, a nuclear receptor, changes IOP through ABCA1 regulated aqueous humour dynamic alterations and SEPT9, a septin protein, acts through cytoskeletal alterations [2]. In the eye, genes could specifically act at certain parts, like trabecular meshwork (LMX1B, ABCA1), ciliary body (LMX1B), lamina cribrosa (ELN), superficial retinal nerve fibre layer (NR1H3, ABCA1, MADD, ASAP1, ATOH7) and prelaminar region (SEPT9) region [88]. LMX1B mutations have been associated with nail-patella syndrome (nail dysplasia, the patella is absent or is hypoplastic, chronic kidney disease) and a third of these patients develop glaucoma, due to increased IOP [89].

There are several genes significantly associated with CDR, namely, as cited alphabetically by Zukerman et al., – *ABCA1* (ATP-Binding Cassette, Sub-Family A (ABC1), Member 1), *ABG*, *ADAMTS8* (ADAM Metallopeptidase With Thrombospondin Type 1 Motif 8), *ASAP1* (ArfGAP With SH3 Domain, Ankyrin Repeat And PH Domain 1), *ASB7* (Ankyrin Repeat And SOCS Box Containing 7), *ATOH7* (Atonal BHLH Transcription Factor 7), *ATOH7-PBLD* (Atonal BHLH Transcription Factor 7- Phenazine Biosynthesis Like Protein Domain Containing), *BMP2* (Bone Morphogenetic Protein 2), *CARD10* (Caspase Recruitment Domain Family Member 10), *CDC7-TGFBR3* (Cell Division Cycle 7- Transforming Growth Factor Beta Receptor 3), *CDKN2B* (Cyclin Dependent Kinase Inhibitor 2B), *CDKN2B-CDKN2BAS* (Cyclin Dependent Kinase Inhibitor 2B-CDKN2B Antisense RNA 1), *CHEK2* (Checkpoint Kinase 2), *COL8A1* (Collagen Type VIII Alpha 1 Chain), *CRISPLD1* (Cysteine Rich Secretory Protein LCCL Domain Containing 1), *DCLK1* (Doublecortin Like Kinase 1), *DGKB* (Diacylglycerol Kinase Beta), *DUSP1* (Dual Specificity Phosphatase 1), *ELN* (Elastin), *ENO4* (Enolase 4), *EXOC2* (Exocyst Complex Component 2), *F5* (Coagulation Factor V), *FAM101A* (Family With Sequence Similarity 101, Member A), *GAS7* (Growth Arrest Specific 7), *HSF2* (Heat Shock Transcription Factor 2), *PDZD2* (PDZ Domain Containing 2), *PLCE1* (Phospholipase C Epsilon 1), *PSCA* (Prostate Stem Cell Antigen), *RARB* (Retinoic Acid Receptor Beta), *RERE* (Arginine-Glutamic Acid Dipeptide Repeats), *RPAP3* (RNA Polymerase II Associated Protein 3), *RPE65* (Retinoid Isomerohydrolase RPE65), *RREB1* (Ras Responsive Element Binding Protein 1), *SALL1* (Spalt Like Transcription Factor 1), *SCYL1* (SCY1 Like Pseudokinase 1),

SIX1 (SIX Homeobox 1), *SIX6* (SIX Homeobox 6), *SSSCA1* (Sjogren'S Syndrome/ Scleroderma Autoantigen 1), *TMTC2* (Transmembrane O-Mannosyltransferase Targeting Cadherins 2), and *VCAN* (Versican) [90]. Some of them have been linked with both CDR and IOP - *ABCA1, ABG, AFAP1, CAV1, GAS7* and *LMX1B* [2, 91]. RPE65 gene mutations result in Leber congenital amaurosis and early childhood onset retinitis pigmentosa [92]. ABCA1 is associated with cholesterol metabolism and liver function and is associated with retinal ganglion cell death and normal physiology [91]. ELN modifies the normal activity of elastin resulting in optic nerve head degeneration; ASAP1 is associated with giant cell medicated retinal ganglion cell loss and ATOH7 is connected with Muller cell differentiation and retinal ganglion cell genesis [90]. The degenerative patterns are seen in different structures of the RGC—soma atrophy, nuclear shrinkage axonic insult, and deteriorating changes in the synapses and dendrites, finally extending to the amacrine and bipolar cells [87]. Adding to the complexity, a transcriptome wide association studies identified SIX6 and CDKN2A/B to be associated with POAG and these are also linked to cardiovascular diseases and cancer [93]. The mitogen activated protein kinase p38 and Jun N terminal kinases are activated through several signalling pathways which initiate the degeneration of the soma of the RGC [94]. Subsequently, activation of the apoptotic pathway is triggered and the BCL2 gene family BAX is prompted in monkeys, rabbits and humans as well [95, 96].

6. Neuroprotection & neurodegeneration genomics in glaucoma

Glaucoma is nowadays considered to be a chronic neurodegenerative disorder which has decreased sensitivity to colour and contrast, blurry vision and reducing the field of vision with nil signs or symptoms [45]. The transcription factors, transporters, glycosylation proteins, and mutations will result in loss of function, low-risk variants gene expression modifications due to RNA splicing and transcription activities. Epigenetic activities like DNA methylation, histone body acetylation, deacetylation, structural chromatin modification and transcription. Micro RNAs miR24, miR29, miR204, miR146a [45]. In mice with optic nerve crush and glaucomatous damage could be rescued with miR-194 and miR-644-2 inhibitors provided neuroprotection and miR-181a and miR-181d-5p mimics showed neuritogenesis in retinal ganglion cells [97].

Optic nerve head is the primary critical site of degeneration in glaucoma. Axonal deprivation of neurotrophins like brain derived neurotrophic factors and mitochondrial dysfunction leads to axon transport failure [98]. There are other stakeholders in axonal degeneration of RGCs, like reduced blood flow, extracellular matrix remodelling, oxidative stress and reactive gliosis [99]. The Rho/ROCK signalling pathway prevents central nervous system regeneration through transducing inhibitory signals and is a good target for intervention in axon regeneration in glaucoma [100]. P13K/Akt pathway facilitates axonal growth and regeneration by converting PIP2 (phosphatidylinositol bisphosphate) to PIP3 (phosphatidylinositol trisphosphate) which in turn activates protein kinase Akt. This action results in phosphorylation and activation of mTOR (rapamycin), which promotes protein synthesis, motility, cell growth and survival [101]. Jak/STAT is involved in axonal regeneration by the binding of cytokines to the extracellular receptors associated with protein kinase JAK, which activates and phosphorylates the STATs. Axon regeneration is inhibited by the suppressor of cytokine signalling (SOCS) suppressing the Jak/STAT signalling [101]. Interestingly, in an immunoreactive male Lewis rats for S100B protein (the antibody which is found in high titre in glaucoma patients) showed 43 proteins were dysregulated in the retina, out of which alpha-2 macroglobulin increase was significantly associated with heat shock protein 60, showcasing the role of immunological factors in glaucoma [102].

Glaucomatous pressure leads to the progressive death of the retinal ganglion cells (RGCs), degeneration of the optic nerve and loss of peripheral vision, though normal tension glaucoma happens with the same pathological mechanism, questioning the role of intraocular pressure in the process. The trabecular meshwork is the seat of the pathology with a number of influencing factors like ageing, genetics, mechanical and oxidative stress, all collectively inhibiting the neurotrophic molecules nourishing the RGCs.

Neuroprotection of the retinal ganglion cells is critical for cell survival since several signalling pathways play the role, like JAK/STAT, MAPK, TrkA, TrkB and clinical trials with CNTF (ciliary neurotrophic factor and NGF [nerve growth factor] are in vogue [103]. CNTF is a neuropoietic cytokine belonging to IL6, which binds to the receptor of gp130 to activate JAK/STAT and MAPK to neuroprotect the RGCs [103]. NGF is secreted by nerve tissue (neurons, oligodendrocytes, Schwann cells), immune cells (T cells, mast cells, macrophages), skin cells (fibroblasts, keratinocytes, melanocytes) and smooth cells, which regulate apoptosis, neuronal plasticity, neurogenesis and neuroinflammation [103]. BDNF (brain-derived nerve growth factor), VEGF (vascular endothelial growth factor), PEDG (pigment epithelium-derived factor), GDNF (glial cell line derived neurotrophic factor) and Norrin are some of the other RGC neuroprotective proteins [103].

Epithelial cells, glial cells, leukocytes and neurons produce various neuroprotective factors like brain-derived neurotrophic factor, ciliary neurotrophic factor, glial cell line derived neurotrophic factor, nerve growth factor, norrin, pigment epithelium-derived factor, vascular endothelial growth factor and each in an exceptional way prevent RGC damage which is triggered by the ischaemic neuropathy, glaucoma, ocular hypertension and oxygen-induced retinopathy and the survival is achieved by interventional strategy through activating a variety of signalling pathways like JAK/STAT, MAPK, TrkA and TrKB [103].

The cell and tissue stakeholders in glaucoma are trabecular meshwork, retinal ganglion cell layer, retinal nerve fibre layer, cells in the optic nerve head (lamina cribrosa, optic nerve head astrocytes) and peripapillary sclera around the optic nerve head [104]. These components react to biomechanical stress like compression and stretching and the cell structures that respond are the cell membrane, cytoskeleton (actin microfilaments and tubules), extracellular matrix and nucleus. Gene expression, hence, in these cells are altered with copious TGFbeta2 synthesis in glaucoma models [104].

6.1 Biomarker genomics in glaucoma

Protein biomarkers have been identified in various parts of the eye structure associated with glaucoma, as explained in the review by Cueto et al. [1]. However, caution has to be adopted while interpreting the protein biomarker studies, due to the nature of these studies where different clinical and laboratory methodologies with variable sensitivity and specificity techniques and equipments were used, the sample sizes were too small, many studies are not validated, there are conflicting reports of dysregulation and there is poor consensus, no data between, the aqueous humour, tears, serum and vitreous samples. However, overexpression of the biomarkers could become neurotoxic and down-regulation and lack of or less expression of neuroprotectors will lead to degeneration of the retinal ganglion cells via the TrkA receptor pathway. Biomarkers could provide early screening and detection of glaucoma in the target population, diagnosis and prognostication. The biomarkers upstream or downstream could be novel targets for therapeutic interventions and visual stability or recovery. Accumulation of biomarkers will distort the blood aqueous barrier due to the inflammation and dysregulation of the extracellular matrix tissue

Serial number	Biomarkers type	Biomarkers
1	Inflammatory biomarkers	Increased: TGFB2, CD44, erythropoietin, TNFA, IL8, serum amyloid A, *CXCL13, CXCL16, CCL13, CCL15, CCL22, CCL24, IL-4, IL-16 (PXFG); autotoxin, Growth differentiation protein 15 and endothelin, Proatrial natriuretic peptide (regulates vascular/neural integrity of adult retina), IL-5, IL-12, IL-15, interferon gamma, fibroblast growth factor, vascular endothelial growth* Decreased: *Secreted frizzled related protein-1, klotho (ageing protein),*
2.	Oxidative stress related biomarkers	Increased: *superoxide dismutase, glutathione peroxidase, malondialdehyde, nitric oxide synthase, carbonyl, hydrogen peroxide, advanced glycation end products.* Decreased: Catalase, vitamins C/E
3.	Extracellular matrix related biomarkers	Increased: Fibronectin; clusterin; periostin Decreased: Hyaluronic acid, fibulin-7, Variably expressed: Connective tissue growth factor, gelatinase. Under regulated: Cystatin C, osteopontin,
4.	*Immune-response-, neurodegeneration-, and apoptosis-related markers*	Increased: Heat shock protein-70, vimentin; heat shock protein-27, transthyretin; *prostaglandin H2 D-isomerase, caspase 14 precursor, CysC, albumin precursor, transferrin; apolipoprotein A4, ALB, antithrombin 3 (SERPINC1),* CD14, CD59, complement factor D, APOA4, chromogranin A, MYB, TIMP1, microfibril-associated glycoprotein 4, agrin, and apolipoprotein C-III, Ig j chain C region, inter-a-trypsin inhibitor heavy chain 4, isocitrate dehydrogenase (NAD) subunit α, ALB, CysC, TIMP2, A2M, PGTDS, NPP2, apolipoprotein A1, APOC3, apolipoprotein E, transthyretin, and α2-macroglobulin, vitronectin, complement factors (C3a, C5b-9), Decreased: *α-enolase (ENO1), actin, and glyceraldehyde-3-phosphate dehydrogenase (POAG, PEXG), transthyretin, prostaglandin H2D isomerase, opticin, interphotoreceptor retinoid-binding protein, apolipoprotein D, SOD1,*
5.	Metabolite based biomarkers	Increased: Homocysteine, diadenosine tetraphosphate, MDA, creatinine, carnitines, aminoacids (glutamine, glycine, alanine, leucine, isoleucine, hydroxyproline, acetylornithine), several phosphatidylcholines, lysophosphatidylcholines, sphingomyelin, glycine (significantly different), pelargonic acid and galactose 1, glucose-1 phosphate, sorbitol, spermidine 2, betaine, taurine, glutamate, Decreased: Adenosine triphosphate/ Adenosine diphosphate, taurine, spermine
6.	Lipid metabolism	Increased: palmitoleic acid, gamma-linolenic acid, arachidonic acid, adrenic acid, hydroxylinoleate, hydroxyarachidonate isomers Decreased: eicosapentaenoic fatty acid, DHA, total ω3 long-chain polyunsaturated fatty acid

Table 1.
Dysregulation of gene expression and biomarkers in primary open angle glaucoma, primary closed-angle glaucoma, primary congenital glaucoma, pseudo-exfoliation glaucoma and neovascular glaucoma are summarised. Please refer to Ceutu et al., for further details [1].

physiology. Similarly, the biomarkers will intervene in the autonomic regulation of the sympathetic system affecting the ciliary body and trabecular meshwork physiological architecture. To date, over 450 biomarkers have been identified which have never been validated across large sample size patients and controls, not across different populations in the world and have not entered the arena of clinical practice, keeping the research door wide open.

Biomarkers have been identified in aqueous humour, optic nerve, retina, trabecular meshwork, tears, vitreous body, serum and blood. Besides, there are biomarkers related to apoptosis, inflammation, oxidative stress, extracellular matrix, immune response, neuroprotection, and neurodegeneration. A fairly extensive list of the biomarkers in glaucoma is provided in **Table 1**, please refer to Cueto et al., for detailed information [1].

6.2 Recent advances of genomic interventional strategies & glaucoma

Gene therapy in glaucoma is promising and is tackled by neuroprotection of the focusing on prevention of neuronal cell soma and axon loss. Another method is of optic nerve axonic regeneration [87]. In neuroprotection gene therapy, mostly in animal studies, what is addressed are overexpressing of growth and neurotrophic factors (brain-derived neurotrophic factor, fibroblast growth factor, ciliary neurotrophic factor), antiapoptotic factors (BAG1, Bcl-X, BIRC4/XIAP), transcription factors (ATF3, Brn3b, CREB, NMDA, KLF7), oxidative stress components (catalase, NRF2, SOD2), Rho/ROCK pathway (exoenzyme C3, RhoA, ROCK2), mitochondrial targets (NMNAT1, DBA2J, OPA1) and other targets (ABCA1, MCT2, Hsp70, MEK1, ULK1, miRNAs) [87]. On the axon regeneration gene therapy, what is targeted are either by overexpression or silencing in the optic nerve, optic chiasma, optic tract - PI3K/Akt pathway (PTEN, P13K, cRHEB, S6K1, GSK3, eIF2B, FGF2, IGF1, neuretin), Jak/STAT pathway (CNTF, IL6, IL22, STAT3, SOCS4, Pim1), Rho/ROCK pathway (RhoA, ROCK2, LIMK-1, LOTUS, PirB), transcription factors (KLF9, c-myc, KLF4, p53, SOX11) and other targets (many including, Lin28, HDAC5, melanopsin, TIMP2, PRPH). The gene and molecules list are selective and not exhaustive. These therapies could also be given in a combinatorial manner. Many of these molecules are awaiting the approval of the FDA, USA for clinical trials [87].

7. Experimental bioinformatics analysis

We used a bioinformatic analysis to arrive at the exhaustive list of genes or genetic factors associated with glaucoma. Genes and variants associated with different types of glaucoma were mined by using the DisGeNET Cytoscape App (version 7.0) [105].

Gene	Gene_Full_Name	Protein_Class
CYP1B1	Cytochrome P450 family 1 subfamily B member 1	Enzyme
LTBP2	Latent transforming growth factor beta binding protein 2	Calcium-binding protein
MYOC	Myocilin	Cellular structure

Table 2.
Genes associated with Juvenile open-angle glaucoma.

The DisGeNET database, retrieves gene-disease and variant-disease associations from curated databases. Analysis was performed for "Gene Disease Networks" and "Variant Disease Network", by selecting "curated" as source and "Eye diseases" as disease class and "Glaucoma" as disease. The plethora list of genes and genetic factors are provided according to the type of glaucoma in **Tables 2–9**.

Gene	Variant	Chr	Position	Consequence	Alleles	Class
CYP1B1	rs104893629	2	38071087	missense variant	T/A	snv

Table 3.
Variants associated with Juvenile open-angle glaucoma.

Gene	Gene Full Name	Protein Class
ADAMTSL1	ADAMTS like 1	Enzyme
ADRB2	Adrenoceptor beta 2	G-protein coupled receptor
ANGPT1	Angiopoietin 1	Signaling
ARSD	Arylsulfatase D	Enzyme
COL1A1	Collagen type I alpha 1 chain	
CYP1B1	Cytochrome P450 family 1 subfamily B member 1	Enzyme
CYP2B6	Cytochrome P450 family 2 subfamily B member 6	
FOXC1	Forkhead box C1	Transcription factor
GLC3B	Glaucoma 3, primary infantile, B	
GLC3C	Glaucoma 3, primary congenital, C	
HTC2	Hypertrichosis 2 (generalized, congenital)	
KIF1B	Kinesin family member 1B	Cellular structure
LOC110599580	CYP1B1 promoter	
LOXL1	Lysyl oxidase like 1	
LTBP2	Latent transforming growth factor beta binding protein 2	Calcium-binding protein
MFN2	Mitofusin 2	Enzyme
MYOC	Myocilin	Cellular structure
PGC	Progastricsin	Enzyme
PLXNA2	Plexin A2	
SH3PXD2B	SH3 and PX domains 2B	
SLC4A4	Solute carrier family 4 member 4	Transporter
STATH	Statherin	
TEK	TEK receptor tyrosine kinase	Kinase
TYR	Tyrosinase	Enzyme

Literature suggests that the inheritance of PCG includes an autosomal-recessive and sex-associated element with variable penetrance. Over 150 variants identified in CYP1B1 gene are responsible for the of PCG. Various studies showed the genes (CYP1B1, LTBP2, MYOC, COL1A1, FOXC1, ANGTP1, TEK) associated with the pathogenesis of PCG.

Table 4.
Genes associated with primary congenital glaucoma.

Gene	Variant	Chr	Position	Consequence	Alleles	Class
ADRB2	rs1042714	5	148826910	Stop gained	G/C;T	snv
ADRB2	rs1800888	5	148827322	Missense variant	C/T	snv
COL1A1	rs72645318	17	50197057	Stop gained	G/A	snv
COL1A1	rs72651658	17	50190861	Missense variant	C/T	snv
CYP1B1	rs79204362	2	38071251	Missense variant	C/T	snv
CYP1B1	rs104893622	2	38071234	Missense variant	C/T	snv
CYP1B1	rs1800440	2	38070996	Missense variant	T/C;G	snv
CYP1B1	rs55989760	2	38071195	Missense variant	C/G;T	snv
CYP1B1	rs56010818	2	38071185	Missense variant	C/T	snv
CYP1B1	rs72549379	2	38071264	Missense variant	C/T	snv
CYP1B1;CYP1B1-AS1	rs28936700	2	38075207	Missense variant	C/G;T	snv
CYP1B1;CYP1B1-AS1	rs104893623	2	38075219	Stop gained	C/T	snv
CYP1B1;CYP1B1-AS1	rs1272655298	2	38074527	Missense variant	C/G;T	snv
CYP1B1;CYP1B1-AS1	rs2567206	2	38076389	Non coding transcript exon variant	G/A	snv
CYP1B1;CYP1B1-AS1	rs72481807	2	38074872	Stop gained	C/A;T	snv
CYP1B1;CYP1B1-AS1	rs9282671	2	38075148	Missense variant	A/T	snv
CYP1B1-AS1;CYP1B1	rs57865060	2	38074704	Missense variant	C/T	snv
CYP1B1-AS1;CYP1B1	rs72549387	2	38075218	Stop gained	C/G;T	snv
FN1	rs1277989297	2	215428270	Stop gained	G/A	snv
LTBP2	rs121918355	14	74555629	Stop gained	G/A;T	snv
LTBP2	rs3742793	14	74603790	Intron variant	G/C	snv
LTBP2	rs61738025	14	74552299	Synonymous variant	C/T	snv
MYOC	rs74315339	1	171652468	Missense variant	C/A	snv
MYOC;MYOCOS	rs752829138	1	171638607	Frameshift variant	TC/-	delins
PAX6	rs121907917	11	31794079	Stop gained	G/A	snv

Table 5.
Variants associated with primary congenital glaucoma.

Gene	Gene_Full_Name	Protein_Class
ABCA1	ATP binding cassette subfamily A member 1	Transporter
ABCB1	ATP binding cassette subfamily B member 1	Transporter
ABCC4	ATP binding cassette subfamily C member 4	Transporter
ABO	ABO, alpha 1-3-N-acetylgalactosaminyltransferase and alpha 1-3-galactosyltransferase	Enzyme
ACE	Angiotensin I converting enzyme	Enzyme
ACOT7	Acyl-CoA thioesterase 7	Enzyme
ACTB	Actin beta	Cellular structure

Gene	Gene_Full_Name	Protein_Class
ACTBL2	Actin beta like 2	
ACTG1	Actin gamma 1	Cellular structure
ACTG2	Actin gamma 2, smooth muscle	Cellular structure
ADAMTS10	ADAM metallopeptidase with thrombospondin type 1 motif 10	Enzyme
ADAMTS17	ADAM metallopeptidase with thrombospondin type 1 motif 17	Enzyme
ADAMTSL3	ADAMTS like 3	Enzyme
ADRB2	Adrenoceptor beta 2	G-protein coupled receptor
AFAP1	Actin filament associated protein 1	
AGBL2	ATP/GTP binding protein like 2	Enzyme
AGER	Advanced glycosylation end-product specific receptor	Receptor
AKT1	AKT serine/threonine kinase 1	Kinase
ALB	Albumin	Transporter
ANGPT2	Angiopoietin 2	Signaling
ANGPTL7	Angiopoietin like 7	Signaling
ANXA5	Annexin A5	
APBB2	Amyloid beta precursor protein binding family B member 2	
APEX1	Apurinic/apyrimidinic endodeoxyribonuclease 1	
APOC3	Apolipoprotein C3	
APOE	Apolipoprotein E	
APP	Amyloid beta precursor protein	Enzyme modulator
AQP1	Aquaporin 1 (Colton blood group)	Ion channel
ARHGEF12	Rho guanine nucleotide exchange factor 12	
ARHGEF7	Rho guanine nucleotide exchange factor 7	
ARSD	Arylsulfatase D	Enzyme
ASB10	Ankyrin repeat and SOCS box containing 10	
ASCC1	Activating signal cointegrator 1 complex subunit 1	
ASCC2	Activating signal cointegrator 1 complex subunit 2	
ATOH7	Atonal bHLH transcription factor 7	Enzyme
ATP10A	ATPase phospholipid transporting 10A (putative)	Transporter
ATXN2	ataxin 2	Nucleic acid binding
AXL	AXL receptor tyrosine kinase	Kinase
B4GALT3	Beta-1,4-galactosyltransferase 3	Enzyme
BAK1	BCL2 antagonist/killer 1	Signaling
BDNF	Brain derived neurotrophic factor	Signaling
BIRC6	Baculoviral IAP repeat containing 6	
BMP4	Bone morphogenetic protein 4	Signaling
BRCA1	BRCA1 DNA repair associated	Enzyme

Gene	Gene_Full_Name	Protein_Class
C1QBP	Complement C1q binding protein	
C3	Complement C3	Enzyme modulator
CACNA1C	Calcium voltage-gated channel subunit alpha1 C	Ion channel
CACNA2D1	Calcium voltage-gated channel auxiliary subunit alpha2delta 1	Ion channel
CALCA	Calcitonin related polypeptide alpha	Signaling
CALCRL	Calcitonin receptor like receptor	G-protein coupled receptor
CARD10	Caspase recruitment domain family member 10	
CAT	Catalase	Enzyme
CAV1	caveolin 1	Enzyme modulator
CAV2	caveolin 2	Enzyme modulator
CCHCR1	Coiled-coil alpha-helical rod protein 1	
CCL16	C-C motif chemokine ligand 16	Signaling
CCL2	C-C motif chemokine ligand 2	Signaling
CCL4	C-C motif chemokine ligand 4	Signaling
CCL4L1	C-C motif chemokine ligand 4 like 1	
CCL4L2	C-C motif chemokine ligand 4 like 2	
CCN2	Cellular communication network factor 2	Signaling
CD40	CD40 molecule	
CDC7	Cell division cycle 7	Kinase
CDH1	Cadherin 1	
CDH5	Cadherin 5	
CDK9	Cyclin dependent kinase 9	Kinase
CDKN1A	Cyclin dependent kinase inhibitor 1A	
CDKN2A	Cyclin dependent kinase inhibitor 2A	
CDKN2B	Cyclin dependent kinase inhibitor 2B	
CDKN2B-AS1	CDKN2B antisense RNA 1	
CDX2	Caudal type homeobox 2	Transcription factor
CHDH	Choline dehydrogenase	Enzyme
CIAO3	Cytosolic iron-sulfur assembly component 3	Enzyme
CLCN2	Chloride voltage-gated channel 2	Ion channel
CLU	Clusterin	
CNTF	Ciliary neurotrophic factor	
CNTN4	Contactin 4	Receptor
CNTNAP4	Contactin associated protein family member 4	
COCH	Cochlin	Receptor
COL11A1	Collagen type XI alpha 1 chain	
COL15A1	Collagen type XV alpha 1 chain	

Gene	Gene_Full_Name	Protein_Class
COL18A1	Collagen type XVIII alpha 1 chain	
COL1A1	Collagen type I alpha 1 chain	
COL5A1	Collagen type V alpha 1 chain	
COL5A2	Collagen type V alpha 2 chain	
COL8A1	Collagen type VIII alpha 1 chain	Extracellular structure
COL8A2	Collagen type VIII alpha 2 chain	Extracellular structure
COX1	Cytochrome c oxidase subunit I	Enzyme
COX2	Cytochrome c oxidase subunit II	Enzyme
CRISP2	Cysteine rich secretory protein 2	Immune response
CRYAB	Crystallin alpha B	
CST3	Cystatin C	
CTSD	Cathepsin D	Enzyme
CUX1	Cut like homeobox 1	Transcription factor
CXCL5	C-X-C motif chemokine ligand 5	Signaling
CXCR3	C-X-C motif chemokine receptor 3	G-protein coupled receptor
CYP1A1	Cytochrome p450 family 1 subfamily a member 1	Enzyme
CYP1B1	Cytochrome p450 family 1 subfamily b member 1	Enzyme
CYP27A1	Cytochrome p450 family 27 subfamily a member 1	Enzyme
CYP2C19	Cytochrome p450 family 2 subfamily c member 19	
CYP2D6	Cytochrome p450 family 2 subfamily d member 6	
CYP46A1	Cytochrome p450 family 46 subfamily a member 1	Enzyme
DBN1	Drebrin 1	Cellular structure
DCLK1	Doublecortin like kinase 1	Kinase
DCN	Decorin	
DDIT3	DNA damage inducible transcript 3	
DDX20	DEAD-box helicase 20	
DDX3X	DEAD-box helicase 3 X-linked	
DLG2	Discs large MAGUK scaffold protein 2	Receptor
DNASE1L3	Deoxyribonuclease 1 like 3	
EBF1	EBF transcription factor 1	
EDN1	Endothelin 1	Signaling
EDNRA	Endothelin receptor type A	G-protein coupled receptor
EFEMP1	EGF containing fibulin extracellular matrix protein 1	Extracellular structure
EGFR	Epidermal growth factor receptor	Kinase
EGR1	Early growth response 1	Nucleic acid binding

Gene	Gene_Full_Name	Protein_Class
EIF2D	Eukaryotic translation initiation factor 2D	Receptor
ELN	Elastin	
ELOVL5	ELOVL fatty acid elongase 5	Enzyme
ESR1	Estrogen receptor 1	Nuclear receptor
ESR2	Estrogen receptor 2	Nuclear receptor
FASTKD1	FAST kinase domains 1	
FBLN1	Fibulin 1	
FBLN5	Fibulin 5	Calcium-binding protein
FBLN7	Fibulin 7	
FBN1	Fibrillin 1	Calcium-binding protein
FHL5	Four and a half LIM domains 5	Transcription factor
FLNB	Filamin B	
FLOT1	Flotillin 1	
FN1	Fibronectin 1	Signaling
FNDC3B	Fibronectin type III domain containing 3B	
FOXC1	Forkhead box C1	Transcription factor
FUT7	Fucosyltransferase 7	Enzyme
FZR1	Fizzy and cell division cycle 20 related 1	Enzyme modulator
GALC	Galactosylceramidase	
GAS1	Growth arrest specific 1	
GAS7	Growth arrest specific 7	
GDF15	Growth differentiation factor 15	Signaling
GJA1	Gap junction protein alpha 1	Cell-cell junction
GLB1	Galactosidase beta 1	Enzyme
GLC1B	Glaucoma 1, open angle, B (adult-onset)	
GLC1C	Glaucoma 1, open angle, C	
GLC1D	Glaucoma 1, open angle, D (adult-onset)	
GLC1H	Glaucoma 1, open angle, H (adult-onset)	
GLC1J	Glaucoma 1, open angle, J (juvenile-onset)	
GLC1K	Glaucoma 1, open angle, K (juvenile-onset)	
GLC1N	Glaucoma 1, open angle, N (juvenile-onset)	
GLC3B	Glaucoma 3, primary infantile, B	
GLCCI1	Glucocorticoid induced 1	
GMDS	GDP-mannose 4,6-dehydratase	Enzyme
GRIN2B	Glutamate ionotropic receptor NMDA type subunit 2B	Ion channel
GSTK1	Glutathione S-transferase kappa 1	
GSTM1	Glutathione S-transferase mu 1	

Gene	Gene_Full_Name	Protein_Class
GSTM2	Glutathione S-transferase mu 2	
GSTP1	Glutathione S-transferase pi 1	
GSTT1	Glutathione S-transferase theta 1	
GUCY1A1	Guanylate cyclase 1 soluble subunit alpha 1	
H3P40	H3 histone pseudogene 40	
HAS2	Hyaluronan synthase 2	
HDAC6	Histone deacetylase 6	Epigenetic regulator
HES1	Hes family bHLH transcription factor 1	Transcription factor
HEYL	Hes related family bHLH transcription factor with YRPW motif like	Transcription factor
HK2	Hexokinase 2	Kinase
HLA-A	Major histocompatibility complex, class I, A	
HLA-DQB1	Major histocompatibility complex, class II, DQ beta 1	Immune response
HLA-DRB1	Major histocompatibility complex, class II, DR beta 1	Immune response
HPGDS	Hematopoietic prostaglandin D synthase	
HSPA14	Heat shock protein family A (Hsp70) member 14	
HSPA1A	Heat shock protein family A (Hsp70) member 1A	
HSPA1B	Heat shock protein family A (Hsp70) member 1B	
HSPA4	Heat shock protein family A (Hsp70) member 4	
HSPA5	Heat shock protein family A (Hsp70) member 5	
HSPB1	Heat shock protein family B (small) member 1	
HSPB2	Heat shock protein family B (small) member 2	
HSPB3	Heat shock protein family B (small) member 3	
HSPD1	Heat shock protein family D (Hsp60) member 1	
HTC2	Hypertrichosis 2 (generalized, congenital)	
HYAL3	Hyaluronidase 3 hyaluronidase 3	Enzyme
ICA1	Islet cell autoantigen 1	
IDH3A	Isocitrate dehydrogenase (NAD(+)) 3 catalytic subunit alpha	Enzyme
IFNG	Interferon gamma	
IGF2	Insulin like growth factor 2	
IGFALS	Insulin like growth factor binding protein acid labile subunit	Receptor
IGKC	Immunoglobulin kappa constant	
IL10	Interleukin 10	
IL17B	Interleukin 17B	
IL1A	Interleukin 1 alpha	
IL1B	Interleukin 1 beta	
IL1RN	Interleukin 1 receptor antagonist	
IL2	Interleukin 2	

Gene	Gene_Full_Name	Protein_Class
IL20	Interleukin 20	
IL20RB	Interleukin 20 receptor subunit beta	Receptor
IL2RA	Interleukin 2 receptor subunit alpha	Receptor
IL6	Interleukin 6	
IL7	Interleukin 7	
IL9	Interleukin 9	
ISG20	Interferon stimulated exonuclease gene 20	
ITGA5	Integrin subunit alpha 5	
ITGAV	Integrin subunit alpha V	
ITIH4	Inter-alpha-trypsin inhibitor heavy chain 4	Enzyme modulator
ITPR3	Inositol 1,4,5-trisphosphate receptor type 3	Ion channel
KDR	Kinase insert domain receptor	Kinase
LDLR	Low density lipoprotein receptor	
LGALS14	Galectin 14	Signaling
LGTN	Ligatin	
LHCGR	Luteinizing hormone/choriogonadotropin receptor	G-protein coupled receptor
LINC02605	Long intergenic non-protein coding RNA 2605	
LMX1B	LIM homeobox transcription factor 1 beta	Nucleic acid binding
LOC110599580	CYP1B1 promoter	
LOXL1	Lysyl oxidase like 1	
LOXL2	Lysyl oxidase like 2	
LTBP2	Latent transforming growth factor beta binding protein 2	Calcium-binding protein
MAP3K1	Mitogen-activated protein kinase kinase kinase 1	Kinase
MAP3K8	Mitogen-activated protein kinase kinase kinase 8	Kinase
MARCHF8	Membrane associated ring-CH-type finger 8	
MARCHF9	Membrane associated ring-CH-type finger 9	
MBL2	Mannose binding lectin 2	Receptor
MBP	Myelin basic protein	
MFGE8	Milk fat globule-EGF factor 8 protein	Enzyme
MINDY4	MINDY lysine 48 deubiquitinase 4	
MIR182	microRNA 182	
MIR210	microRNA 210	
MIR302D	microRNA 302d	
MIR34B	microRNA 34b	
MIR630	microRNA 630	
MLXIP	MLX interacting protein	
MMP1	Matrix metallopeptidase 1	Enzyme

Gene	Gene_Full_Name	Protein_Class
MMP12	Matrix metallopeptidase 12	Enzyme
MMP2	Matrix metallopeptidase 2	Enzyme
MMP3	Matrix metallopeptidase 3	Enzyme
MMP9	Matrix metallopeptidase 9	Enzyme
MMRN1	Multimerin 1	
MPO	Myeloperoxidase	Enzyme
MPP7	Membrane palmitoylated protein 7	Enzyme
MT1A	Metallothionein 1A	
MT1B	Metallothionein 1B	
MT1E	Metallothionein 1E	
MT1F	Metallothionein 1F	
MT1G	Metallothionein 1G	
MT1H	Metallothionein 1H	
MT1IP	Metallothionein 1I, pseudogene	
MT1JP	Metallothionein 1J, pseudogene	
MT1L	Metallothionein 1L, pseudogene	
MT1M	Metallothionein 1M	
MT1X	Metallothionein 1X	
MTCO2P12	MT-CO2 pseudogene 12	
MTHFR	Methylenetetrahydrofolate reductase	
MTNR1A	Melatonin receptor 1A	G-protein coupled receptor
MUTYH	mutY DNA glycosylase	Enzyme
MVB12B	Multivesicular body subunit 12B	
MYLIP	Myosin regulatory light chain interacting protein	
MYOC	Myocilin	Cellular structure
MYOCOS	Myocilin opposite strand	
MZB1	Marginal zone B and B1 cell specific protein	
NANOS2	Nanos C2HC-type zinc finger 2	
ND2	MTND2	
NFKB1	Nuclear factor kappa B subunit 1	Transcription factor
NFKB2	Nuclear factor kappa B subunit 2	Transcription factor
NOS2	Nitric oxide synthase 2	
NOS3	Nitric oxide synthase 3	
NPPA	Natriuretic peptide A	
NPPC	Natriuretic peptide C	Signaling
NR3C1	Nuclear receptor subfamily 3 group C member 1	Nuclear receptor
NTF4	Neurotrophin 4	Signaling

Gene	Gene_Full_Name	Protein_Class
NTM	Neurotrimin	
NXF1	Nuclear RNA export factor 1	Nucleic acid binding
OAS3	2'-5'-oligoadenylate synthetase 3	Enzyme
OGG1	8-oxoguanine DNA glycosylase	
OGN	Osteoglycin	
OPA1	OPA1 mitochondrial dynamin like GTPase	Enzyme modulator
OPTC	Opticin	Receptor
OPTN	Optineurin	
PADI2	Peptidyl arginine deiminase 2	
PAH	Phenylalanine hydroxylase	
PARP1	Poly(ADP-ribose) polymerase 1	
PCOLCE2	Procollagen C-endopeptidase enhancer 2	
PDE5A	Phosphodiesterase 5A	
PDIA5	Protein disulfide isomerase family A member 5	
PEX5	Peroxisomal biogenesis factor 5	Transporter
PITX2	Paired like homeodomain 2	
PKHD1	PKHD1 ciliary IPT domain containing fibrocystin/polyductin	
PLA2G4A	Phospholipase A2 group IVA	Enzyme
PLB1	Phospholipase B1	
PLG	Plasminogen	Enzyme
PLXDC2	Plexin domain containing 2	
PLXNA2	Plexin A2	
PMEL	Premelanosome protein	Signaling
POTEKP	POTE ankyrin domain family member K, pseudogene	
POTEM	POTE ankyrin domain family member M	
PPID	Peptidylprolyl isomerase D	
PPIF	Peptidylprolyl isomerase F	
PRDM5	PR/SET domain 5	
PRKAA1	Protein kinase AMP-activated catalytic subunit alpha 1	Kinase
PRNP	Prion protein	
PRPF8	Pre-mRNA processing factor 8	Nucleic acid binding
PRS	Prieto X-linked mental retardation syndrome	
PRSS55	Serine protease 55	Enzyme
PSD	Pleckstrin and Sec7 domain containing	
PTEN	Phosphatase and tensin homolog	Enzyme
PTGFR	Prostaglandin F receptor	G-protein coupled receptor
PTGS1	Prostaglandin-endoperoxide synthase 1	Enzyme

Gene	Gene_Full_Name	Protein_Class
PTGS2	Prostaglandin-endoperoxide synthase 2	Enzyme
PTPRJ	Protein tyrosine phosphatase receptor type J	Enzyme
RAMP2	Receptor activity modifying protein 2	Receptor
RAN	RAN, member RAS oncogene family	Enzyme modulator
RBP1	Retinol binding protein 1	
RHOA	ras homolog family member A	Enzyme modulator
RHOD	ras homolog family member D	Enzyme modulator
RNR2	l-rRNA	
ROCK1	Rho associated coiled-coil containing protein kinase 1	Kinase
ROCK2	Rho associated coiled-coil containing protein kinase 2	Kinase
ROS1	ROS proto-oncogene 1, receptor tyrosine kinase	Kinase
RPGRIP1	RPGR interacting protein 1	Enzyme modulator
RPN2	Ribophorin II	Enzyme
RTCA	RNA 3'-terminal phosphate cyclase	Enzyme
SART3	Spliceosome associated factor 3, U4/U6 recycling protein	Nucleic acid binding
SCGB1A1	Secretoglobin family 1A member 1	Signaling
SEC14L2	SEC14 like lipid binding 2	
SELENBP1	Selenium binding protein 1	Immune response
SEMA6A	Semaphorin 6A	Signaling
SERPINA3	Serpin family A member 3	Enzyme modulator
SERPINE1	Serpin family E member 1	Enzyme modulator
SFRP1	Secreted frizzled related protein 1	
SH3PXD2B	SH3 and PX domains 2B	
SHBG	Sex hormone binding globulin	
SIRT1	Sirtuin 1	Epigenetic regulator
SIX1	SIX homeobox 1	Transcription factor
SIX6	SIX homeobox 6	Transcription factor
SLC23A1	Solute carrier family 23 member 1	Transporter
SLC23A2	Solute carrier family 23 member 2	Transporter
SLC4A10	Solute carrier family 4 member 10	Transporter
SLCO6A1	Solute carrier organic anion transporter family member 6A1	Transporter
SND1	Staphylococcal nuclease and tudor domain containing 1	Transcription factor
SOAT1	Sterol O-acyltransferase 1	Enzyme
SOD1	Superoxide dismutase 1	Enzyme
SOD2	Superoxide dismutase 2	Enzyme
SPARC	Secreted protein acidic and cysteine rich	Signaling
SPOCK1	SPARC (osteonectin), cwcv and kazal like domains proteoglycan 1	Enzyme modulator

Gene	Gene_Full_Name	Protein_Class
SPP1	Secreted phosphoprotein 1	
SPRR2A	Small proline rich protein 2A	
SPZ1	Spermatogenic leucine zipper 1	
SRBD1	S1 RNA binding domain 1	Nucleic acid binding
SRL	Sarcalumenin	Enzyme modulator
SRSF3	Serine and arginine rich splicing factor 3	Nucleic acid binding
STIP1	Stress induced phosphoprotein 1	
SULT1E1	Sulfotransferase family 1E member 1	
TAP1	Transporter 1, ATP binding cassette subfamily B member	Transporter
TBK1	TANK binding kinase 1	Kinase
TEK	TEK receptor tyrosine kinase	Kinase
TGFB1	Transforming growth factor beta 1	Signaling
TGFB2	Transforming growth factor beta 2	Signaling
TGFB3	Transforming growth factor beta 3	Signaling
TGFBR3	Transforming growth factor beta receptor 3	
TGM2	Transglutaminase 2	Enzyme
THBS1	Thrombospondin 1	
THBS2	Thrombospondin 2	
TIMP1	TIMP metallopeptidase inhibitor 1	Enzyme modulator
TIMP2	TIMP metallopeptidase inhibitor 2	Enzyme modulator
TIMP3	TIMP metallopeptidase inhibitor 3	Enzyme modulator
TIMP4	TIMP metallopeptidase inhibitor 4	Enzyme modulator
TLR2	Toll like receptor 2	
TLR4	Toll like receptor 4	
TMCO1	Transmembrane and coiled-coil domains 1	
TMTC2	Transmembrane O-mannosyltransferase targeting cadherins 2	
TNF	Tumor necrosis factor	Signaling
TNNT1	Troponin T1, slow skeletal type	Cellular structure
TP53	Tumor protein p53	Transcription factor
TP53BP2	Tumor protein p53 binding protein 2	Enzyme modulator
TPX2	TPX2 microtubule nucleation factor	Cellular structure
TRPM5	Transient receptor potential cation channel subfamily M member 5	Ion channel
TXNRD2	Thioredoxin reductase 2	Enzyme
UROD	Uroporphyrinogen decarboxylase	
USO1	USO1 vesicle transport factor	Transporter
VAV2	Vav guanine nucleotide exchange factor 2	
VAV3	Vav guanine nucleotide exchange factor 3	

Gene	Gene_Full_Name	Protein_Class
VDR	Vitamin D receptor	Nuclear receptor
VEGFA	Vascular endothelial growth factor A	Signaling
VEGFC	Vascular endothelial growth factor C	Signaling
WDR36	WD repeat domain 36	
XRCC1	X-ray repair cross complementing 1	
ZNF410	Zinc finger protein 410	Transcription factor
ZNF469	Zinc finger protein 469	
ZP4	Zona pellucida glycoprotein 4	

Literature reports that the potential therapeutic targets based on the molecular and cellular alterations caused by MYOC, OPTN and TBK1 mutations. Additionally, GWAS study performed in adult-onset glaucoma have identified novel loci for POAG (primary open-angle glaucoma) in CAV1/CAV2, CDKN2BAS, TMCO1, SIX6, 8q22(NTG), ABCA1, AFAP1, GMDS, PMM2, TGFBR3, FNDC3B, ARHGEF12, GAS7, FOXC1, ATXN2, TXNRD2, OPTC, MPP7 genes. Additionally, Single SNPs in the MYOC, COL8A2, COL1A1 and ZNF469 gene regions were reported by the study conducted in South Africa in POAG subjects.

Table 6.
Primary open angle glaucoma associated genes.

Gene	Variant	Chr	Position	Consequence	Alleles	Class
ABCB1	rs74315329	7	87509329	Synonymous variant	A/G;T	snv
ABO	rs28939688	9	133262254	Intron variant	C/T	snv
ADAMTS10	rs75654767	19	8589505	Missense variant	C/T	snv
ADRB2	rs1057519378	5	148826910	Stop gained	G/C;T	snv
ADRB2	rs1346865805	5	148827322	Missense variant	C/T	snv
AGER	rs137854858	6	32183666	Missense variant	C/T	snv
APBB2	rs137854860	4	40995241	Intron variant	T/C	snv
APEX1	rs137854863	14	20456995	Missense variant	T/A;C;G	snv
ASB10	rs139006752	7	151181233	Synonymous variant	G/A	snv
ASB10	rs1553534421	7	151181278	Synonymous variant	G/A	snv
ASB10	rs1555954284	7	151181173	Synonymous variant	C/A;G;T	snv
ATOH7	rs1564354968	10	68231992	5 prime UTR variant	T/G	snv
ATOH7	rs200148764	10	68232096	5 prime UTR variant	A/G	snv
B4GALT3;PPOX	rs200710076	1	161175160	Missense variant	C/T	snv
BIRC6	rs201794655	2	32545090	Intron variant	A/T	snv
C14orf39;SIX6	rs373425395	14	60509819	Missense variant	C/A;G	snv
C14orf39;SIX6	rs750643216	14	60509783	Missense variant	G/A	snv
C1orf112;SELE	rs878854408	1	169728058	Missense variant	C/A;T	snv
CARD10	rs1217691063	22	37516037	Missense variant	C/A;T	snv
CARD10	rs2165241	22	37508609	Missense variant	G/A	snv
CARD10	rs33912345	22	37508568	Missense variant	C/T	snv

Gene	Variant	Chr	Position	Consequence	Alleles	Class
CARD10	rs3825942	22	37492794	Missense variant	G/A	snv
CARD10	rs1048661	22	37506365	Missense variant	G/A	snv
CAT	rs566289099	11	34438684	Upstream gene variant	C/T	snv
CAT	rs1063192	11	34461361	Synonymous variant	C/T	snv
CAT	rs11258194	11	34438925	Upstream gene variant	A/T	snv
CAV1	rs74315330	7	116550415	Intron variant	G/A	snv
CAV2	rs1042522	7	116508316	3 prime UTR variant	T/C;G	snv
CD48	rs12994401	1	160681172	Frameshift variant	C/-;CC;CCC	delins
CD48	rs137853277	1	160681173	Frameshift variant	-/T	ins
CDKN2B;CDKN2B-AS1	rs2149356	9	22003368	3 prime UTR variant	G/A;T	snv
CDKN2B-AS1	rs4986791	9	22056500	Intron variant	G/A	snv
CDKN2B-AS1	rs74315337	9	22033367	Non coding transcript exon variant	C/T	snv
CDKN2B-AS1	rs10120688	9	22062135	Intron variant	G/T	snv
CDKN2B-AS1	rs1131691014	9	22055049	Intron variant	A/G;T	snv
CDKN2B-AS1	rs145285325	9	22019130	Intron variant	A/G	snv
CDKN2B-AS1	rs2157719	9	22028802	Intron variant	A/G	snv
CNTNAP4	rs2234926	16	76307609	Intron variant	A/G	snv
COL8A2	rs25487	1	36099217	Missense variant	C/G;T	snv
COX1;COX2	rs367923973	MT	6150	Missense variant	G/A	snv
COX2;COX1	rs4898	MT	6253	Missense variant	T/C	snv
COX2;COX1;ATP8	rs4986790	MT	6480	Missense variant	G/A	snv
CYP1B1	rs74315328	2	38071060	Missense variant	G/C	snv
CYP1B1	rs74315332	2	38071007	Missense variant	A/G;T	snv
CYP1B1	rs74315339	2	38070996	Missense variant	T/C;G	snv
CYP1B1;CYP1B1-AS1	rs781662103	2	38075034	Missense variant	C/A	snv
CYP1B1;CYP1B1-AS1	rs878854066	2	38075247	Missense variant	G/C	snv
CYP1B1;CYP1B1-AS1	rs1001179	2	38076389	Non coding transcript exon variant	G/A	snv
CYP1B1;CYP1B1-AS1	rs10202118	2	38075148	Missense variant	A/T	snv
CYP1B1-AS1;CYP1B1	rs1056827	2	38074704	Missense variant	C/T	snv
CYP46A1	rs11656696	14	99691630	Non coding transcript exon variant	A/G	snv
DCLK1	rs1279683	13	36078480	Intron variant	T/C	snv
DDX3X	rs1533428	X	41346607	Missense variant	C/T	snv
EDNRA	rs16947	4	147542688	3 prime UTR variant	G/A;C	snv
ENO4	rs17576	10	116864069	Intron variant	G/A	snv
ESR1	rs1799750	6	151929945	Intron variant	C/A	snv

Gene	Variant	Chr	Position	Consequence	Alleles	Class
ESR1	rs1799983	6	151970431	Intron variant	C/A	snv
ESR2	rs180040	14	64279461	Intron variant	G/A;T	snv
ESR2	rs1900004	14	64292158	Intron variant	C/T	snv
FASLG	rs199752860	1	172658358	Upstream gene variant	C/T	snv
FASTKD1	rs2234927	2	169531449	Missense variant	A/T	snv
FDXR	rs267606929	17	74872110	Stop gained	G/A;C	snv
FDXR	rs3219489	17	74863112	Missense variant	C/A;G;T	snv
FNDC3B	rs369410616	3	172315221	Intron variant	C/G	snv
FNDC3B	rs3918188	3	172274597	Intron variant	G/A	snv
GAS7	rs397507444	17	10130362	Intron variant	C/A	snv
GCM1	rs74315334	6	53258320	Regulatory region variant	T/C	snv
GPX4	rs74315336	19	1101993	Upstream gene variant	A/G	snv
GSTP1	rs74315338	11	67585218	Missense variant	A/G	snv
HSP90AA1	rs754203	14	102083827	Missense variant	T/C	snv
IL20RA	rs754237376	6	137008718	Missense variant	G/A	snv
IL20RB-AS1;IL20RB	rs10012	3	136982255	Missense variant	C/T	snv
INKA2;DDX20; LOC101928718	rs10038177	1	111754860	Non coding transcript exon variant	A/T	snv
KCNQ4	rs10063949	1	40814886	Intron variant	C/T	snv
KLC3;ERCC2	rs1011970	19	45351661	Stop gained	T/A;G	snv
LINC02640	rs1042714	10	68241124	Intron variant	C/T	snv
LOC102724808;OPA1	rs10451941	3	193647160	Missense variant	A/G	snv
LOC105376196	rs1045642	9	104933567	Downstream gene variant	G/A	snv
LOC107986513;GMDS	rs104886478	6	1707020	Intron variant	C/T	snv
LOC112268121;EDNRB-AS1	rs1051993	13	77800045	Intron variant	A/T	snv
LOC730100	rs1052133	2	51845108	Intron variant	C/T	snv
LOC730100	rs1052990	2	51723186	Intron variant	C/T	snv
LOC730100	rs1056836	2	51732120	Intron variant	T/A;C	snv
LOC730100	rs1056837	2	51725011	Intron variant	G/A	snv
LOXL1;LOXL1-AS1	rs11125375	15	73927241	Missense variant	G/A;C;T	snv
LOXL1-AS1;LOXL1	rs111698934	15	73929861	Intron variant	T/C	snv
LOXL1-AS1;LOXL1	rs11241095	15	73927205	Missense variant	G/T	snv
LTBP2	rs112983858	14	74551266	Missense variant	C/A;T	snv
LTBP2	rs1130409	14	74502911	Missense variant	C/G;T	snv
LTBP2	rs1135840	14	74505102	Missense variant	T/C	snv
MIR182;LOC105375501	rs11536889	7	129770387	Non coding transcript exon variant	C/G;T	snv

Gene	Variant	Chr	Position	Consequence	Alleles	Class
MIR34C;BTG4;MIR34B; LOC728196	rs11568658	11	111511840	Intron variant	T/C	snv
MMP9	rs11669977	20	46011586	Missense variant	A/G	snv
MPP7	rs1171063544	10	28116482	Intron variant	G/C;T	snv
MTHFR	rs11720822	1	11796309	Missense variant	A/G	snv
MTHFR	rs11771443	1	11794407	Missense variant	T/G	snv
MUL1	rs12025126	1	20503285	Missense variant	C/T	snv
MUTYH	rs12154178	1	45331833	Missense variant	C/A;G	snv
MUTYH	rs121909194	1	45329400	Missense variant	C/T	snv
MYOC	rs12377632	1	171652476	Stop gained	G/A;C;T	snv
MYOC	rs1255428605	1	171652385	Missense variant	C/T	snv
MYOC	rs1256031	1	171652468	Missense variant	C/A	snv
MYOC	rs1268656	1	171652578	Missense variant	C/G	snv
MYOC	rs1270841723	1	171652341	Stop gained	G/A	snv
MYOC	rs12789379	1	171652139	Missense variant	C/G;T	snv
MYOC	rs1279386	1	171652539	Missense variant	A/G	snv
MYOC;MYOCOS	rs1315538274	1	171636338	Stop gained	G/A	snv
MYOC;MYOCOS	rs13181	1	171636382	Missense variant	G/A	snv
MYOC;MYOCOS	rs13186912	1	171636131	Missense variant	A/G	snv
MYOC;MYOCOS	rs14035	1	171636143	Missense variant	A/G	snv
MYOC;MYOCOS	rs1428758	1	171636161	Missense variant	C/T	snv
MYOC;MYOCOS	rs143413116	1	171636302	Missense variant	C/G	snv
MYOC;MYOCOS	rs144249808	1	171636185	Missense variant	T/C	snv
MYOC;MYOCOS	rs145437203	1	171636010	Missense variant	A/C;T	snv
MYOC;MYOCOS	rs1463461589	1	171636686	Missense variant	C/T	snv
MYOC;MYOCOS	rs1466441587	1	171636542	Missense variant	C/T	snv
MYOCOS;MYOC	rs146737847	1	171636329	Missense variant	A/G	snv
MYOCOS;MYOC	rs166850	1	171636310	Missense variant	G/A	snv
MYOCOS;MYOC	rs1695	1	171636331	Missense variant	G/A	snv
MYOCOS;MYOC	rs16984299	1	171636000	Missense variant	G/T	snv
MYOCOS;MYOC	rs1799782	1	171638703	Missense variant	G/A;C	snv
MYOCOS;MYOC	rs1800440	1	171636341	Missense variant	C/T	snv
MYOCOS;MYOC	rs1800779	1	171636173	Missense variant	T/C	snv
MYOCOS;MYOC	rs1800888	1	171638675	Missense variant	C/T	snv
MYOCOS;MYOC	rs184561087	1	171636028	Missense variant	T/C	snv
MYOCOS;MYOC	rs185815146	1	171635999	Missense variant	G/A	snv
NCKAP5	rs1884054	2	133605461	Regulatory region variant	T/A;C;G	snv

Gene	Variant	Chr	Position	Consequence	Alleles	Class
ND2;RNR2;ND1	rs1926320	MT	3010	Non coding transcript exon variant	G/A	snv
NDUFA6-DT;CYP2D6	rs1927911	22	42127941	Missense variant	G/A;T	snv
NDUFA6-DT;CYP2D6	rs197388	22	42126611	Missense variant	C/G	snv
NOS3	rs199476128	7	150999023	Missense variant	T/A;G	snv
NOS3	rs199746824	7	151005693	Intron variant	C/A;T	snv
NOS3	rs200165736	7	150990599	Upstream gene variant	C/T	snv
NOS3	rs200547613	7	150992855	Intron variant	G/A;C	snv
NOS3	rs2070600	7	150998107	Intron variant	G/A	snv
NOS3;ATG9B	rs2156323	7	151012483	3 prime UTR variant	G/T	snv
NRP1	rs2253592	10	33221802	Missense variant	A/G	snv
NTF4	rs2383204	19	49060867	Non coding transcript exon variant	A/G	snv
NTF4	rs2472493	19	49061660	Missense variant	A/G	snv
NTF4	rs2567206	19	49061735	Missense variant	G/A	snv
NTF4	rs2754511	19	49061453	Missense variant	G/A	snv
NTM	rs2801219	11	131422069	Intron variant	A/G;T	snv
OGG1	rs28358580	3	9756778	Missense variant	C/T	snv
OGG1;CAMK1	rs2842980	3	9757089	Missense variant	C/G	snv
OPA1	rs34551253	3	193637313	Intron variant	T/A;C	snv
OPA1	rs34595252	3	193637285	Splice region variant	T/A;C	snv
OPTN	rs3766355	10	13109270	Missense variant	G/A	snv
OPTN	rs3793342	10	13136766	Missense variant	G/A	snv
OPTN	rs3801994	10	13110416	Missense variant	G/C	snv
OPTN	rs386741044	10	13109279	Frameshift variant	-/AGCT	delins
OPTN	rs3928306	10	13109198	Missense variant	C/A;G;T	snv
OPTN	rs4880	10	13132122	Missense variant	A/G	snv
OPTN	rs4938723	10	13110400	Missense variant	T/A	snv
OPTN	rs523096	10	13132098	Missense variant	A/G	snv
OPTN	rs523747	10	13110394	Missense variant	G/A;T	snv
OPTN	rs5335	10	13124076	Missense variant	G/A;C	snv
OPTN	rs537516822	10	13124076	Missense variant	G/A;C	snv
PBX2;AGER	rs547984	6	32185657	3 prime UTR variant	C/A	snv
PDIA5	rs554235897	3	123150194	Intron variant	C/T	snv
PRPF8	rs571448378	17	1684534	Missense variant	G/A	snv
PRPF8	rs5743704	17	1684498	Missense variant	A/G	snv
PTGFR	rs5746136	1	78491756	Intron variant	C/A;T	snv
RAN	rs576499843	12	130876696	3 prime UTR variant	C/T	snv
RERE	rs5773704	1	8699495	Intron variant	T/C	snv

Gene	Variant	Chr	Position	Consequence	Alleles	Class
RFTN1;OXNAD1	rs57865060	3	16354161	Intron variant	C/G;T	snv
RHOA	rs59892895	3	49363049	Intron variant	T/C	snv
RNR2;ND1	rs61732310	MT	2416	Non coding transcript exon variant	T/C	snv
SEC14L2	rs61854782	22	30406040	Intron variant	C/A;G;T	snv
SLC23A1	rs6445055	5	139383837	Intron variant	T/C	snv
SLC23A2	rs690037	20	5002446	Intron variant	G/A;C	snv
SNORD13G;ABCC4	rs6917589	13	95210754	Missense variant	C/A	snv
SOD2	rs693421	6	159679084	3 prime UTR variant	A/T	snv
SOD2	rs6994076	6	159692840	Missense variant	A/G	snv
SOD2	rs7037117	6	159682052	3 prime UTR variant	C/T	snv
SOD2	rs7049105	6	159678228	3 prime UTR variant	T/C	snv
STIP1	rs7159462	11	64195658	Missense variant	C/A;G	snv
STIP1	rs735860	11	64203143	Missense variant	A/G	snv
SYNE2;ESR2	rs737723	14	64180928	Intron variant	T/G	snv
TIMP1;SYN1;MIR4769	rs74315331	X	47585586	Synonymous variant	T/C	snv
TLR2	rs74315341	4	153704799	Missense variant	C/A	snv
TLR4	rs746418406	9	117711921	Intron variant	T/G	snv
TLR4	rs746702110	9	117713324	Missense variant	C/T	snv
TLR4	rs747058633	9	117713024	Missense variant	A/G;T	snv
TLR4	rs747782	9	117715853	3 prime UTR variant	G/C	snv
TLR4	rs7481514	9	117710452	Intron variant	T/A;C	snv
TLR4	rs748621461	9	117707776	Intron variant	A/G	snv
TLR4	rs748899944	9	117721385	3 prime UTR variant	A/G	snv
TMTC2	rs751417985	12	82698057	Intron variant	G/A	snv
TP53	rs751497460	17	7676154	Missense variant	G/C;T	snv
TP53	rs754829637	17	7676154	Frameshift variant	-/C	ins
TP53	rs755246983	17	7676153	Missense variant	GG/AC	mnv
TRPM5	rs757228	11	2415234	Missense variant	C/A;T	snv
TTPA	rs75864656	8	63087002	Upstream gene variant	A/T	snv
TXNRD2	rs7588567	22	19876070	3 prime UTR variant	T/C	snv
VAV2	rs761875612	9	133855699	Intron variant	G/A	snv
VAV3	rs763068244	1	107874935	Missense variant	G/A	snv
VAV3	rs763110	1	107959790	Intron variant	C/A	snv
VAV3	rs76481776	1	107617607	Missense variant	A/C;G	snv
WDR36	rs766147142	5	111100751	Intron variant	C/T	snv
WDR36	rs769217	5	111103810	Missense variant	A/C;G	snv
WDR36	rs782006965	5	111121006	Synonymous variant	A/T	snv

Gene	Variant	Chr	Position	Consequence	Alleles	Class
WDR36	rs7830	5	111092362	Missense variant	T/C	snv
WDR36	rs7916697	5	111119021	Missense variant	A/G	snv
WTAPP1;MMP1	rs7916852	11	102797141	Synonymous variant	A/G	snv
WTAPP1;MMP1	rs7943316	11	102799765	Intron variant	C/-	delins
XRCC1	rs7961953	19	43551574	Missense variant	T/C	snv
XRCC1	rs8176693	19	43553422	Missense variant	G/A	snv
	rs879053914	15	97027933	Intergenic variant	T/C	snv
	rs9282671	1	237933586	Intergenic variant	A/C	snv
	rs9503012	1	237935790	Downstream gene variant	T/A;G	snv
	rs974495	11	47919373	Intergenic variant	T/C	snv

Table 7.
Variants associated with primary open angle glaucoma.

Gene	Gene_Full_Name	Protein_Class
ABCA1	ATP binding cassette subfamily A member 1	Transporter
ABCC5	ATP binding cassette subfamily C member 5	Transporter
ACD	ACD shelterin complex subunit and telomerase recruitment factor	
AKR1C4	Aldo-keto reductase family 1 member C4	Enzyme
APOE	Apolipoprotein E	
AQP1	Aquaporin 1 (Colton blood group)	Ion channel
ATOH7	Atonal bHLH transcription factor 7	Enzyme
BIRC6	Baculoviral IAP repeat containing 6	
BRCA1	BRCA1 DNA repair associated	Enzyme
C10orf53	Chromosome 10 open reading frame 53	
C3	Complement C3	Enzyme modulator
CALCRL	Calcitonin receptor like receptor	G-protein coupled receptor
CAT	Catalase	Enzyme
CCL2	C-C motif chemokine ligand 2	Signaling
CCN2	Cellular communication network factor 2	Signaling
CDC42	Cell division cycle 42	Enzyme modulator
CDR1	Cerebellar degeneration related protein 1	
CHAT	Choline O-acetyltransferase	Enzyme
CIAO3	Cytosolic iron-sulfur assembly component 3	Enzyme
COL11A1	Collagen type XI alpha 1 chain	
COL1A1	Collagen type I alpha 1 chain	

Gene	Gene_Full_Name	Protein_Class
CST3	Cystatin C	
CTSD	Cathepsin D	Enzyme
CYP1B1	Cytochrome P450 family 1 subfamily B member 1	Enzyme
CYP2B6	Cytochrome P450 family 2 subfamily B member 6	
DBN1	Drebrin 1	Cellular structure
DCN	Decorin	
DPM2	Dolichyl-phosphate mannosyltransferase subunit 2, regulatory	
EIF2D	Eukaryotic translation initiation factor 2D	Receptor
ELN	Elastin	
EPDR1	Ependymin related 1	
F2	Coagulation factor II, thrombin	Enzyme
FAM102A	Family with sequence similarity 102 member A	
FBLN7	Fibulin 7	
FERMT2	Fermitin family member 2	
GLIS3	GLIS family zinc finger 3	
GSTM1	Glutathione S-transferase mu 1	
HGF	Hepatocyte growth factor	Enzyme
HLA-DPA1	Major histocompatibility complex, class II, DP alpha 1	Immune response
HSPA4	Heat shock protein family A (Hsp70) member 4	
HTR3C	5-hydroxytryptamine receptor 3C	Ion channel
HTR3D	5-hydroxytryptamine receptor 3D	Ion channel
IL1A	Interleukin 1 alpha	
IL1B	Interleukin 1 beta	
KDR	Kinase insert domain receptor	Kinase
KERA	Keratocan	
LGTN	Ligatin	
LOC110599580	CYP1B1 promoter	
LOX	Lysyl oxidase	
LOXL1	Lysyl oxidase like 1	
LOXL2	Lysyl oxidase like 2	
MFRP	Membrane frizzled-related protein	Enzyme
MINDY4	MINDY lysine 48 deubiquitinase 4	
MMP1	Matrix metallopeptidase 1	Enzyme
MMP9	Matrix metallopeptidase 9	Enzyme
MTHFR	Methylenetetrahydrofolate reductase	
MYOC	Myocilin	Cellular structure

Gene	Gene_Full_Name	Protein_Class
NEB	Nebulin	
NOS3	Nitric oxide synthase 3	
NT5E	5'-nucleotidase ecto	Enzyme
NTF4	Neurotrophin 4	Signaling
OGG1	8-oxoguanine DNA glycosylase	
OPA3	Outer mitochondrial membrane lipid metabolism regulator OPA3	
OPTN	Optineurin	
PACC1	Proton activated chloride channel 1	
PARL	Presenilin associated rhomboid like	Enzyme
PCMTD1	Protein-L-isoaspartate (D-aspartate) O-methyltransferase domain containing 1	Enzyme
PDE5A	Phosphodiesterase 5A	
PDIA5	Protein disulfide isomerase family A member 5	
PLEKHA7	Pleckstrin homology domain containing A7	
PLXNA2	Plexin A2	
PRSS56	Serine protease 56	
RAC1	Rac family small GTPase 1	Enzyme modulator
RUNX1T1	RUNX1 partner transcriptional co-repressor 1	Transcription factor
SFRP4	Secreted frizzled related protein 4	
SOD2	Superoxide dismutase 2	Enzyme
SPARC	Secreted protein acidic and cysteine rich	Signaling
SPP1	Secreted phosphoprotein 1	
ST18	ST18 C2H2C-type zinc finger transcription factor	Transcription factor
TGFB1	Transforming growth factor beta 1	Signaling
TGFB2	Transforming growth factor beta 2	Signaling
THBS1	Thrombospondin 1	
TMCO1	Transmembrane and coiled-coil domains 1	
TP53	Tumor protein p53	Transcription factor
TXNRD2	Thioredoxin reductase 2	Enzyme
VSX2	Visual system homeobox 2	
ZNRF3	Zinc and ring finger 3	

The inheritance pattern of angle closure causing mutations in COL18A1 *was autosomal dominant. PACG (primary angle-closure glaucoma (EPDR1, CHAT, GLIS3, FERMT2, DPM2-FAM102); and exfoliation syndrome (XFS) glaucoma (CACNA1A). Additionally, it has been reported that the most significant GWAS in the Asian population were identified in SNPs of rs11024102 (PLEKHA7; 11p15.1), rs3753841 (COL11A1; 1p21.1), and rs1015213 (8q11.23).*

Table 8.
Genes associated with primary angle closure glaucoma.

Gene	Variant	Chr	Position	Consequence	Alleles	Class
ABCC5	rs1132776	3	183978614	Synonymous variant	A/G	snv
ABCC5	rs939336	3	183967746	Stop gained	A/G;T	snv
BIRC6	rs2754511	2	32545090	Intron variant	A/T	snv
C10orf53	rs1258267	10	49687724	Intron variant	G/A	snv
CALCRL; LOC105373786	rs1157699	2	187394177	Intron variant	C/G;T	snv
CAT	rs1001179	11	34438684	Upstream gene variant	C/T	snv
COL11A1	rs3753841	1	102914362	Missense variant	G/A	snv
COL11A1	rs12138977	1	102927901	Intron variant	C/T	snv
COL11A1	rs1676486	1	102888582	Missense variant	A/G;T	snv
DPM2;FAM102A	rs3739821	9	127940198	Non coding transcript exon variant	A/G	snv
EPDR1;SFRP4	rs3816415	7	37948709	Intron variant	G/A	snv
FERMT2	rs7494379	14	52944673	Intron variant	C/G;T	snv
GLIS3	rs736893	9	4217028	Intron variant	G/A;C	snv
HGF	rs17427817	7	81735119	Intron variant	C/A;G; T	snv
HGF	rs12540393	7	81734871	Intron variant	C/T	snv
HGF	rs3735520	7	81771623	Upstream gene variant	G/A;T	snv
HGF	rs5745718	7	81718232	Intron variant	T/G	snv
HSPA1L;HSPA1A	rs1043618	6	31815730	5 prime UTR variant	G/A;C; T	snv
HTR3D	rs12493550	3	184034985	Intron variant	G/A	snv
LINC02640	rs1900004	10	68241124	Intron variant	C/T	snv
LOC105373786; CALCRL	rs6759535	2	187373374	Intron variant	T/C	snv
LOC105373786; CALCRL	rs840617	2	187365606	Intron variant	A/T	snv
LOC107985096	rs1676484	1	102839465	Intron variant	A/C	snv
LOXL1;LOXL1-AS1	rs3825942	15	73927241	Missense variant	G/A;C; T	snv
LOXL1-AS1;LOXL1	rs2165241	15	73929861	Intron variant	T/C	snv
MMP1;WTAPP1	rs756459094	11	102795237	Missense variant	T/A;C; G	snv
MMP9	rs17576	20	46011586	Missense variant	A/G	snv
MMP9	rs2664538	20	46011586	Missense variant	A/G	snv
MMP9	rs3918249	20	46009497	Intron variant	T/C	snv
MTHFR	rs1217691063	1	11796309	Missense variant	A/G	snv
MYOC	rs183532	1	171640341	Intron variant	T/A;C	snv
MYOC	rs235875	1	171644616	Intron variant	C/T	snv
MYOC	rs235913	1	171649516	Intron variant	T/C;G	snv

Gene	Variant	Chr	Position	Consequence	Alleles	Class
NOS3	rs3793342	7	150998107	Intron variant	G/A	snv
NTF4	rs11669977	19	49060867	Non coding transcript exon variant	A/G	snv
NTF4	rs61732310	19	49061735	Missense variant	G/A	snv
PDIA5	rs11720822	3	123150194	Intron variant	C/T	snv
PLEKHA7	rs11024102	11	16987058	Intron variant	T/C	snv
PLEKHA7	rs216489	11	16802189	Intron variant	G/A;T	snv
SLC12A5-AS1;MMP9	rs2250889	20	46013767	Missense variant	G/C;T	snv
SLC12A5-AS1;MMP9	rs17577	20	46014472	Missense variant	G/A;C	snv
SLC38A4	rs983667	12	46769523	Intron variant	C/T	snv
SOD2	rs4880	6	159692840	Missense variant	A/G	snv
TP53	rs1042522	17	7676154	Missense variant	G/C;T	snv
TP53	rs1131691014	17	7676154	Frameshift variant	-/C	ins
TP53	rs878854066	17	7676153	Missense variant	GG/AC	mnv
TXNRD2	rs3788317	22	19902302	Intron variant	G/T	snv
VAV2	rs2156323	9	133855699	Intron variant	G/A	snv
VAV3	rs1466441587	1	107874935	Missense variant	G/A	snv
VAV3	rs2801219	1	107959790	Intron variant	C/A	snv
VAV3	rs576499843	1	107617607	Missense variant	A/C;G	snv
WTAPP1;MMP1	rs1799750	11	102799765	Intron variant	C/-	delins
ZNRF3	rs7290117	22	29054868	3 prime UTR variant	C/G;T	snv
	rs1015213	8	51974981	Intron variant	C/T	snv
	rs4656461	1	165717968	TF binding site variant		G/A

Table 9.
Variants associated with primary angle closure glaucoma.

8. Conclusions

Glaucoma genetics and genomics have to be assessed with the larger picture of visual impairment, disease prevalence, comorbidities, genetics, genomics, disease mechanisms, mechanical stress, neuroprotection, neurodegeneration, apoptosis, and immune imbalance. Few single causative genes, but multiple genes' dysregulated expressions at several tissues' sites of the eye like ciliary body, trabecular meshwork, lamina cribrosa, retina and optic nerve determine the spectrum of phenomics in glaucoma (**Figure 1**). This has led to the identification of neurotrophic factors, and anti-apoptotic molecules to prevent further neurodegeneration of RGCs and loss of vision. The complex nature of the disease and the discovery of several hundred genes and molecules is a boon and a bane at the same time. This status needs further research to focus and identify a battery of few molecules that could be used, individually or as a cocktail, in a majority of patients with glaucoma. However, it looks like the field may move towards a cocktail of molecular therapy based on personalised medicine and the individuals' genetic signature pattern and phenomics.

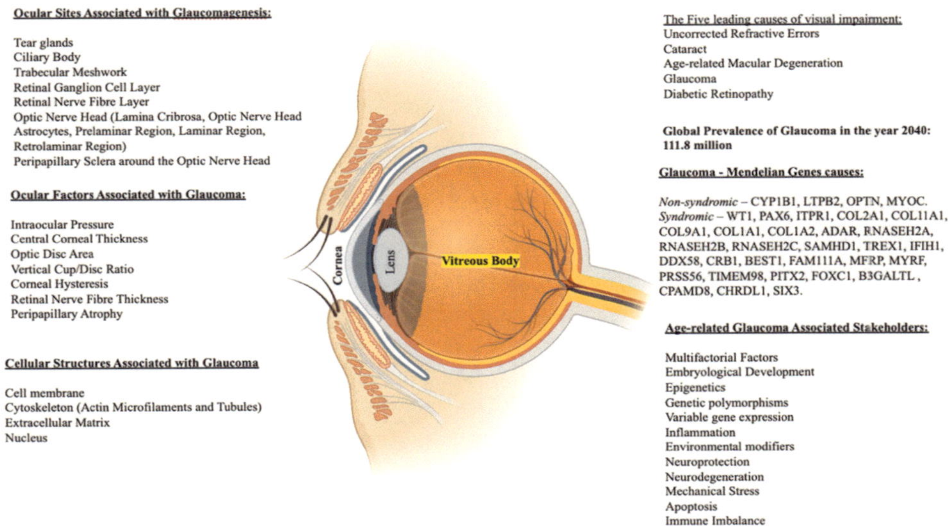

Figure 1.
The ocular tissues, genomics and biomechanisms of glaucoma.

Author details

Govindasamy Kumaramanickavel[1*], Siddhita Jadhav[1,2], Sugirdhana Parthiban Ramsait[1] and Pinakin Gunvant Davey[3]

1 Counselling in Medical Genetics Unit, GenVams Trust, GenVamsalya, Chennai, India

2 University Eye Clinic Maastricht, Maastricht University Medical Center, Maastricht, The Netherlands

3 College of Optometry, Western University of Health Sciences, Pomona, California, United States of America

*Address all correspondence to: gkumarmvel@gmail.com

References

[1] Cueto AFV, Álvarez L, García M, Álvarez-barrios A, Artime E, Cueto LFV, et al. Candidate glaucoma biomarkers: From proteins to metabolites, and the pitfalls to clinical applications. Biology. 2021;**10**:763

[2] Zukerman R, Harris A, Oddone F, Siesky B, Verticchio Vercellin A, Ciulla TA. Glaucoma heritability: Molecular mechanisms of disease. Genes (Basel). 2021;**12**:8

[3] Roughead EE, Kalisch LM, Pratt NL, Killer G, Barnard A, Gilbert AL. Managing glaucoma in those with co-morbidity: Not as easy as it seems. Biology. 2021;**19**:74

[4] Flaxman SR, Bourne RRA, Resnikoff S, Ackland P, Braithwaite T, Cicinelli M V, et al. Articles Global causes of blindness and distance vision impairment 1990-2020: A systematic review and meta-analysis. 2017. Available from: www.thelancet.com/lancetgh

[5] (17) (PDF) World blindness and visual impairment: Despite many successes, the problem is growing [Internet]. [cited 2020 Apr 6]. Available from: https://www.researchgate.net/publication/323435449_World_blindness_and_visual_impairment_despite_many_successes_the_problem_is_growing

[6] Gordois A, Cutler H, Pezzullo L, Gordon K, Cruess A, Winyard S, et al. An estimation of the worldwide economic and health burden of visual impairment. Global Public Health. 2012;**7**(5):465-481

[7] Wittenborn JS, Zhang X, Feagan CW, et al. The economic burden of vision loss and eye disorders among the United States population younger than 40 years. Ophthalmology. 2013;**120**(9):1728-1735

[8] Bourne RR, Stevens GA, White RA, et al. Causes of vision loss worldwide, 1990-2010: A systematic analysis. Lancet Global Health. 2013;**1**(6):e339-e349

[9] Khanna RC, Marmamula S, Rao GN. International vision care: Issues and approaches. Annual Review of Visual Science. 2017;**3**(1):53-68

[10] Raman R, Rani PK, Reddi Rachepalle S, et al. Prevalence of diabetic retinopathy in India: Sankara Nethralaya diabetic retinopathy epidemiology and molecular genetics study report 2. Ophthalmology. 2009;**116**(2):311-318

[11] Zetterberg M. Age-Related Eye Disease and Gender. Maturitas: Elsevier Ireland Ltd; 2016. pp. 19-26

[12] Stevens GA, White RA, Flaxman SR, Price H, Jonas JB, Keeffe J, et al. Global prevalence of vision impairment and blindness: Magnitude and temporal trends, 1990-2010. Ophthalmology. 2013;**120**(12):2377-2384

[13] Reitmeir P, Linkohr B, Heier M, Molnos S, Strobl R, Schulz H, et al. Common eye diseases in older adults of southern Germany: results from the KORA-Age study. National Health Aging Trends in Study Pain. 2011;**154**(12):481-486

[14] Wong TY, Loon SC, Saw SM. The epidemiology of age related eye diseases in Asia [Internet]. British Journal of Ophthalmology. 2006;**90**:506-511

[15] Hashemi H, Khabazkhoob M, Nabovati P, Ostadimoghaddam H, Shafaee S, Doostdar A, et al. The prevalence of age-related eye disease in an elderly population. Ophthalmic Epidemiology. 2017;**24**(4):222-228

[16] Klein R, Klein BEK. The prevalence of age-related eye diseases and visual impairment in aging: Current estimates. Investigative Ophthalmology and Visual Science. 2013;**54**(14):SF5

[17] Maberley DA, Hollands H, Chuo J, et al. The prevalence of low vision and blindness in Canada. Eye (Lond). 2006; **20**(3):341-346. DOI: 10.1038/sj.eye.6701879

[18] Congdon N. Causes and prevalence of visual impairment among adults in the United States. Archives of Ophthalmology. 2004;**122**(4):477-485

[19] Chou R, Dana T, Bougatsos C, Grusing S, Blazina I. Screening for impaired visual acuity in older adults: Updated evidence report and systematic review for the US preventive services task force. JAMA. 2016;**315**(9):915-933

[20] Prasad S, Kamath GG, Jones K, Clearkin LG, Phillips RP. Prevalence of blindness and visual impairment in a population of people with diabetes. Eye. 2001;**15**(5):640-643

[21] Sheeladevi S, Seelam B, Nukella P, Borah R, Ali R, Keay L. Prevalence of refractive errors, uncorrected refractive error, and presbyopia in adults in India: A systematic review. Indian Journal of Ophthalmology. 2019;**67**:583-592

[22] Furtado JM, Lansingh VC, Carter MJ, Milanese MF, Peña BN, Ghersi HA, et al. Causes of blindness and visual impairment in Latin America. Survey of Ophthalmology. 2012;**57**(2):149-177

[23] Zheng Y, Lavanya R, Wu R, Wong WL, Wang JJ, Mitchell P, et al. Prevalence and causes of visual impairment and blindness in an urban Indian population: The Singapore Indian eye study. Ophthalmology. 2011;**118**(9): 1798-1804

[24] Liang YB, Friedman DS, Wong TY, et al. Prevalence and causes of low vision and blindness in a rural Chinese adult population: The Handan Eye Study. Ophthalmology. 2008;**115**(11):1965-1972

[25] Chiang PPC, Zheng Y, Wong TY, Lamoureux EL. Vision impairment and major causes of vision loss impacts on vision-specific functioning independent of socioeconomic factors. Ophthalmology. 2013;**120**(2):415-422

[26] Ramke J, Zwi AB, Palagyi A, Blignault I, Gilbert CE. Equity and blindness: Closing evidence gaps to support universal eye health. Ophthalmic Epidemiology. 2015;**22**(5): 297-307

[27] Hashemi N, Moghaddasi H, Rabiei R, Asadi F, Farahi A. Eye health information systems in selected countries. Journal of Ophthalmic Visual Research. 2018;**13**(3):333-338

[28] Boerma T, Eozenou P, Evans D, Evans T, Kieny MP, Wagstaff A. Monitoring progress towards universal health coverage at country and global levels. PLoS Medicine. 2014;**11**(9):e1001731

[29] Yang X, Pan X, Zhao X, Luo J, Xu M, Bai D, et al. Autophagy and Age-Related Eye Diseases. 2019

[30] Paul S, Abraham V. How healthy is our geriatric population? A community-based cross-sectional study. Journal of Family Medicine and Primary Care. 2015;**4**(2):221

[31] Vijaya L, George R, Arvind H, Baskaran M, Raju P, Ramesh SV, et al. Prevalence and causes of blindness in the rural population of the Chennai Glaucoma Study. British Journal of Ophthalmology. 2006;**90**(4):407

[32] Quigley H, Broman AT. The number of people with glaucoma worldwide in

2010 and 2020. The British Journal of Ophthalmology. 2006;**90**:262-267

[33] Tham Y-C, Li X, Wong TY, Quigley HA, Aung T, Cheng C-Y. Global Prevalence of Glaucoma and Projections of Glaucoma Burden through 2040 A Systematic Review and Meta-Analysis. Ophthalmology. 2014;**121**:2081

[34] Bourne RRA. Worldwide glaucoma through the looking glass. The British Journal of Ophthalmology. 2020;**90**: 253-254

[35] Kapetanakis VV, MPY C, Foster PJ, Cook DG, Owen CG, Rudnicka AR. Global variations and time trends in the prevalence of primary open angle glaucoma (POAG): A systematic review and meta-analysis. The British Journal of Ophthalmology. 2016;**100**:86-93

[36] Chiu SL, Chu CL, Muo CH, Chen CL, Lan SJ. The prevalence and the incidence of diagnosed open-angle glaucoma and diagnosed angle-closure glaucoma: Changes from 2001 to 2010. Journal of Glaucoma. 2016;**25**(5):e514-e519

[37] George R, Ve RS, Vijaya L. Glaucoma in India: Estimated burden of disease. Journal of Glaucoma. 2010;**19**(6):391-397

[38] Rein DB, Zhang P, Wirth KE, Lee PP, Hoerger TJ, McCall N, et al. The economic burden of major adult visual disorders in the United States. Archives of Ophthalmology. 2006;**124**(12): 1754-1760

[39] Leffler CT, Schwartz SG, Giliberti FM, Young MT, Bermudez D. What was Glaucoma Called before the 20th Century?: 2015

[40] Teikari JM. Genetic factors in open-angle (simple and capsular) glaucoma: A population-based twin study. Acta Ophthalmologica. 1987;**65**(6):715-720

[41] Cuellar-Partida G, Craig JE, Burdon KP, Wang JJ, Vote BJ, Souzeau E, et al. Assessment of polygenic effects links primary open-angle glaucoma and age-related macular degeneration. Scientific Reports. 2016;**31**:6

[42] Ge T, Chen C-Y, Neale BM, Sabuncu MR, Smoller JW. Phenome-wide heritability analysis of the UK Biobank. PLOS Genetics. 2017;**13**(4):e1006711

[43] Weinreb RN, Leung CK, Crowston JG, et al. Primary open-angle glaucoma. Nature Reviews Disease Primers. 2016;**2**:16067

[44] Asefa NG, Neustaeter A, Jansonius NM, Snieder H. Heritability of glaucoma and glaucoma-related endophenotypes: Systematic review and meta-analysis. Survive in Ophthalmology. 2019;**64**(6):835-851

[45] Cascella R, Strafella C, Germani C, et al. The genetics and the genomics of primary congenital Glaucoma. BioMed Research International. 2015;**2015**:321291

[46] Sripriya S, George R, Vijaya L, Kumaramanickavel G. Basic science: Understanding the biology of Glaucoma: The current scenario. Current Journal of Glaucoma. 2007;**1**(1):7-16

[47] Plášilová M, Stoilov I, Sarfarazi M, Kádasi L, Feráková E, Ferák V. Identification of a single ancestral CYP1B1 mutation in Slovak Gypsies (Roms) affected with primary congenital glaucoma. Journal of Medical Genetics. 1999;**36**(4):290-294

[48] Dandona L, Williams JD, Williams BCRG. Population-based assessment of childhood blindness in southern India. Archives of Ophthalmology. 1998;**116**:545-546

[49] Ramprasad VL, George RJ, Sripriya S, Nirmaladevi J, Vijaya L, Kumaramanickavel G. Molecular genetic

analysis of a consanguineous south Indian family with congenital glaucoma: Relevance of genetic testing and counseling. Ophthalmic Genetics. 2007; **28**(1):17-24

[50] Sripriya S, Nirmaladevi J, George R, et al. OPTN gene: Profile of patients with glaucoma from India. Molecular Vision. 2006;**12**:816-820

[51] Stone EM, Fingert JH, Alward WLM, Nguyen TD, Polansky JR, Sunden SLF, et al. Identification of a gene that causes primary open angle glaucoma. Science. 1997;**275**(5300):668-670

[52] Sripriya S, Uthra S, Sangeetha R, George RJ, Hemmamalini A, Paul PG, et al. Low frequency of myocilin mutations in Indian primary open-angle glaucoma patients. Clinical Genetics. 2004;**65**(4):333-337

[53] Quigley HA, Stone EM, Fingert JH. Familial glaucoma—A pedigree revisited with genetic testing after 70 years. JAMA Ophthalmology. 2022; **140**(5):543-544

[54] Cunha DL, Arno G, Corton M, Moosajee M. The spectrum of PAX6 mutations and genotype-phenotype correlations in the eye. Genes. 2019; **10**(12):1050

[55] Wallace DJ, Chau FY, Santiago-Turla C, Hauser M, Challa P, Lee PP, et al. Osteogenesis imperfecta and primary open angle glaucoma: Genotypic analysis of a new phenotypic association. Molecular Visual. 2014;**20**:1174

[56] Balikov DA, Jacobson A, Prasov L. Glaucoma syndromes: Insights into glaucoma genetics and pathogenesis from monogenic syndromic disorders. Genes. 2021;**12**:9

[57] Souma T, Tompson SW, Thomson BR, Siggs OM, Kizhatil K, Yamaguchi S, et al. Angiopoietin receptor TEK mutations underlie primary congenital glaucoma with variable expressivity. Journal of Clinical Investment. 2016;**126**(7):2575

[58] Berry FB, Lines MA, Oas JM, Footz T, Underhill DA, Gage PJ, et al. Functional interactions between FOXC1 and PITX2 underlie the sensitivity to FOXC1 gene dose in Axenfeld–Rieger syndrome and anterior segment dysgenesis. Human Molecular Genetics. 2006;**15**(6):905-919

[59] Graw J. The genetic and molecular basis of congenital eye defects. Nature Reviews. Genetics. 2003;**4**(11):876-888

[60] Ragge NK, Lorenz B, Schneider A, Bushby K, De Sanctis L, De Sanctis U, et al. SOX2 anophthalmia syndrome. American Journal of Medical Genetetics. 2005;**135**:1-7

[61] Davidson AE, Cheong SS, Hysi PG, Venturini C, Plagnol V, Ruddle JB, et al. Association of CHRDL1 mutations and variants with X-linked Megalocornea, Neuhäuser syndrome and central corneal thickness. PLoS One. 2014;**9**: 2012-2016

[62] Shetty R, Nuijts RM, Nanaiah SG, et al. Two novel missense substitutions in the VSX1 gene: Clinical and genetic analysis of families with Keratoconus from India. BMC Medical Genetics. 2015; **16**:33

[63] Reis LM, Semina EV. Genetics of anterior segment dysgenesis disorders. Current Opinion in Ophthalmology. 2011;**22**(5):314-324

[64] DeJesus Y, Moreno Ceballos G. A timeline of discovery and current research on primary open-angle glaucoma and emergence of potentially permanent treatment solutions. Spectra

Undergraduate Research Journal. 2021; **1**(2):24-35

[65] Sudlow C, Gallacher J, Allen N, et al. UK Biobank: An open access resource for identifying the causes of a wide range of complex Diseases of middle and old Age. PLoS Medicine. 2015;**12**(3):e1001779

[66] Choquet H, Paylakhi S, Kneeland SC, Thai KK, Hoffmann TJ, Yin J, et al. A multiethnic genome-wide association study of primary open-angle glaucoma identifies novel risk loci. Nature Communications. 2018;**9**(1):1-14

[67] Burdon KP. Genome-wide association studies in the hunt for genes causing primary open-angle glaucoma: a review. Clinical Experiment Ophthalmology. 2012;**40**(4):358-363

[68] Abu-Amero K, Kondkar A, Chalam K. An updated review on the genetics of primary open angle glaucoma. International Journal of Molecular Science. 2015;**16**(2): 28886-28911

[69] Miller MA, Fingert JH, Bettis DI. Genetics and genetic testing for glaucoma. Current Opinion in Ophthalmology. 2017;**28**:133-138

[70] Liu Y, Allingham RR. Molecular genetics in glaucoma. Experimental Eye Research. Oct 2011;**93**(4):331-339

[71] Wiggs JL, Hauser MA, Abdrabou W, Allingham RR, Budenz DL, Delbono E, et al. The NEIGHBOR consortium primary open angle Glaucoma genome-wide association study: Rationale, study design and clinical variables. Journal of Glaucoma. 2013;**22**(7):517

[72] Verma SS, Cooke Bailey JN, Lucas A, Bradford Y, Linneman JG, Hauser MA, et al. Epistatic gene-based interaction analyses for Glaucoma in eMERGE and NEIGHBOR consortium. PLoS Genetics. 2016;**12**(9)

[73] Sripriya S, George R, Arvind H, et al. Transforming growth factor beta-1 -509C>T polymorphism in Indian patients with primary open angle glaucoma. Molecular Diagnosis Therapy. 2007;**11**(3):151-154

[74] Nair KS, Srivastava C, Brown RV, Koli S, Choquet H, Kang HS, et al. GLIS1 regulates trabecular meshwork function and intraocular pressure and is associated with glaucoma in humans. Nature Communication. 2021;**12**(1):15

[75] Quigley HA, Congdon NG, Friedman DS. Glaucoma in China (and worldwide): Changes in established thinking will decrease preventable blindness. The British Journal of Ophthalmology. 2001;**85**:1271-1272

[76] Vithana EN, Khor CC, Qiao C, Nongpiur ME, George R, Chen LJ, et al. Genome-wide association analyses identify three new susceptibility loci for primary angle closure glaucoma. Nature Genetics. 2012;**44**(10):1142-1146

[77] Ahram DF, Alward WL, Kuehn MH. The genetic mechanisms of primary angle closure glaucoma. Eye. 2015; **29**(10):1251

[78] Wiggs JL, Pasquale LR. Genetics of glaucoma. Human Molecular Genetics. 2017;**26**(R1):R21

[79] Inamori Y, Ota M, Inoko H, Okada E, Nishizaki R, Shiota T, et al. The COL1A1 gene and high myopia susceptibility in Japanese. Human Genetics. 2007;**122**(2):151-157

[80] Zhang D, Shi Y, Gong B, He F, Lu F, Lin H, et al. An association study of the COL1A1 gene and high myopia in a Han Chinese population. 2022

[81] Aboobakar IF, Wiggs JL. The genetics of glaucoma: Disease associations, personalised risk assessment and therapeutic opportunities-A review. Clinical Experiment in Ophthalmology. 2022; **50**(2):143-162

[82] Thorleifsson G, Magnusson KP, Sulem P, Walters GB, Gudbjartsson DF, Stefansson H, et al. Common sequence variants in the LOXL1 gene confer susceptibility to exfoliation glaucoma. Science. 2007;**317**(5843):1397-1400

[83] Ramprasad VL, George R, Soumittra N, Sharmila F, Vijaya L, Kumaramanickavel G. Association of non-synonymous single nucleotide polymorphisms in the LOXL1 gene with pseudoexfoliation syndrome in India. Molecular Vision. 9 Feb 2008;**14**:318-322

[84] Aboobakar IF, Johnson WM, Stamer WD, Hauser MA, Allingham RR. Major review: Exfoliation syndrome; advances in disease genetics, molecular biology, and epidemiology. Experimental Eye Research. 2017;**154**:88-103

[85] Tian Y, Li J, Su S, Cao Y, Wang Z, Zhao S, et al. PCOS-GWAS susceptibility variants in THADA, INSR, TOX3, and DENND1A are associated with metabolic syndrome or insulin resistance in women with PCOS. Frontier in Endocrinology. 2020;**11**:274

[86] Weinreb RN, Aung T, Medeiros FA. The pathophysiology and treatment of glaucoma: A review. JAMA. 2014; **311**(18):1901-1911

[87] Dias MS, Araujo VG de, Lani-Louzada R, Linden R, Ribas VT, Petrs-Silva H. Perspective on Gene Therapy for Glaucoma. 2022

[88] Prada D, Harris A, Guidoboni G, Siesky B, Huang AM, Arciero J. Autoregulation and neurovascular coupling in the optic nerve head. Survive in Ophthalmology. 2016;**61**(2):164-186

[89] Haro E, Petit F, Pira CU, Spady CD, Lucas-Toca S, Yorozuya LI, et al. Identification of limb-specific Lmx1b auto-regulatory modules with Nail-patella syndrome pathogenicity. Natural Communication. 2021;**12**(1):1-11

[90] Zukerman R, Harris A, Oddone F, Siesky B, Verticchio Vercellin A, Ciulla TA. Glaucoma heritability: Molecular mechanisms of disease. Genes. 2021;**12**(8):1135

[91] Springelkamp H, Höhn R, Mishra A, Hysi PG, Khor CC, Loomis SJ, et al. Meta-analysis of genome-wide association studies identifies novel loci that influence cupping and the glaucomatous process. Nature Communication. 2014;**5**:47

[92] Mamatha G, Srilekha S, Meenakshi S, Kumaramanickavel G. Screening of the RPE65 gene in the Asian Indian patients with leber congenital amaurosis. Ophthalmic Genetics. 2008; **29**(2):73-78

[93] Faro V, Bhattacharya A, Zhou W, Zhou D, Wang Y, Läll K, et al. Genome-wide association meta-analysis identifies novel ancestry-specific primary open-angle glaucoma loci and shared biology with vascular mechanisms and cell proliferation. medRxiv. 2021;**2021**:10

[94] Nickells RW. The cell and molecular biology of Glaucoma: Mechanisms of retinal ganglion cell death. Investigative Ophthalmology & Visual Science. 2012; **53**(5):2476-2481

[95] Quigley HA, Nickells RW, Kerrigan LA, Pease ME, Thibault DJ, Zack DJ. Retinal ganglion cell death in experimental glaucoma and after

axotomy occurs by apoptosis. Investigative Ophthalmology & Visual Science. 1995;**36**(5):774-786

[96] Cordeiro MF, Normando EM, Cardoso MJ, Miodragovic S, Jeylani S, Davis BM, et al. Real-time imaging of single neuronal cell apoptosis in patients with glaucoma. Brain. 2017;**140**(6): 1757-1767

[97] Mead B, Kerr A, Nakaya N, Tomarev SI. miRNA changes in retinal ganglion cells after optic nerve crush and glaucomatous damage. Cells. 2021;**10**(7): 1757

[98] Pernet V, Di Polo A. BDNF promotes robust survival of retinal ganglion cells but not axon regeneration within the Adult rat optic nerve. Investigative Ophthalmology & Visual Science. 2003; **44**(13):136

[99] R Z, A H, AV V, B S, LR P, TA C. Molecular genetics of glaucoma: Subtype and ethnicity considerations. Genes. 2020;**12**(1):1-36

[100] Liu J, Gao HY, Wang XF. The role of the Rho/ROCK signaling pathway in inhibiting axonal regeneration in the central nervous system. Neural Regeneration Research. 2015;**10**(11):1892

[101] Barros Ribeiro Da Silva V, Porcionatto M, Toledo Ribas V. The rise of molecules able to regenerate the central nervous system. Journal of Medical Chemistry. 2022;**63**(2):490-511

[102] Reinehr S, Guntermann A, Theile J, Benning L, Grotegut P, Kuehn S, et al. Proteomic analysis of retinal tissue in an S100B autoimmune glaucoma model. Biology. 2021;**11**(1):16

[103] Fudalej E, Justyniarska M, Kasarełło K, Dziedziak J, Szaflik JP, Cudnoch-Jędrzejewska A. Neuroprotective factors of the retina and their role in promoting survival of retinal ganglion cells: A review. Ophthalmic Research. 2021;**64**(3):345-355

[104] Clark AF. The cell and molecular biology of Glaucoma: Biomechanical factors in Glaucoma. Investigative Ophthalmology & Visual Science. 2012; **53**(5):2473-2475

[105] Piñero J, Saüch J, Sanz F, Furlong LI. The DisGeNET cytoscape app: Exploring and visualizing disease genomics data. Computational and Structural Biotechnology Journal. 2021; **19**:2960-2967

Chapter 7

Perspective on Gene Therapy for Glaucoma

Mariana Santana Dias, Victor Guedes de Araujo, Rafael Lani-Louzada, Rafael Linden, Vinicius Toledo Ribas and Hilda Petrs-Silva

Abstract

Glaucoma is a chronic and multifactorial neurodegenerative disease marked by structural damage to the optic nerve with axonal loss, progressive retinal ganglion cell degeneration, and optic disc excavation. Both high intraocular pressure and aging are important risk factors, but not essential to the progression of glaucomatous neurodegeneration. Current treatments are based on controlling intraocular pressure, which is not always effective in avoiding the progression of visual loss. In this sense, novel therapeutic strategies to glaucoma should aim to promote the neuroprotection of both the cell soma of retinal ganglion cells and the axons of the optic nerve. Gene therapy is a new therapeutical approach to glaucoma with a great capacity to overcome neurodegeneration. It consists of the transfer of exogenous genetic material to target cells with a therapeutic purpose. Gene therapy strategies for glaucoma include both the neuroprotection aiming to prevent cell soma and axonal loss and the regeneration of optic nerve axons. In this chapter, we review the most promising current gene therapies for glaucoma that address the various aspects of glaucoma pathology. We also discuss the potential of combining neuroprotective and regenerative strategies to reach a synergic effect for the treatment of glaucoma.

Keywords: glaucoma, retinal ganglion cell, optic nerve, gene therapy, neuroprotection, neuroregeneration

1. Introduction

Glaucoma is a heterogeneous group of highly prevalent ocular disorders that can progress to blindness, impacting functional capacity, social relations, and quality of life. It is now the leading cause of irreversible blindness in the world [1]. Furthermore, it affects mainly the elderly, and its prevalence is expected to increase in the next decades, in parallel with the progressive aging of the world population [2]. The high incidence of glaucoma with continuous growth, combined with its outcome of progressive and irreversible blindness, makes this disease a major public health problem. The pathophysiology of glaucoma is still not completely understood, and the disease has no cure. Glaucoma is a multifactorial, chronic disease characterized by structural damage to the optic nerve, thinning of the nerve fiber layer, and the degeneration of retinal ganglion cells (RGCs). These changes result in corresponding visual field impairment that progresses to complete vision loss. RGCs transmit visual information to the brain through the axons of the optic nerve. RGC axons converge to the optic disc and exit the globe through the lamina cribrosa to form the optic nerve. In glaucoma, the progressive cupping of the optic disc occurs due to damage to the lamina cribrosa and loss of RGC axons [3]. Long-standing evidence describes elevated intraocular pressure (IOP) and aging as the most prevalent stressors for RGCs in glaucoma. However, glaucomatous optic neuropathy may also develop in normal IOP conditions, in which damage occurs to the optic nerve without eye pressure exceeding the normal range [4].

Current treatments for glaucoma are related to IOP reduction, since high IOP is a manageable known risk factor. The procedure uses hypotensive eye drops or surgical interventions [5]. However, such approaches are often not sufficient to impair the death of RGCs and the progression of blindness, which may affect about half of the treated individuals [6, 7]. Recently, novel therapeutic approaches have searched for an efficient way to overcome neurodegeneration, focusing directly on preventing cell death and ensuring axonal integrity, including promising strategies based on gene therapy. This method consists of the transfer and expression of exogenous genetic material to cells and was originally developed to correct genetic diseases by supplying the cells with a normal copy of a defective gene [8]. Advances in the safety and efficacy of viral vectors capable to deliver therapeutic genetic material, as well as the recent approval of gene-based medicines by regulatory agencies of various countries, put gene therapy on center stage. A widespread panel of possible applications includes studies aimed at the treatment of complex, multifactorial diseases, such as glaucoma. Gene therapy strategies for glaucoma include the manipulation of a variety of intra- and extracellular factors involved in different cellular processes, such as apoptosis, metabolism, and axonal regeneration pathways. Such approaches may prevent neurodegeneration, and promising preclinical results strongly suggest translational potential.

2. Glaucoma: a neurodegenerative disease with early axonal damage

RGC cell death is the common outcome in glaucomatous neuropathies. It is believed to be a consequence of chronic stress, such as caused by IOP, which is expected to affect mainly the unmyelinated, initial portion of the RGC axons located in the optic nerve head (ONH). Such stress is associated with axon dysfunction, such as the biomechanical interruption of axonal transport [9]. Clinical and experimental evidence identified factors that may contribute to optic nerve head damage, such as mitochondrial dysfunction, oxidative stress, excitotoxicity, deprivation of neurotrophic factors, genetic susceptibility, reduced blood flow, vascular dysregulation, and neuroinflammation [9–11]. These alterations form an interconnected network of pathogenic processes that culminate in the degeneration of RGCs. However, each part of the RGC structure—soma, axon, and synapses—shows both the temporally and mechanically distinct degenerative patterns [12].

The degeneration of RGCs can be influenced by damage that affects their synapses and dendrites, as well as by signs from an axonal insult [13]. Early-onset modifications in dying RGCs include the silencing of RGC-specific gene expression, which precedes loss of neurons in certain animal models of glaucoma [14]. The pruning of RGC dendritic trees, cell body atrophy, nuclear shrinkage, and loss of RGC synapses with amacrine and bipolar cells are also among the initial changes detected in the glaucomatous retina [15]. These events activate several signaling pathways, such as those involving the mitogen-activated protein kinase p38 and Jun N-terminal kinases, which transmit the degeneration message to RGC soma [16]. As a key mechanism of RGC death in glaucoma, programmed cell death by apoptosis has been demonstrated in different species, such as rodents [17], nonhuman primates [18], and humans [19]. The cell death pathway is mediated by protein interactions of the BCL2 gene family, such as BAX or BAK, stimulators of apoptosis, while others, such as BCL-X and BCL2, have antiapoptotic functions. Activated BAX protein aggregates in the outer mitochondrial membrane and induces membrane instability and permeabilization, leading to the release in the cell cytoplasm of cytochrome c, which activates a cascade of caspases to induce cell death. On the other hand, BCL-X inhibits the mitochondrial activation of BAX, keeping the latter in the cytosol. RGC apoptosis depend on the activation of BAX, with the participation of mitochondrial components. BAX knockout animals ($BAX^{-/}$) submitted to acute optic nerve injuries are resistant to cell death by apoptosis, although BAX deficiency is not sufficient to prevent the axonal dysfunction of RGCs [20], suggesting that the mechanisms of cell death and axon degeneration are independent. RGC body loss, however, follows a spatially defined pattern. In rodents subjected to IOP by either a genetic or experimental approach, an asynchronous degeneration of individual RGCs leads to a sectorial pattern of neuron loss [21]. These experimental observations are akin to the pathological and clinical studies of glaucomatous humans, who show localized abnormalities and remodeling of the inner plexiform layer of the retina, correlated with a reduction in visual field function usually seen in early disease stages [9].

The ONH is considered the primary site of damage to RGCs in glaucoma. Despite the difference in lamina composition between humans and rodents, either IOP-dependent or IOP-independent insults to ONH can give rise to distal and proximal signs for the axonal degeneration of RGCs [12]. Among molecular changes triggered in this region, axonal transport failure due to mitochondrial dysfunction and an unbalanced axonal supply of neurotrophins such as brain-derived neurotrophic factor (BDNF) by oligodendrocytes stand out [13, 22]. Decreased blood flow, oxidative stress, reactive gliosis, and extracellular matrix remodeling are also molecular actors that regulate axonal degeneration in glaucomatous retina [9]. However, the exact contribution of each factor to RGC degeneration in glaucoma is not well established. Damaged axons in the optic nerve undergo degeneration, alter functional connectivity of neural circuits, and, consequently, cause a progressive loss of visual function. Axonal degeneration can be classified according to distinct parameters, such as the spatial relationship with the site of damage (proximal vs. distal) and time course (acute vs. chronic). Traumatic damage, as mimicked by optic nerve crush (ONC), results in complete axon degeneration through a series of well-defined events. First, there is acute axonal degeneration (AAD) close to the injury site, where rapid axon disintegration occurs at up to about 500 μm distal and proximal to injury site. This initial process of AAD is followed by a latency period of several hours, in which the rest of the injured axon remains unchanged. Then, two distinct degeneration processes begin: (i) abrupt granular disintegration of axon distal portion, a process known as Wallerian degeneration (WD), where there is cytoskeleton breakdown and organelle destruction; (ii) retrograde degeneration of the axon proximal portion (dying back). In addition, there may be secondary degeneration of cells not affected by the initial injury [23, 24]. In contrast with acute injuries, in chronic conditions, axons gradually degenerate toward a death process that progresses in a distal-to-proximal pattern from the synaptic region to the cell body. In the experimental models of glaucoma, both dying back and WD have been proposed as the mechanisms of axonal loss, while the role of AAD in glaucomatous degeneration is not understood. The heterogeneity of lesion sites highlights the need for further studies to better understand the time course and the complex processes of anterograde and retrograde degeneration of different subcellular regions of RGCs in experimental glaucoma [12].

An aggravating factor of neuronal degeneration in the adult central nervous system (CNS) of mammals is its low regenerative capacity. Once an injury occurs, damaged axons cannot regenerate and recover their integrity to prevent neuron death, therefore resulting in irreversible deficits. For this reason, numerous studies investigate the inhibition mechanisms of axonal regeneration in the CNS. The manipulation of these events can mediate the regrowth of axons and potentially benefit individuals affected either by acute injuries in the CNS or by neurodegenerative diseases associated with axonal dysfunctions, such as glaucoma.

3. Gene therapy for glaucoma

3.1 Strategies for neuroprotection

Over the past few decades, several strategies for neuroprotection of RGCs have been explored. Among those, gene therapy techniques have been developed and refined to allow an efficient targeting of this cell type. Considering RGC death, the critical cellular event of glaucomatous degeneration, the main targets of gene therapy strategies rely on antiapoptotic approaches, as well as on neurotrophic factors, Rho/Rho-associated protein kinase (ROCK) pathway, and mitochondrial disbalance, as summarized in **Table 1**.

Neurotrophic factors, such as brain-derived neurotrophic factor (BDNF), are essential for neuronal survival in the CNS, including RGCs. Acting through Tropomyosin receptor kinase B (TrkB) receptor, present on RGC dendrites and cell bodies, the BDNF can activate metabolic pathways for cell survival. Unbalanced physiological BDNF levels or its receptor have been shown in the experimental animal models of glaucoma as well as in patients [25], providing the rationale for new therapies based on BDNF supplementation. The viral vector-mediated overexpression of BDNF promoted robust neuroprotection in a variety of experimental glaucoma models, including acute injuries by NMDA injection [26], ischemia/reperfusion induced by an abrupt elevation of IOP [27], partial optic nerve transection [28], and surgically induced chronic OHT [29]. However, a sustained expression of exogenous BDNF has proved neurotoxic and led to downregulation of its high-affinity TrkB receptor, thus reducing BDNF/TrkB downstream signaling and therapeutical efficacy [30]. To overcome this transient effect, a simultaneous gene therapy with BDNF and TrkB receptor transgenes was tested. After a single intravitreal (IVT) injection, axonal transport was enhanced, and visual functional recovery was achieved in a laser-induced ocular hypertension rat model [31]. Ciliary neurotrophic factor (CNTF) is another well-characterized neurotrophic factor with neuroprotective effects demonstrated when overexpressed by different viral vector platforms in multiple RGC degeneration models, such as ONC [32], vascular occlusion [33], and OHT-induced models [34].

Rho/ROCK signaling pathway plays an important role in the pathogenesis of glaucoma and has been studied as a possible target to promote the neuroprotection of RGCs [35]. This pathway regulates several cellular processes, including cytoskeletal

Target	Mechanism of action	Animal models
1. Growth and neurotrophic factors		
BDNF	Overexpression of neurotrophic factor BDNF	ON transection; photocoagulation of TM; NMDA ivt.; cannulation of AC; partial ON transection
BDNF + TrkB	Overexpression of BDNF + receptor	ONC; photocoagulation of TM
BMP4	Overexpression of growth factor BMP4	Microbeads
FGF2	Overexpression of neurotrophic factor FGF	ON transection; NMDA ivt.
CNTF	Overexpression of the cytokine CNTF	ON transection; ONC; focal crush + retinal vessels occlusion; photocoagulation of TM
GDNF	Overexpression of neurotrophic factor GDNF	ON transection
GDNF + BIRC4	Overexpression of GDNF + caspase inhibitor BIRC4	ON transection
PEDF	Overexpression of PEDF	Cannulation of AC; NMDA ivt.
VEGFD	Overexpression of growth factor VEGFD	NMDA ivt.
2. Antiapoptotic factors		
BAG1	Overexpression of co-chaperone BAG1	ON transection; ONC
Bcl-X_L	Overexpression of antiapoptotic factor Bcl-X_L	Hypertonic saline injection in episcleral vein; DBA2J mouse
BIRC4/XIAP	Overexpression of caspase inhibitor BIRC4	Hypertonic saline injection in episcleral vein; ON transection; microbeads
sFasL	Overexpression of antiapoptotic factor FasL	DBA2J mouse; microbeads
3. Transcription factors		
ATF3	Overexpression of ATF3	ONC
Brn3b	Overexpression ofBrn3b	Hypertonic saline injection in episcleral vein
CREB	Overexpression of a constitutively active variant of CREB	NMDA ivt.
KLF7	Overexpression of KLF7	Cannulation of AC
4. Oxidative stress components		
Catalase	Overexpression of antioxidant enzyme, scavenger of hydrogen peroxid	Cannulation of AC
NRF2	Overexpression of transcription factor NRF2, which mediates transcription of several antioxidant elements	ONC
SOD2	Overexpression of antioxidant enzyme SOD2	Cannulation of AC
SOD2 + Catalase	Overexpression of SOD2 + catalase	ONC
5. Rho/ROCK pathway		
Exoenzyme C3	Overexpression of an inhibitor of Rho proteins	Cannulation of AC

Target	Mechanism of action	Animal models
RhoA	Silencing of RhoA	ONC
ROCK2	Silencing of ROCK2	ONC
6. Mitochondria-related targets		
NMNAT1	Overexpression of NAD production related enzyme	DBA2J mouse
OPA1	Overexpression of mitochondrial fusion protein OPA1	DBA2J mouse
Neuroglobin	Overexpression of the hemoprotein neuroglobin	DBA2J mouse
8. Other targets		
ABCA1	Overexpression of ABCA1 phospholipid transporter	Cannulation of AC
MCT2	Overexpression of monocarboxylate transporter MCT2	DBA2J mouse; microbeads
CaMKII	Overexpression of constitutively active CaMKII, enzyme in the Ca^{+2} signaling pathway	NMDA ivt.; ONC; microbeads; Glast-deficient mice
S100A4	Overexpression of S100A4, a Ca^{+2} binding protein	Cannulation of AC
CR2-Crry	Overexpression of complement inhibitor CR2-Crry	DBA2J mouse
CRMP2	Overexpression of CRMP2, a cytoskeleton regulator	Partial ON transection
Hsp70	Overexpression of chaperone Hsp70	ONC
MEK1	Overexpression of MEK1, an ERK1/2 activator	ON transection; hypertonic saline injection in episcleral vein
Shp2	Silencing of protein-tyrosine phosphatase shp2	Microbeads
ULK1	Overexpression of a dominant-negative form of autophagy activating kinase 1	ONC
miRs-17-5p + 30c-2 + 92a	Delivery of multiple miRNAs with a variety of targets	ONC
miRs-92a + 292 + 182		

Note: OHT: Ocular hypertension; I/R: Ischemia/reperfusion; ON: Optic nerve; TM: Trabecular meshwork; AC: Anterior chamber; ONC: Optic nerve crush; ivt: Intravitreal.

Table 1.
Gene therapy strategies for neuroprotection.

remodeling and synthesis of extracellular matrix components. Intravitreal injections of rAAV2 vectors carrying shRNA to knockdown RhoA expression can protect RGC from death caused by optic nerve injury [36]. In a similar study, the rAAV2-mediated knockdown of another member of this pathway, such as ROCK2, confers structural neuroprotection to RGC soma and axons after ONC [37]. Moreover, the inhibition of ROCK by the overexpression of BAG1 [38], an inhibitor of Rho/Rock signaling, can rescue RGC from apoptosis induced by axon injuries.

The modulation of apoptotic pathways has also been explored with gene therapy platforms. The overexpression of Bcl-XL, an antiapoptotic member of the Bcl-2 protein family, using an rAAV2 vector with phosphoglycerate kinase gene promoter (Pgk), robustly ameliorated RGC soma pathology and axonal degeneration in the chronic OHT mouse model, DBA/2 J, and provided a long-term somal neuroprotection after acute ONC [39]. Mechanisms involved in this therapy rely on blocking apoptosis induced by the activation of BAX, limiting its fusion to the mitochondria compartment. Alternatively, the overexpression of caspase inhibitor BIRC4 using rAAVs led to neuroprotection in a glaucoma model of OHT induced by the injection of magnetic microbeads in the anterior chamber, showing the preservation of RGC function as evaluated by pattern electroretinogram (PERG), and axonal integrity in the optic nerve [40]. Additionally, apoptosis in neuronal cells has been associated with the subcellular localization of Annexin A1 (ANXA1), since the nuclear localization of this molecule can modulate transcriptional factors such as p53 and p65 and trigger this type of cell death. As related to this pathway, Luo et al. described a strong neuroprotective action mediated by the overexpression of ATP-binding cassette (ABC) transporter A1 (ABCA1), which reduced the nuclear localization of ANXA1, and was associated with robust RGC survival in an I/R model induced by the cannulation of the anterior chamber [41].

A known outcome of RGC injury is the disruption of intracellular Ca^{+2} homeostasis, an ion that acts as an important intracellular signaling molecule [42]. Ca^{+2}/calmodulin-dependent protein kinase II (CaMKII) is a key responder in this pathway and has transcription factor CREB as an important downstream effector [43]. Guo et al. reported a decrease in phosphorylated CaMKII after RGC lesion by NMDA-induced excitotoxicity and ONC, indicating lower protein activity. The reactivation of CaMKII, mediated by the rAAV overexpression of a constitutively active mutant, robustly enhanced RGC survival after NMDA lesion, ONC, glaucoma models of microbead injection and in Glast-deficient mice. CREB activation was necessary and sufficient for the protective action of CaMKII. Furthermore, the neuroprotective effect of CaMKII had a long-lasting effect, was present even if overexpression was induced after the lesion, and led to the preservation of visual function [44].

In addition to those pathways, mitochondria dysfunction is another target explored to slow down glaucoma progression. ONH damage leads to an unbalance of mitochondrial homeostatic activity, compromising oxidative phosphorylation due to the dysregulation of intracellular calcium concentrations, thus contributing to reduced energy availability, increased production of reactive oxygen species (ROS), and activation of RGC apoptosis [45]. Selectively targeting specific ROS-mediated signaling pathways using rAAV2 constructs encoding the transcription factors NRF2 and/or PGC1a promoted the scavenger of ROS and protected RGCs from oxidative stress triggered by ONC [46]. However, the overproduction of stress response transcription factors Nrf2 and PGC1a can be toxic to neurons; therefore, adequate levels of expression are required. Moreover, reduced nicotinamide adenine dinucleotide (NAD) levels have been closely correlated with mitochondrial dysfunction and were implicated in glaucomatous degeneration [47]. NAD is a key component for healthy mitochondrial metabolism and an important redox cofactor essential for RGC function. Intravitreal viral gene therapy overexpressing Nmnat1, the terminal enzyme for NAD production, robustly protected DBA/2 J RGC against neurodegeneration, and prevented several early changes such as axoplasmic transport impairment and decline in RGC functional activity [48].

3.2 Strategies for axonal regeneration

Axonal damage is an early event during RGC degeneration in glaucoma. In this sense, besides preventing cell degeneration, gene therapy strategies to glaucoma should also aim at axonal regrowth after axon loss. However, axonal regeneration in mammalian CNS is not easy, since after development is completed, axons lose their ability to regrow. This is opposed to the peripheral nervous system, in which after axon damage, the distal portion of the lesion, not connected to cell body, degenerates, but a growth cone may develop in the axon's proximal part, which will regrow again. In this case, successful axonal regeneration leads to target reconnection, and usually, the neuron does not die. In the CNS, a scar develops in the lesion site, axons do not regenerate, and the neuros eventually die [49, 50]. This inability to regenerate has been associated with a few different factors, divided into two major groups known as cell intrinsic and cell extrinsic. Cell intrinsic factors include mostly genes related to axonal growth, which have their expression modulated after development, comprising several transcriptional factors as well as components of signaling pathways such as phosphoinositide 3-kinase (PI3K)/Akt (PI3K/Akt) and Janus kinase/signal transducer and activator of transcription protein (Jak/STAT) [51]. Cell extrinsic factors are mostly molecules associated with astrocytes and oligodendrocytes, such as chondroitin sulfate proteoglycans (CSPGs), NOGO myelin-associated glycoprotein (MAG), and oligodendrocyte myelin glycoprotein (OMGp), which are present in the glial scar and act as inhibitors of axonal regeneration. Yet, such molecules activate the Rho/Rho-associated protein kinase (Rho/ROCK) intracellular pathway, which mediates the intracellular responses to the extrinsic inhibitor molecules [52].

Numerous strategies have been tested for the regeneration of RGC axons. All used the ONC model to induce rapid axonal degeneration followed by RGC death, where axons completely degenerate distal to the injury site, thus facilitating the identification of regrown axons [53]. A handful of those approaches include gene transfer by viral vectors promoting the overexpression of proregenerative genes or, alternatively, silencing of antiregenerative ones. Gene manipulations that are capable of inducing axon regrowth are, in general, related to either intrinsic or extrinsic mechanisms that impair axonal regeneration, with a great diversity of targets. An overview of the mechanisms identified to date to enhance axonal regeneration based on viral vector delivery to the optic nerve is presented in **Table 2**.

PI3K/Akt is a well-known pathway related to axonal growth, and modifying different steps of it can lead to axonal regeneration. The activation of PI3-K converts phosphatidylinositol (4,5) bisphosphate (PIP2) into phosphatidylinositol (3,4,5) trisphosphate (PIP3), which activates the protein kinase Akt. One of the main consequences of Akt activation is phosphorylation and activation of mechanistic target of rapamycin (mTOR), a protein involved in a high diversity of cellular processes, including cell growth, motility, survival, and protein synthesis [52]. One of the first identified strategies to promote axonal regeneration is the inhibition of phosphatase and tensin homolog (PTEN). PTEN is a protein phosphatase that converts PIP3 into PIP2 and, therefore, inhibits Akt/mTOR, opposing the action of PI3K. The silencing of PTEN gene mediated by an intravitreal injection of rAAV-shRNA.PTEN vectors promotes axonal regeneration in the optic nerve [54]. This strategy was especially effective when used with a mutant capsid designed to enhance transduction. The intravitreal injection of rAAV2(Y444F)-shRNA.PTEN led to robust axonal regeneration, with some axons found all the way through the optic nerve, past the chiasma and into the optic tract [55]. The manipulation of several other targets in PI3K/Akt/

Target	Mechanism of action	Extent
1. PI3K/Akt pathway		
PTEN	**Silencing of an inhibitor of PI3K/Akt pathway**	**OT**
PI3K	Overexpression of a catalytic subunit of PI3K	ON
Akt	Overexpression of a constitutively active form of Akt	ON
cRHEB	Overexpression of a positive regulator of mTOR signaling	ON
S6K1	Overexpression of a downstream effector of mTOR	ON
GSK3	Overexpression of dominant negative form of GSK3β	ON
eIF2B	Overexpression of a constitutively active mutant of eIF2Bε	ON
FGF2	Overexpression of growth factor FGF2	ON
IGF1	Overexpression of growth factor IGF1	ON
Neuritin	Overexpression of neurotrophic factor neuritin	ON
2. Jak/STAT pathway		
CNTF	**Overexpression of a mutant peptide with higher affinity for CNTFRα**	**OT**
IL-6	**Overexpression of a hyperactive form of IL-6**	**CH**
IL-22	Silencing of IL22, a cytokine	ON
STAT3	Overexpression of constitutively active variants of STAT3	ON
SOCS4	Silencing of a suppressor of cytokine signaling	ON
Pim1	Overexpression of a downstream effector molecule of Jak/STAT	ON
3. Rho/ROCK pathway		
RhoA	Silencing of RhoA	ON
ROCK2	Silencing of ROCK2	ON
LIMK-1	Silencing of a downstream target of ROCK2	ON
LOTUS	Overexpression of a Nogo receptor antagonist	ON
PirB	Silencing of a receptor of myelin-associated inhibitors (MAIs)	ON
4. Transcription Factors		
KLF9	**Silencing of KLF9**	**CH**
c-myc	Overexpression of c-myc	ON
KLF4	Delivery of miRNA-135 s, which targets KLF4	ON
p53	Overexpression of p53	ON
SOX 11	Overexpression of SOX 11	ON
5. Other targets		
Lin 28	**Overexpression of Lin 28, an RNA-binding protein**	**CH**
Cpeb1	Overexpression of Cpeb1, an RNA-binding protein	ON
Armcx1	Overexpression of Armcx1, a mitochondrial protein	ON
BAG 1	Overexpression of co-chaperone BAG1	ON
DCLK2	Overexpression of DCLK2, a cytoskeleton regulator	ON
HDAC5	Overexpression of histone deacetylase HDAC5	ON
Set-β	Overexpression of Set-β, a transcriptional regulator	ON
Tceal3	Overexpression of Tceal3, a transcriptional regulator	ON

Target	Mechanism of action	Extent
Melanopsin	Overexpression of photopigment melanopsin, a G-protein coupled receptor	ON
Lipin1	Silencing of Lipin1 (biosynthesis of triglycerides)	ON
Pcyt1a	Overexpression of constitutively active Pcyt1 (biosynthesis of phospholipids)	ON
Pcyt2	Overexpression of Pcyt2 (biosynthesis of phospholipids)	ON
ULK1	Overexpression of a dominant-negative form of autophagy activating kinase 1	ON
MLP*	Overexpression of MLP, a cysteine-rich protein	ON
NDNF*	Overexpression of NDNF, a neurotrophic factor	ON
PRPH*	Overexpression of PRPH, a neuronal intermediate filament protein	ON
TIMP2*	Overexpression of TIMP2, tissue inhibitor of metalloproteinases 2	ON
UCN*	Overexpression of UCN, corticotropin-releasing factor	ON
THBS1*	Overexpression of THBS1, a secreted glycoprotein	ON
RASSF3*	Silencing of Rassf3, associated with the Ras family	ON
TBC1D22B*	Silencing of Tbc1d22b, a GTPase-activating protein for Rab family	ON

**identified by large-scale screening; OT: Optic tract; ON: Optic nerve; CH: Optic chiasma.*

Table 2.
Gene therapy strategies for axonal regeneration. Targets and most efficient strategy for each one after ONC.

mTOR pathway with the use of gene therapy vectors also led to axonal regeneration, even though restricted to the optic nerve. Strategies included the use of rAAVs to overexpress a constitutively active form of Akt [56], the catalytic subunit of protein kinase PI3K [57], and ras-homolog-enriched-in-brain 1 (Rheb1), a positive regulator of mTOR signaling [58]. The activation of Akt also leads to phosphorylation and inhibition of glycogen synthase kinase 3 (GSK3). GSK3, on the other hand, leads to the inhibition of translation initiation factor 2B epsilon (eIF2Bε). Using rAAVs to overexpress either a dominant negative form of GSK3β or a constitutively active eIF2Bε mutant also led to axonal regeneration [59].

Another common signaling pathway related to axonal regeneration is Jak/STAT. This pathway is usually activated after cytokine biding to extracellular receptors associated with protein kinases JAKs, leading to its activation and phosphorylation of STATs. An important negative feedback mechanism of this pathway is mediated by the proteins of the suppressor of cytokine signaling (SOCS) family, which inhibits Jak/STAT signaling [52]. Two highly efficient rAAV-mediated regenerative strategies involve the overexpression of two of the major cytokines that can activate the Jak/STAT pathway, interleukin 6 (IL-6) and ciliary neurotrophic factor (CNTF). When the overexpression of mutant CNTF peptide exhibiting a higher affinity for CNTF receptor alfa (CNTFRα) was driven by a ShH10 vector, an rAAV variant that preferentially infects Müller glia in mice, axonal regeneration was identified all the way into the optic tract [60]. The overexpression of a designer, hyperactive, form of IL-6 led to axonal regeneration until the chiasma [61]. Other successful strategies related to Jak/STAT and regeneration of the optic nerve involved the overexpression of a constitutively active variants of STAT3 [62] and the inhibition of SOCS4 with shRNA [63].

Furthermore, several transcriptional factors are associated with regenerative pathways and have been so far studied with gene therapy platforms. Among strategies for high-distance regeneration, silencing of KLF9 using rAAV-KLF9.shRNA mediated axonal regeneration up to the chiasm after intravitreal injection in rats [64]. The manipulation of other transcriptional factors led to regeneration in the optic nerve, including rAAV-mediated overexpression of SRY-box transcription factor 11 (SOX 11) [65, 66] and c-myc [67].

Rho/ROCK pathway is also important in the control of axonal regeneration. It is a convergence pathway activated in response of receptor binding of extrinsic inhibitory factors, that activates RhoA and its downstream target ROCK, the activation of which led to the collapse of the growth cone and impaired axonal growth [52]. The intravitreal injection of rAAVs associated with either RhoA-shRNA, ROCK2-shRNA, or LIMK-1-shRNA, targeting LIM domain kinase (LIMK), a downstream target of ROCK2, led to enhanced axonal regeneration in the optic nerve [36, 37]. Similarly, the overexpression of BAG 1, which inhibits ROCK2 activity, increased regeneration [38].

Some other proregenerative manipulations have also been described, which are not directly linked to the above-mentioned pathways. An especially robust strategy was the overexpression of Lin 28, an RNA-binding protein that is expressed mainly during early embryogenesis in mammals and the reactivation of which is associated with tissue repair mechanisms. Axonal regeneration after the intravitreal injection of rAAV-Lin28a in mice was identified until the chiasma [68].

Recently, many novel targets for axonal regeneration have been described based on large-scale screenings, capable of identifying a myriad of potential genes associated with this mechanism. Those studies were based on the transcriptional profiling of RGC subtypes with a higher regenerative ability, or under conditions in which a regenerative response was favored, or alternatively, in a genome-wide loss of function *in vitro* screen using an shRNA library [69–72].

The most efficient proregenerative strategies identified so far are related to the manipulation of more than one factor. In fact, several combinatorial strategies using rAAVs have been reported to lead to long-distance axonal regeneration. The overexpression of four transcriptional factors, Oct4/Pou5f1, Sox2, and Klf4 genes combined within a same rAAV particle, led to efficient axonal regeneration up to the chiasma [73]. Another successful example is combining KLF9 knockdown by rAAV-KLF-9shRNA and injection of PTEN, a chelator of mobile zinc, which mediated high-distance axonal regeneration until the optic tract [74]. Similarly, using the combination of PTEN silencing by rAAV- shPTEN4, CNTF overexpression using rAAV-CNTF, and injection of a cAMP analog, some axons reached the chiasm and followed along the contralateral nerve, reaching central nervous system targets [54]. A combination of cRheb1 overexpression and induction of neuronal activity by visual stimulation even partially recovered visual function of injured animals, leading to robust axonal regeneration and enabling reinnervation of central targets with a partial recovery of optokinetic reflex after ONC [58].

3.3 Combinatorial gene therapy

Pathways to promote RGC survival and axonal regeneration are not usually overlapping. As discussed above, different signaling pathways and regulatory molecules seem to be critical for either promoting neuroprotection or inducing axonal regeneration. In this sense, a combination of both strategies in a single-gene therapy approach would likely be highly beneficial for glaucoma. With an efficient neuroprotective approach, more RGCs will survive the injury and, thus, be available to successfully regenerate their axons in response to a proregenerative stimulus. On the other hand, an effective regenerative approach will guarantee the integrity of the axons of RGCs that have been already partially or completely lost, with the potential to recover neuronal function and favor cell survival at a long term, inclusive of retrograde neurotrophic support from the axonal targets. There is evidence that neuroprotective and regenerative pathways do not always overlap, and gene manipulation strategies can even have opposite consequences in each one. Clear examples are the genetic manipulation of apoptosis-related genes BAX and Bcl-2. The gene knockout of the proapoptotic protein BAX and the constitutive overexpression of the antiapoptotic protein Bcl-2 are very efficient strategies to prevent the neurodegeneration of RGCs, with survival of almost all cells in the ganglion cell layer of the retina but cannot efficiently regenerate their axons [75, 76]. Yet, dual leucine zipper kinase (DLK/MAP3K12), sphingosine 1-phosphate receptor 1 (S1PR1), and BDNF have neuroprotective properties, although they act as the inhibitors of axonal regeneration [77–79]. The transcriptional factor Sox 11, on the other hand, has been associated with both the proregenerative and prodeath responses [80]. Examples mentioned above depict well the complexity of the neurodegenerative and regenerative responses of RGCs, which needs to be considered when designing a gene therapy strategy to glaucoma. Still, some studies highlight the potential of combining neuroprotective and proregenerative strategies. For example, the intravitreal injection of rAAV-CNTF or rAAV-THBS is more efficient in promoting axonal regeneration when BAX protein is depleted [70, 76]. Similarly, the overexpression of CNTF in mice engineered to overexpress Bcl-2 had a stronger effect over axonal regeneration than in wild-type mice [32]. These examples of combined genetic manipulations show the potential of such strategies. However, they remain to be further explored in a gene therapy approach.

3.4 Challenges

Gene therapy involves the transfer and expression of exogenous genetic material in target cells for therapeutic purposes. Currently, gene therapy trials are on the rise, with more than six products reaching commercial approval by regulatory agencies such as U.S. Food and Drug Administration (FDA) and European Medicines Agency (EMA), and more than 40 products, targeting a variety of pathological conditions, are expected to be approved for clinical use in next decade [81]. Besides the latest growth in the field, gene therapy products are still very expensive, especially because of high manufacturing costs combined to the fact that most current gene therapy products treat rare diseases and benefit a restricted number of patients [81]. Expansion in gene therapy research, including other targets and high prevalent diseases, such as glaucoma, might contribute to decrease costs in the long run.

Recent successes in ocular gene therapy with LUXTURNA—a gene therapy product to improve and maintain vision in patients with Leber's congenital amaurosis—have paved the path for more studies in the field [82]. Ideally, for a therapy to be successful, the transduction of target cells involved in the pathology must occur. Thus, gene therapy studies for glaucoma need to efficiently transduce RGCs and reach the therapeutic level of gene expression. The transfer of genetic material to cells depends on the use of carriers that facilitate the entry of nucleic acid into target cells. In the retina, recombinant viral vectors derived from AAV have been the most efficient tool for gene transfer *in vivo* [83]. Despite recent evidence of genotoxicity mediated by rAAV vectors due to insertional mutagenesis into genomic DNA that culminated in tumor generation and alteration in liver function [84], no adverse effects of this magnitude have been described to date, after several safety ophthalmological clinical trials [85].

The delivery of gene therapy vectors to the retina may follow two major intraocular injection routes, namely subretinal (SR) for retinal epithelial cells and photoreceptors transduction and intravitreal (IVT), reaching preferentially the ganglion cell layer [86]. In higher species, both the SR and IVT injections induce mild and transient inflammatory responses [87], which are stronger when the doses of injected vector are increased. Inflammation can result in the clearance of transduced cells by cytotoxic T-cells, thus reducing therapy efficacy and worsening patient condition. Cellular immune responses prevent vector readministration due to the generation of neutralizing antibodies against rAAV capsid [88]. Other factors can influence ocular immunogenicity, such as rAAV cassette elements. rAAV incorporating ubiquitous promoters derived from viral sequences, such as CMV or CAG, led to microglia activation and inflammatory cytokine expression, triggering RPE and photoreceptor death after subretinal injections, while photoreceptor-specific promoters were not toxic to these cells even when higher doses were administered [89]. Further studies conducted in large animals, using other cell-type-specific promoters and a wider range of doses, will provide more insight into the correlation between toxicity and genetic material.

In small animals, the IVT injection of rAAV vectors efficiently transduces RGCs, but in nonhuman primates, the transduction is very inefficient [90]. This may be related to physical and biological barriers, such as the large size of primate eye when compared with rodents, which causes a significant dilution of the injected vector, as well as the thickness of the internal limiting membrane that hinders the passage of vectors to the retina [91]. These barriers make it difficult to translate preclinical studies to humans. Several recent studies have tried to enhance rAAV transduction efficiency after IVT injections, especially the use of mutant rAAV capsids [92]. However, the translation of these strategies to larger animals is still a challenge. Tyrosine-mutant rAAV vectors were not as efficient in dogs as they were in mice [93]. Digestion of ILM [94] and subILM injections [95] are also proposed strategies to increase transduction in primates through vitreous. However, until now, efficient and widespread transduction of nonhuman primates' RGCs after IVT injection has not been achieved.

Although the route of vector administration is important for directing gene expression in the region of interest, retinal tissue is complex, with a wide variety of cell types and rAAV vectors have been shown to transduce all of those. The use of an RGC-specific promoter can restrict gene expression to target cells, thus reducing unwanted off-target effects. For example, a Thy1 promoter confers high expression levels with some selectivity for RGCs; however, owing to its size of more than 6 kB, it is not suitable for rAAV [96]. A promoter less than 200 bp of NEFH gene, on the other hand, showed a more restricted expression to this cell type, and owing to its small size, it may serve as a tool for the insertion of genes or larger regulatory sequences in space-constrained vectors [97]. Moreover, hSYN promoter, despite being very efficient in mice, were shown to be inefficient by IVT in primates, making it difficult to translate its use [90]. Recently, PLE345 (NEFL)showed robust expression in RGC bodies and nerve fibers primarily at the injection site, with patches in the periphery, and with a small number of cells of the inner nuclear layer [98]. Still, a promoter based on the regulatory region of the gamma-synuclein gene (SNCG) drove strong expression in RGCs in both mice and primates, allowing gene editing on this cell type and optogenetic restoration of vision [99, 100]. Those promoters may benefit future gene therapy applications in the path to clinical translation.

4. Conclusions

Despite the different subtypes of glaucoma, such as open-angle, angle-closure, pseudoexfoliative, and normal-tension, among others, the common outcome converges to RGC death. In the past two decades, promising gene therapy strategies to glaucoma have been developed, focusing on both the neuroprotective and proregenerative mechanisms to overcome RGC degeneration, and, in theory, will be able to cover all the glaucoma subtypes. However, the translation to clinic is far much complex. For example, animal models do not cover the pathophysiology aspects of the different subtypes of glaucoma, and a lot of animal studies do not predict with sufficient certainty what will happen in humans. Finding a successful strategy is still a big challenge. An ideal gene therapy approach still needs to surpass issues related to vector delivery platforms, such as safety and efficacy, besides efficient promotion of long-term cell survival and axonal regrowth. For this, the manipulation of a single gene will most likely not be enough and will probably require the combinatorial use of distinct strategies.

Acknowledgements

This work was financially supported by CAPES/Financ. Code 001; CNPq and FAPERJ.

Conflict of interest

Authors declare no conflict of interest.

Author details

Mariana Santana Dias[1], Victor Guedes de Araujo[1], Rafael Lani-Louzada[2,3], Rafael Linden[2], Vinicius Toledo Ribas[4] and Hilda Petrs-Silva[1*]

1 Laboratory of Gene Therapy and Viral Vectors, Carlos Chagas Filho Institute of Biophysics, Federal University of Rio de Janeiro, Rio de Janeiro, Brazil

2 Laboratory of Neurogenesis, Carlos Chagas Filho Institute of Biophysics, Federal University of Rio de Janeiro, Rio de Janeiro, Brazil

3 Hospital Nossa Senhora da Saúde, Santa Casa da Misericórdia do Rio de Janeiro (Gamboa's Hospital), Institute of Ophthalmology of Rio de Janeiro, Rio de Janeiro, Brazil

4 Laboratory of Neurobiology, Department of Morphology, Institute of Biological Sciences, Federal University of Minas Gerais, Belo Horizonte, Brazil

*Address all correspondence to: hilda@biof.ufrj.br

References

[1] WHO - World Health Organization. Global data on visual impairment [Internet]. 2021. Available from: https://www.who.int/news-room/fact-sheets/detail/blindness-and-visual-impairment [Accessed: December 13, 2021]

[2] Tham YC, Li X, Wong TY, Quigley HA, Aung T, Cheng CY. Global prevalence of glaucoma and projections of glaucoma burden through 2040: A systematic review and meta-analysis. Ophthalmology. 2014;**121**(11):2081-2090. DOI: 10.1016/j.ophtha.2014.05.013

[3] Weinreb RN, Aung T, Medeiros FA. The pathophysiology and treatment of glaucoma: A review. Journal of the American Medical Association. 2014;**311**(18):1901-1911. DOI: 10.1001/jama.2014.3192

[4] Killer HE, Pircher A. Normal tension glaucoma: Review of current understanding and mechanisms of the pathogenesis. Eye (London, England). 2018;**32**(5):924-930. DOI: 10.1038/s41433-018-0042-2

[5] Meier-Gibbons F, Berlin MS, Töteberg-Harms M. Influence of new treatment modalities on adherence in glaucoma. Current Opinion in Ophthalmology. 2019;**30**(2):104-109. DOI: 10.1097/ICU.0000000000000551

[6] Heijl A, Buchholz P, Norrgren G, Bengtsson B. Rates of visual field progression in clinical glaucoma care. Acta Ophthalmologica. 2013;**91**(5):406-412. DOI: 10.1111/j.1755-3768.2012.02492.x

[7] Rossetti L, Digiuni M, Montesano G, Centofanti M, Fea AM, Iester M, et al. Blindness and Glaucoma: A Multicenter data review from 7 academic eye clinics. PLoS One. 2015;**10**(8):e0136632. DOI: 10.1371/journal.pone.0136632

[8] Sheridan C. Gene therapy finds its niche. Nature Biotechnology. 2011;**29**(2):121-128. DOI: 10.1038/nbt.1769

[9] Weinreb RN, Leung CKS, Crowston JG, Medeiros FA, Friedman DS, Wiggs JL, et al. Primary open-angle glaucoma. Nature Reviews. Disease Primers. 2016;**2**:16067. DOI: 10.1038/nrdp.2016.67

[10] Zukerman R, Harris A, Vercellin AV, Siesky B, Pasquale LR, Ciulla TA. Molecular genetics of Glaucoma: Subtype and ethnicity considerations. Genes (Basel). 2020;**12**(1):55. DOI: 10.3390/genes12010055

[11] Kamel K, Farrell M, O'Brien C. Mitochondrial dysfunction in ocular disease: Focus on glaucoma. Mitochondrion. 2017;**35**:44-53. DOI: 10.1016/j.mito.2017.05.004

[12] Tezel G. Multifactorial pathogenic processes of retinal ganglion cell degeneration in Glaucoma towards multi-target strategies for broader treatment effects. Cell. 2021;**10**(6):1372. DOI: 10.3390/cells10061372

[13] Munemasa Y, Kitaoka Y. Molecular mechanisms of retinal ganglion cell degeneration in glaucoma and future prospects for cell body and axonal protection. Frontiers in Cellular Neuroscience. 2013;**6**:60. DOI: 10.3389/fncel.2012.00060

[14] Pelzel HR, Schlamp CL, Waclawski M, Shaw MK, Nickells RW. Silencing of Fem1cR3 gene expression

in the DBA/2J mouse precedes retinal ganglion cell death and is associated with histone deacetylase activity. Investigative Ophthalmology & Visual Science. 2012;**53**(3):1428-1435. DOI: 10.1167/iovs.11-8872

[15] Williams PA, Howell GR, Barbay JM, Braine CE, Sousa GL, John SW, et al. Retinal ganglion cell dendritic atrophy in DBA/2J glaucoma. PLoS One. 2013;**8**(8):e72282. DOI: 10.1371/journal.pone.0072282

[16] Nickells RW. The cell and molecular biology of glaucoma: Mechanisms of retinal ganglion cell death. Investigative Ophthalmology & Visual Science. 2012;**53**(5):2476-2481. DOI: 10.1167/iovs.12-9483h

[17] Cordeiro MF, Guo L, Luong V, Harding G, Wang W, Jones HE, et al. Real-time imaging of single nerve cell apoptosis in retinal neurodegeneration. Proceedings of the National Academy of Sciences of the United States of America. 2004;**101**(36):13352-13356. DOI: 10.1073/pnas.0405479101

[18] Quigley HA, Nickells RW, Kerrigan LA, Pease ME, Thibault DJ, Zack DJ. Retinal ganglion cell death in experimental glaucoma and after axotomy occurs by apoptosis. Investigative Ophthalmology & Visual Science. 1995;**36**(5):774-786

[19] Cordeiro MF, Normando EM, Cardoso MJ, Miodragovic S, Jeylani S, Davis BM, et al. Real-time imaging of single neuronal cell apoptosis in patients with glaucoma. Brain. 2017;**140**(6):1757-1767. DOI: 10.1093/brain/awx088

[20] Libby RT, Li Y, Savinova O v, Barter J, Smith RS, Nickells RW, et al. Susceptibility to neurodegeneration in a glaucoma is modified by Bax gene dosage. PLoS Genetics 2005;**1**(1):17-26

[21] Vidal-Sanz M, Salinas-Navarro M, Nadal-Nicolás FM, Alarcón-Martínez L, Valiente-Soriano FJ, de Imperial JM, et al. Understanding glaucomatous damage: Anatomical and functional data from ocular hypertensive rodent retinas. Progress in Retinal and Eye Research. 2012;**31**(1):1-27

[22] Vrabec JP, Levin LA. The neurobiology of cell death in glaucoma. Eye (London, England). 2007;**21** (Suppl. 1):S11-S14. DOI: 10.1038/sj.eye.6702880

[23] Knöferle J, Koch JC, Ostendorf T, Michel U, Planchamp V, Vutova P, et al. Mechanisms of acute axonal degeneration in the optic nerve in vivo. Proceedings of the National Academy of Sciences of the United States of America. 2010;**107**(13):6064-6069. DOI: 10.1073/pnas.0909794107

[24] Ribas VT, Lingor P. Calcium channel inhibition-mediated axonal stabilization improves axonal regeneration after optic nerve crush. Neural Regeneration Research. 2016;**11**(8):1245-1246. DOI: 10.4103/1673-5374.189184

[25] Gupta V, You Y, Li J, Gupta V, Golzan M, Klistorner A, et al. BDNF impairment is associated with age-related changes in the inner retina and exacerbates experimental glaucoma. Biochimica et Biophysica Acta. 2014;**1842**(9):1567-1578. DOI: 10.1016/j.bbadis.2014.05.026

[26] Shiozawa AL, Igarashi T, Kobayashi M, Nakamoto K, Kameya S, Fujishita S, et al. Tyrosine triple mutated AAV2-BDNF gene therapy in an inner retinal injury model induced by intravitreal injection of N-methyl-D-aspartate (NMDA). Molecular Vision. 2020;**26**:409-422

[27] Igarashi T, Miyake K, Kobayashi M, Kameya S, Fujimoto C, Nakamoto K,

et al. Tyrosine triple mutated AAV2-BDNF gene therapy in a rat model of transient IOP elevation. Molecular Vision. 2016;**22**:816-826

[28] Chiha W, Bartlett CA, Petratos S, Fitzgerald M, Harvey AR. Intravitreal application of AAV-BDNF or mutant AAV-CRMP2 protects retinal ganglion cells and stabilizes axons and myelin after partial optic nerve injury. Experimental Neurology. 2020;**326**:113167. DOI: 10.1016/j.expneurol.2019.113167

[29] Martin KRG, Quigley HA, Zack DJ, Levkovitch-Verbin H, Kielczewski J, Valenta D, et al. Gene therapy with brain-derived neurotrophic factor as a protection: Retinal ganglion cells in a rat glaucoma model. Investigative Ophthalmology & Visual Science. 2003;**44**(10):4357-4365. DOI: 10.1167/iovs.02-1332

[30] Wójcik-Gryciuk A, Gajewska-Woźniak O, Kordecka K, Boguszewski PM, Waleszczyk W, Skup M. Neuroprotection of retinal ganglion cells with AAV2-BDNF Pretreatment restoring Normal TrkB receptor protein levels in Glaucoma. International Journal of Molecular Sciences. 2020;**21**(17):6262. DOI: 10.3390/ijms21176262

[31] Khatib TZ, Osborne A, Yang S, Ali Z, Jia W, Manyakin I, et al. Receptor-ligand supplementation via a self-cleaving 2A peptide-based gene therapy promotes CNS axonal transport with functional recovery. Science Advances. 2021;**7**(14):eabd2590. DOI: 10.1126/sciadv.abd2590

[32] Leaver SG, Cui Q, Bernard O, Harvey AR. Cooperative effects of bcl-2 and AAV-mediated expression of CNTF on retinal ganglion cell survival and axonal regeneration in adult transgenic mice. The European Journal of Neuroscience. 2006;**24**(12):3323-3332. DOI: 10.1111/j.1460-9568.2006.05230.x

[33] MacLaren RE, Buch PK, Smith AJ, Balaggan KS, MacNeil A, Taylor JS, et al. CNTF gene transfer protects ganglion cells in rat retinae undergoing focal injury and branch vessel occlusion. Experimental Eye Research. 2006;**83**(5): 1118-1127. DOI: 10.1016/j.exer.2006.05.019

[34] Pease ME, Zack DJ, Berlinicke C, Bloom K, Cone F, Wang Y, et al. Effect of CNTF on retinal ganglion cell survival in experimental glaucoma. Investigative Ophthalmology & Visual Science. 2009;**50**(5):2194-2200. DOI: 10.1167/iovs.08-3013

[35] Wang J, Liu X, Zhong Y. Rho/rho-associated kinase pathway in glaucoma (review). International Journal of Oncology. 2013;**43**(5):1357-1367. DOI: 10.3892/ijo.2013.2100

[36] Koch JC, Tönges L, Michel U, Bähr M, Lingor P. Viral vector-mediated downregulation of RhoA increases survival and axonal regeneration of retinal ganglion cells. Frontiers in Cellular Neuroscience. 2014;**8**:273. DOI: 10.3389/fncel.2014.00273

[37] Koch JC, Tönges L, Barski E, Michel U, Bähr M, Lingor P. ROCK2 is a major regulator of axonal degeneration, neuronal death and axonal regeneration in the CNS. Cell Death & Disease. 2014;**5**(5):e1225. DOI: 10.1038/cddis.2014.191

[38] Planchamp V, Bermel C, Tönges L, Ostendorf T, Kügler S, Reed JC, et al. BAG1 promotes axonal outgrowth and regeneration in vivo via Raf-1 and reduction of ROCK activity. Brain. 2008;**131**(Pt 10):2606-2619. DOI: 10.1093/brain/awn196

[39] Donahue RJ, Fehrman RL, Gustafson JR, Nickells RW. BCLXL gene therapy moderates neuropathology

in the DBA/2J mouse model of inherited glaucoma. Cell Death & Disease. 2021;**12**(8):781. DOI: 10.1038/s41419-021-04068-x

[40] Visuvanathan S, Baker AN, Lagali PS, Coupland SG, Miller G, Hauswirth WW, et al. XIAP gene therapy effects on retinal ganglion cell structure and function in a mouse model of glaucoma. Gene Therapy. 2021:1-10. DOI: 10.1038/s41434-021-00281-7

[41] Luo J, Wang S, Zhou Z, Zhao Y. Ad- and AAV8-mediated ABCA1 gene therapy in a murine model with retinal ischemia/reperfusion injuries. Molecular Therapy-Methods & Clinical Development. 2021;**20**:551-558. DOI: 10.1016/j.omtm.2021.01.012

[42] Prilloff S, Noblejas MI, Chedhomme V, Sabel BA. Two faces of calcium activation after optic nerve trauma: Life or death of retinal ganglion cells in vivo depends on calcium dynamics. The European Journal of Neuroscience. 2007;**25**(11):3339-3346. DOI: 10.1111/j.1460-9568.2007.05550.x

[43] Ma H, Groth RD, Cohen SM, Emery JF, Li B, Hoedt E, et al. γCaMKII shuttles Ca^{2+}/CaM to the nucleus to trigger CREB phosphorylation and gene expression. Cell. 2014;**159**(2):281-294. DOI: 10.1016/j.cell.2014.09.019

[44] Guo X, Zhou J, Starr C, Mohns EJ, Li Y, Chen EP, et al. Preservation of vision after CaMKII-mediated protection of retinal ganglion cells. Cell. 2021;**184**(16):4299-4314.e12. DOI: 10.1016/j.cell.2021.06.031

[45] Osborne NN, Núñez-Álvarez C, Joglar B, del Olmo-Aguado S. Glaucoma: Focus on mitochondria in relation to pathogenesis and neuroprotection. European Journal of Pharmacology. 2016;**787**:127-133. DOI: 10.1016/j.ejphar.2016.04.032

[46] Xiong W, MacColl Garfinkel AE, Li Y, Benowitz LI, Cepko CL. NRF2 promotes neuronal survival in neurodegeneration and acute nerve damage. The Journal of Clinical Investigation. 2015;**125**(4):1433-1445. DOI: 10.1172/JCI79735

[47] Petriti B, Williams PA, Lascaratos G, Chau K-Y, Garway-Heath DF. Neuroprotection in Glaucoma: NAD+/NADH redox state as a potential biomarker and therapeutic target. Cell. 2021;**10**(6):1402. DOI: 10.3390/cells10061402

[48] Williams PA, Harder JM, Foxworth NE, Cochran KE, Philip VM, Porciatti V, et al. Vitamin B3 modulates mitochondrial vulnerability and prevents glaucoma in aged mice. Science. 2017;**355**(6326):756-760. DOI: 10.1126/science.aal0092

[49] Smith TP, Sahoo PK, Kar AN, Twiss JL. Intra-axonal mechanisms driving axon regeneration. Brain Research. 2020;**1740**:146864. DOI: 10.1016/j.brainres.2020.146864

[50] Yang S-G, Li C-P, Peng X-Q, Teng Z-Q, Liu C-M, Zhou F-Q. Strategies to promote long-distance optic nerve regeneration. Frontiers in Cellular Neuroscience. 2020;**14**:119. DOI: 10.3389/fncel.2020.00119

[51] Ribas VT, Costa MR. Gene manipulation strategies to identify molecular regulators of axon regeneration in the central nervous system. Frontiers in Cellular Neuroscience. 2017;**11**:231. DOI: 10.3389/fncel.2017.00231

[52] Barros Ribeiro da Silva V, Porcionatto M, Toledo Ribas V. The rise of molecules able to regenerate

the central nervous system. Journal of Medicinal Chemistry. 2020;**63**(2):490-511. DOI: 10.1021/acs.jmedchem.9b00863

[53] Coleman MP, Höke A. Programmed axon degeneration: From mouse to mechanism to medicine. Nature Reviews. Neuroscience. 2020;**21**(4):183-196. DOI: 10.1038/s41583-020-0269-3

[54] Yungher BJ, Luo X, Salgueiro Y, Blackmore MG, Park KK. Viral vector-based improvement of optic nerve regeneration: Characterization of individual axons' growth patterns and synaptogenesis in a visual target. Gene Therapy. 2015;**22**(10):811-821. DOI: 10.1038/gt.2015.51

[55] Huang ZR, Chen HY, Hu ZZ, Xie P, Liu QH. PTEN knockdown with the Y444F mutant AAV2 vector promotes axonal regeneration in the adult optic nerve. Neural Regeneration Research. 2018;**13**(1):135-144. DOI: 10.4103/1673-5374.224381

[56] Miao L, Yang L, Huang H, Liang F, Ling C, Hu Y. mTORC1 is necessary but mTORC2 and GSK3β are inhibitory for AKT3-induced axon regeneration in the central nervous system. eLife. 2016;**5**:e14908. DOI: 10.7554/eLife.14908

[57] Nieuwenhuis B, Barber AC, Evans RS, Pearson CS, Fuchs J, MacQueen AR, et al. PI 3-kinase delta enhances axonal PIP3 to support axon regeneration in the adult CNS. EMBO Molecular Medicine. 2020;**12**(8):e11674. DOI: 10.15252/emmm.201911674

[58] Lim J-HA, Stafford BK, Nguyen PL, Lien BV, Wang C, Zukor K, et al. Neural activity promotes long-distance, target-specific regeneration of adult retinal axons. Nature Neuroscience. 2016;**19**(8):1073-1084. DOI: 10.1038/nn.4340

[59] Guo X, Snider WD, Chen B. GSK3β regulates AKT-induced central nervous system axon regeneration via an eIF2Bε-dependent, mTORC1-independent pathway. eLife. 2016;**5**:e11903. DOI: 10.7554/eLife.11903

[60] Pernet V, Joly S, Dalkara D, Jordi N, Schwarz O, Christ F, et al. Long-distance axonal regeneration induced by CNTF gene transfer is impaired by axonal misguidance in the injured adult optic nerve. Neurobiology of Disease. 2013;**51**:202-213. DOI: 10.1016/j.nbd.2012.11.011

[61] Leibinger M, Andreadaki A, Gobrecht P, Levin E, Diekmann H, Fischer D. Boosting central nervous system axon regeneration by circumventing limitations of natural cytokine Signaling. Molecular Therapy. 2016;**24**(10):1712-1725. DOI: 10.1038/mt.2016.102

[62] Pernet V, Joly S, Jordi N, Dalkara D, Guzik-Kornacka A, Flannery JG, et al. Misguidance and modulation of axonal regeneration by Stat3 and rho/ROCK signaling in the transparent optic nerve. Cell Death & Disease. 2013;**4**(7):e734. DOI: 10.1038/cddis.2013.266

[63] Sekine Y, Lin-Moore A, Chenette DM, Wang X, Jiang Z, Cafferty WB, et al. Functional genome-wide screen identifies pathways restricting central nervous system axonal regeneration. Cell Reports. 2018;**23**(2):415-428. DOI: 10.1016/j.celrep.2018.03.058

[64] Apara A, Galvao J, Wang Y, Blackmore M, Trillo A, Iwao K, et al. KLF9 and JNK3 interact to suppress axon regeneration in the adult CNS. The Journal of Neuroscience. 2017;**37**(40):9632-9644. DOI: 10.1523/JNEUROSCI.0643-16.2017

[65] Norsworthy MW, Bei F, Kawaguchi R, Wang Q, Tran NM, Li Y, et al. Sox11 expression promotes regeneration of some retinal ganglion cell types but kills others. Neuron. 2017;**94**(6):1112-1120.e4. DOI: 10.1016/j.neuron.2017.05.035

[66] Chang K-C, Bian M, Xia X, Madaan A, Sun C, Wang Q, et al. Posttranslational modification of Sox11 regulates RGC survival and axon regeneration. eNeuro. 2021;**8**(1):1-8. ENEURO.0358-20.2020. DOI: 10.1523/ENEURO.0358-20.2020

[67] Belin S, Nawabi H, Wang C, Tang S, Latremoliere A, Warren P, et al. Injury-induced decline of intrinsic regenerative ability revealed by quantitative proteomics. Neuron. 2015;**86**(4):1000-1014. DOI: 10.1016/j.neuron.2015.03.060

[68] Nathan FM, Ohtake Y, Wang S, Jiang X, Sami A, Guo H, et al. Upregulating Lin28a promotes axon regeneration in adult mice with optic nerve and spinal cord injury. Molecular Therapy. 2020;**28**(8):1902-1917. DOI: 10.1016/j.ymthe.2020.04.010

[69] Lindborg JA, Tran NM, Chenette DM, DeLuca K, Foli Y, Kannan R, et al. Optic nerve regeneration screen identifies multiple genes restricting adult neural repair. Cell Reports. 2021;**34**(9):108777. DOI: 10.1016/j.celrep.2021.108777

[70] Bray ER, Yungher BJ, Levay K, Ribeiro M, Dvoryanchikov G, Ayupe AC, et al. Thrombospondin-1 mediates axon regeneration in retinal ganglion cells. Neuron. 2019;**103**(4):642-657.e7. DOI: 10.1016/j.neuron.2019.05.044

[71] Levin E, Leibinger M, Gobrecht P, Hilla A, Andreadaki A, Fischer D. Muscle LIM protein is expressed in the injured adult CNS and promotes axon regeneration. Cell Reports. 2019;**26**(4):1021-1032.e6. DOI: 10.1016/j.celrep.2018.12.026

[72] Tran NM, Shekhar K, Whitney IE, Jacobi A, Benhar I, Hong G, et al. Single-cell profiles of retinal ganglion cells differing in resilience to injury reveal neuroprotective genes. Neuron. 2019;**104**(6):1039-1055.e12. DOI: 10.1016/j.neuron.2019.11.006

[73] Lu Y, Brommer B, Tian X, Krishnan A, Meer M, Wang C, et al. Reprogramming to recover youthful epigenetic information and restore vision. Nature. 2020;**588**(7836):124-129. DOI: 10.1038/s41586-020-2975-4

[74] Trakhtenberg EF, Li Y, Feng Q, Tso J, Rosenberg PA, Goldberg JL, et al. Zinc chelation and Klf9 knockdown cooperatively promote axon regeneration after optic nerve injury. Experimental Neurology. 2018;**300**:22-29. DOI: 10.1016/j.expneurol.2017.10.025

[75] Chierzi S, Strettoi E, Cenni MC, Maffei L. Optic nerve crush: Axonal responses in wild-type and bcl-2 transgenic mice. The Journal of Neuroscience. 1999;**19**(19):8367-8376. DOI: 10.1523/JNEUROSCI.19-19-08367.1999

[76] Yungher BJ, Ribeiro M, Park KK. Regenerative responses and axon pathfinding of retinal ganglion cells in chronically injured mice. Investigative Ophthalmology & Visual Science. 2017;**58**(3):1743-1750. DOI: 10.1167/iovs.16-19873

[77] Watkins TA, Wang B, Huntwork-Rodriguez S, Yang J, Jiang Z, Eastham-Anderson J, et al. DLK initiates a transcriptional program that couples apoptotic and regenerative responses

to axonal injury. Proceedings of the National Academy of Sciences of the United States of America. 2013;**110**(10):4039-4044. DOI: 10.1073/pnas.1211074110

[78] Pernet V, di Polo A. Synergistic action of brain-derived neurotrophic factor and lens injury promotes retinal ganglion cell survival, but leads to optic nerve dystrophy in vivo. Brain. 2006;**129**(Pt 4): 1014-1026. DOI: 10.1093/brain/awl015

[79] Joly S, Dalkara D, Pernet V. Sphingosine 1-phosphate receptor 1 modulates CNTF-induced axonal growth and neuroprotection in the mouse visual system. Neural Plasticity. 2017;**2017**:6818970. DOI: 10.1155/2017/6818970

[80] Li Y, Struebing FL, Wang J, King R, Geisert EE. Different effect of Sox11 in retinal ganglion cells survival and axon regeneration. Frontiers in Genetics. 2018;**9**:633. DOI: 10.3389/fgene.2018.00633

[81] Gene therapies should be for all. Nature Medicine. 2021;**27**(8):1311. DOI: 10.1038/s41591-021-01481-9

[82] Prado DA, Acosta-Acero M, Maldonado RS. Gene therapy beyond luxturna: A new horizon of the treatment for inherited retinal disease. Current Opinion in Ophthalmology. 2020;**31**(3):147-154. DOI: 10.1097/ICU.0000000000000660

[83] Wang D, Tai PWL, Gao G. Adeno-associated virus vector as a platform for gene therapy delivery. Nature Reviews. Drug Discovery. 2019;**18**(5):358-378. DOI: 10.1038/s41573-019-0012-9

[84] Nguyen GN, Everett JK, Kafle S, Roche AM, Raymond HE, Leiby J, et al. A long-term study of AAV gene therapy in dogs with hemophilia a identifies clonal expansions of transduced liver cells. Nature Biotechnology. 2021;**39**(1):47-55. DOI: 10.1038/s41587-020-0741-7

[85] Nuzbrokh Y, Kassotis AS, Ragi SD, Jauregui R, Tsang SH. Treatment-emergent adverse events in gene therapy trials for inherited retinal diseases: A narrative review. Ophthalmology and Therapy. 2020;**9**(4):709-724. DOI: 10.1007/s40123-020-00287-1

[86] Bennett J. Taking stock of retinal gene therapy: Looking Back and moving forward. Molecular Therapy. 2017;**25**(5):1076-1094. DOI: 10.1016/j.ymthe.2017.03.008

[87] Yiu G, Chung SH, Mollhoff IN, Nguyen UT, Thomasy SM, Yoo J, et al. Suprachoroidal and subretinal injections of AAV using Transscleral microneedles for retinal gene delivery in nonhuman Primates. Molecular Therapy-Methods & Clinical Development. 2020;**16**:179-191. DOI: 10.1016/j.omtm.2020.01.002

[88] Martino AT, Markusic DM. Immune response mechanisms against AAV vectors in animal models. Molecular Therapy-Methods & Clinical Development. 2019;**17**:198-208. DOI: 10.1016/j.omtm.2019.12.008

[89] Xiong W, Wu DM, Xue Y, Wang SK, Chung MJ, Ji X, et al. AAV cis-regulatory sequences are correlated with ocular toxicity. Proceedings of the National Academy of Sciences of the United States of America. 2019;**116**(12):5785-5794. DOI: 10.1073/pnas.1821000116

[90] Yin L, Greenberg K, Hunter JJ, Dalkara D, Kolstad KD, Masella BD, et al. Intravitreal injection of AAV2 transduces macaque inner retina. Investigative Ophthalmology & Visual Science. 2011;**52**(5):2775-2783. DOI: 10.1167/iovs.10-6250

[91] Ramachandran PS, Lee V, Wei Z, Song JY, Casal G, Cronin T, et al. Evaluation of dose and safety of AAV7m8 and AAV8BP2 in the non-human primate retina. Human Gene Therapy. 2017;**28**(2):154-167. DOI: 10.1089/hum.2016.111

[92] Petrs-Silva H, Dinculescu A, Li Q, Min S-H, Chiodo V, Pang J-J, et al. High-efficiency transduction of the mouse retina by tyrosine-mutant AAV serotype vectors. Molecular Therapy. 2009;**17**(3):463-471. DOI: 10.1038/mt.2008.269

[93] Mowat FM, Gornik KR, Dinculescu A, Boye SL, Hauswirth WW, Petersen-Jones SM, et al. Tyrosine capsid-mutant AAV vectors for gene delivery to the canine retina from a subretinal or intravitreal approach. Gene Therapy. 2014;**21**(1):96-105. DOI: 10.1038/gt.2013.64

[94] Dalkara D, Kolstad KD, Caporale N, Visel M, Klimczak RR, Schaffer DV, et al. Inner limiting membrane barriers to AAV-mediated retinal transduction from the vitreous. Molecular Therapy. 2009;**17**(12):2096-2102. DOI: 10.1038/mt.2009.181

[95] Gamlin PD, Alexander JJ, Boye SL, Witherspoon CD, Boye SE. SubILM injection of AAV for gene delivery to the retina. Methods in Molecular Biology. 2019;**1950**:249-262. DOI: 10.1007/978-1-4939-9139-6_14

[96] Alić I, Kosi N, Kapuralin K, Gorup D, Gajović S, Pochet R, et al. Neural stem cells from mouse strain Thy1 YFP-16 are a valuable tool to monitor and evaluate neuronal differentiation and morphology. Neuroscience Letters. 2016;**634**:32-41. DOI: 10.1016/j.neulet.2016.10.001

[97] Millington-Ward S, Chadderton N, Berkeley M, Finnegan LK, Hanlon KS, Carrigan M, et al. Novel 199 base pair NEFH promoter drives expression in retinal ganglion cells. Scientific Reports. 2020;**10**(1):16515. DOI: 10.1038/s41598-020-73257-z

[98] Simpson EM, Korecki AJ, Fornes O, McGill TJ, Cueva-Vargas JL, Agostinone J, et al. New MiniPromoter Ple345 (NEFL) drives strong and specific expression in retinal ganglion cells of mouse and primate retina. Human Gene Therapy. 2019;**30**(3):257-272. DOI: 10.1089/hum.2018.118

[99] Chaffiol A, Caplette R, Jaillard C, Brazhnikova E, Desrosiers M, Dubus E, et al. A new promoter allows Optogenetic vision restoration with enhanced sensitivity in macaque retina. Molecular Therapy. 2017;**25**(11):2546-2560. DOI: 10.1016/j.ymthe.2017.07.011

[100] Wang Q, Zhuang P, Huang H, Li L, Liu L, Webber HC, et al. Mouse γ-Synuclein promoter-mediated gene expression and editing in mammalian retinal ganglion cells. The Journal of Neuroscience. 2020;**40**(20):3896-3914. DOI: 10.1523/JNEUROSCI.0102-20.2020